OXFORD MEDICAL PUBLICATIONS

Epilepsy

Oxford Specialist Handbooks in Neurology
Epilepsy

Gonzalo Alarcon

Senior Lecturer and Honorary Consultant in
Clinical Neurophysiology,
Institute of Psychiatry and King's College Hospital,
NHS Foundation Trust, Denmark Hill,
London, UK

Lina Nashef

Consultant Neurologist and Honorary Senior Lecturer,
King's College Hospital NHS Foundation Trust,
Denmark Hill, London, UK

Helen Cross

Prince of Wales's Chair of Childhood Epilepsy,
University College London and Institute of Child Care,
Great Ormond Street Hospital for Children NHS Trust,
London, UK

Jennifer Nightingale

Specialist Epilepsy Nurse,
Barts and The London NHS Trust,
Department of Neurology,
The Royal London Hospital, London, UK,

Stuart Richardson

Lead Clinical Pharmacist, Neurosciences,
Department of Pharmacy,
King's College Hospital NHS Foundation Trust,
London, UK

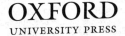

OXFORD
UNIVERSITY PRESS

OXFORD
UNIVERSITY PRESS

Great Clarendon Street, Oxford OX2 6DP

Oxford University Press is a department of the University of Oxford.
It furthers the University's objective of excellence in research, scholarship,
and education by publishing worldwide in

Oxford New York

Auckland Cape Town Dar es Salaam Hong Kong Karachi
Kuala Lumpur Madrid Melbourne Mexico City Nairobi
New Delhi Shanghai Taipei Toronto

With offices in

Argentina Austria Brazil Chile Czech Republic France Greece
Guatemala Hungary Italy Japan Poland Portugal Singapore
South Korea Switzerland Thailand Turkey Ukraine Vietnam

Oxford is a registered trade mark of Oxford University Press
in the UK and in certain other countries

Published in the United States
by Oxford University Press Inc., New York

British Library Cataloguing in Publication Data
Data available

Library of Congress Cataloging-in-Publication Data
Data available

Typeset by Cepha Imaging Private Ltd., Bangalore, India
Printed in Italy
on acid-free paper by
L.E.G.O. S.p.A.—Lavis TN

ISBN 978–0–19–857073–8

10 9 8 7 6 5 4 3 2 1

Foreword

This handbook is remarkable in providing in one volume, both a potential teaching course sufficient to guide the novice from basic neuroscientific and clinical principles to a working knowledge of current epilepsy practice as well as a ready and comprehensive reference for the experienced clinical epileptologist.

Epilepsy is comprehensive and extensively researched. However, it offers more than an aggregation of current knowledge designed for reference. It provides a manual for the clinical management of patients with a distinctive approach. It is, wherever possible, underpinned by evidence from the literature but in the innumerable instances where there is little or none, it gives detailed pragmatic guidance based on the collective experience of the authors, acknowledged standards of good practice, and argument from first principle: in short, the combination of knowledge, experience and common sense that seasoned clinicians employ on a daily basis.

In our climate of evidence-based medicine some may disparage this content but it is, in fact, one of the most valuable aspects of the work. Epilepsy is a huge and evolving field. Most of the big questions remain unanswered and so does an even larger array of smaller ones that arise daily in clinical practice. An epilepsy text book determined not to stray beyond the boundaries of strict evidence-based material would be entirely inadequate in serving patients. Such a work may be a future ideal but at this point in time the epilepsy clinician must master all available approaches based on reason and, with due cynicism, clinicians' experience.

This clinical approach expounded in the book very much reflect clinical practice at King's College Hospital where Gonzalo Alarcon, Lina Nashef and Stuart Richardson are based. It also reflects the strong tradition of epilepsy teaching at King's College Hospital exemplified by the MSc course in epilepsy which is run by Gonzalo Alarcon and attracts a wide range of students internationally. Jennifer Nightingale, is a specialist epilepsy nurse at Barts and the London NHS Trust, who graduated from this course with distinction in 2004. Both clinically and academically, these authors have a rich historical tradition to draw upon. The epilepsy department at King's is descended directly from that at the Maudsley Hospital which stands on the other side of the road to King's; the two institutions retaining close links. At the Maudsley, the neurosurgeon Murray Falconer practised and developed his technique of standard anterior temporal lobectomy in the mid-twentieth century. The utility of this operation is attested by its continued use around the world today. The *en bloc* nature of the resection allowed adequate histopathological study of the temporal lobe, allowing Falconer to recognize the importance of hippocampal sclerosis (HS) in intractable temporal lobe epilepsy (more accurately, mesial temporal sclerosis (MTS): a term coined by Falconer who found that the pathological changes extended to other mesial temporal structures). Anyone even faintly acquainted with the epilepsy literature of the last fifty or so years will realize the importance of this discovery, not just in epilepsy surgery but in triggering a vast amount of scientific work on the role of the hippocampus in epileptogenesis. It should be appreciated that before Falconer's discovery, the importance of HS in epilepsy had been dismissed by the dominant figures in the field. The importance of HS/MTS was rapidly recognized subsequent to Falconer's publication. For example, between 1949 and 1952, Wilder Penfield in Montreal formed eighty-one temporal lobe operations whereas in the preceding ten years he had performed only sixty-eight. As in Falconer's standard operation, Penfield included the uncus, amygdala and the anterolateral temporal lobe in these resections.

The tradition of epilepsy surgery at King's remains strong and vibrant both clinically and academically. The epilepsy surgery programme at the hospital is one of the numerically largest in the UK and certainly the most adventurous in terms of the complexity of its case-mix. Inevitably, this means that a relatively large proportion of patients undergoing assessment for epilepsy surgery at Kings require intracranial electrophysiological exploration and this has provided much opportunity for basic research, not least Gonzalo Alarcon and collaborators' novel work on single-pulse electrical simulation as a tool for indentifying epileptogenic cortex in the presurgical workup.

The historical roots of epileptology at King's, however, penetrate deeper than the twentieth century. Ted Reynolds has, in publications over the last few years, emphasized the great and very early contribution of Robert Bentley Todd at King's College Hospital to the inception of modern epileptology. Todd was appointed to the Chair of Physiology and Morbid Anatomy at King's College in 1836 and in 1840 founded King's College Hospital. He was well aware of Faraday's work on electromagnetism and not only believed that seizures could arise in the cerebral cortex rather than the brainstem, as was the prevailing belief, but saw that the underlying substrate of seizures was an electromagnetism-like phenomenon: *exciting the other parts of the brain and spinal cord with all the violence of the discharge from a highly charged Leyden jar*'.

The book covers all age groups, paediatric epilepsy syndromes and treatment receiving dedicated sections by Helen Cross, Prince of Wales's Chair of childhood epilepsy at UCL-Institute of Child Health, Great Ormond Street Hospital for Children NHS Trust and National Centre for Young People with Epilepsy, Lingfield. In addition to her extensive clinical, teaching and research work, Helen Cross has a wealth of experience in the development of epilepsy services for children. The institutions at which she is based encompass a comprehensive complex epilepsy programme, including the leading paediatric epilepsy surgery unit in the UK. Although epilepsy as part of neurology and neurophysiology has been part of a long tradition at Great Ormond Street Hospital, it was greatly enhanced by the arrival of Brian Neville from Guys in 1989 who not only pushed forward the research programme, but also enhanced the development of assessment services not only for presurgical evaluation but also for children with wider ranging epilepsy related problems, allowing ready translation of research findings into clinical practice.

In the book, there is admittedly a degree of bias towards the practice of epilepsy in the UK, particularly in terms of medicolegal matters, discussion of charitable organizations and national standards of care. However, these parochialisms do not detract from its universal utility and will serve to spark questions of comparison and fundamental principal in readers outside the UK.

Dr Nicholas F Moran
MB ChB MRCP MSc
Consultant Neurologist
Kent & Canterbury Hospital,
and King's College Hospital,
UK

Preface

Epilepsy is one of the most common neurological serious conditions and a frequent cause of disability. The causes, mechanisms, manifestations, and consequences of epilepsy are so diverse that it affects virtually all aspects of patients' lives. Yet misconceptions about epilepsy are common among the general public and health professionals. In-depth understanding of epilepsy requires all facets of modern biomedical science, from basic neurobiology and genetics to social and medico-legal disciplines. Several excellent detailed, lengthy, comprehensive and definitive textbooks are available that cover in-depth most aspects of epileptology. Nevertheless, professionals interested in expanding their academic or practical skills in epilepsy are often confronted with numerous changing classifications, syndromes, terms and concepts that can be difficult to comprehend. Some more basic books exist, which are useful as a first approach to epilepsy but perhaps are too simplistic for those requiring in-depth knowledge or information about specific practical issues.

The present handbook aims at providing in-depth and practical information useful to a wide range of people involved in the management of epilepsy, be they doctors, nurses, pharmacists, researchers, psychologists and others as well as those wishing to specialize in epilepsy. It should also be very useful to neurologists, paediatric neurologists and other epilepsy specialists requiring quick reference to specific points, without lengthy literature reviews or discussions. The volume benefits from the authors' 13-year teaching experience in the MSc in Epilepsy at King's College London (Institute of Psychiatry) to students with a wide range of backgrounds. Numerous bullet points and text boxes are provided to supply quick practical information on issues that are often encountered in practice. We aimed to cover most aspects of epileptology, from basic science to social, economic and legal issues, cross-referenced, as appropriate. Drug management in adults is addressed in more detail in children, where management is most often directly supervised by those with a special interest. In medicine, there are many possible ways to achieve a goal, and often there is not the evidence to support one over another. We very much hope that the book will provide guidance to those still accumulating experience early on in their career, and we also hope that it will encourage others, with more experience, to reflect on advantages and disadvantages of differences in practice.

We are aware that there is a bias towards the situation in the UK and beg the reader's patience where the information provided has no wider relevance, although some may find the information useful for purposes of comparison.

The extent to which this book achieves its goals will depend on how it meets the needs of the reader. We welcome suggestions and constructive criticism, and aim to integrate them in future editions. Please send your comments to: gonzalo.alarcon@iop.kcl.ac.uk. They will be gratefully received.

Gonzalo Alarcon
Lina Nashef
Helen Cross
Jennifer Nightingale
Stuart Richardson

Acknowledgements

The authors would like to express their most sincere gratitude to those who have reviewed all or part of the manuscript for their useful comments, and to the publishers for their well tested patience. In particular, we would like to thank:

Dr I Bodi, for the reviewing the section of the pathology of epilepsy and providing the figures included in this section.

Dr D Berry, for providing the target blood levels for antiepileptic drugs,

Dr F Brunnhuber, for writing the paragraph on activation procedures to induce non-epileptic attacks.

Dr N Ghali (Hindocha), for providing the table on genetic causes for idiopathic epilepsies.

Dr S Goyal, for reviewing the section 'From seizures to syndromes' and providing numerous illustrations.

Dr J Jarosz, for reviewing the sections on neuroimaging.

Ms Helen Liepman, for suggesting the idea of this book, and for her support and patience.

Drs J Mellers and B. Toone, for reviewing the sections on neuropsychiatry.

Prof B Meldrum, for reviewing the section on mechanisms of action of antiepileptic drugs.

Prof C E Polkey and Mr R. Selway, for reviewing the chapter on surgical treatment of epilepsy.

Mr A Reo, for providing information on vitamin D and calcium supplementation.

Dr A Valentín, for writing the section on the mechanisms of epileptogenesis.

In particular, we wish to extend our gratitude to Dr Nicholas Moran, for patiently reviewing the whole manuscript, making numerous suggestions for improving both its content and language, and for writing the foreword.

Acknowledgements

Contents

Symbols and abbreviations

📖	cross reference
>	greater than
<	less than
💾	downloadable document
🖱	website
A&E	Accident & Emergency
ADFLE	autosomal dominant frontal lobe epilepsy
ADHD	attention deficit hyperactivity disorder
AED	antiepileptic drug(s)
AHS	AED hypersensitivity syndrome
BCOS	Benign childhood occipital seizures
bd	twice daily
BECTS	Benign epilepsy of childhood with centro temporal spikes
BMD	bone mineral density
BMEI	benign myoclonic epilepsy of infancy
BNF	British National Formulary
BP	blood pressure
CAE	childhood absence epilepsy
CBT	cognitive behavioural therapy
CGBT	cognitive group behavioural therapy
CI	confidence interval
CNS	central nervous system
CO	carbon monoxide
CPS	complex partial seizure
COC	combined oral contraceptive
CSWS	continuous spike wave of slow sleep
CT	computerized tomography
DBS	deep brain stimulation
DLA	disability living allowance
DNET	dysembryoplastic neuroepithelial tumour
DSM	diagnostic and statistical manual for mental disorders
DTs	Delirium tremens
ECT	Electro convulsive therapy
DTP	diphtheria, tetanus, and whooping cough
DVLA	Driver and Vehicle Licensing Agency
ECG	electrocardiogram
ECoG	electrocorticography

EFS+	epilepsy with febrile seizures plus
EEG	electroencephalogram
EM	erythema multiform
EMG	electromyogram
ESES	electrical status epilepticus in slow-wave sleep
ESN	Epilepsy Specialist Nurse
FBC	full blood count
FDG	fluoro-deoxyglucose
FLAIR	fluid attenuated inversion recovery
FS	febrile seizures
GABA	gamma-aminobutyric acid
GAD	glutamic acid decarboxylase
GEFS+	generalized epilepsy with febrile seizures plus
GFR	glomerular filtration rate
GHB	gamma-hydroxybutyrate
GI	gastrointestinal
GP	general practitioner
GTCS	generalized tonic–clonic seizures
HAD	Hospital Anxiety and Depression Scale
HHE	hemiconvulsion–hemiplegia–epilepsy
HIV	human immunodeficiency virus
HMPAO	hexamethylpropylamine oxime
IBE	International Bureau for Epilepsy
ICU	intensive care unit
IGE	idiopathic generalized epilepsies
ILAE	International League Against Epilepsy
IQ	intelligence quotient
IUD	intra-uterine device
IUS	intra-uterine system
JAE	juvenile absence epilepsy
JEC	Joint Epilepsy Council
JME	juvenile myoclonic epilepsy
LD	learning disability
LH	luteinizing hormone
mcg	microgram/s
MCM	major congenital malformation
MES	maximal electroshock
MELAS	mitochondrial encephalomyopathy with lactic acidosis and stroke-like episodes
MERRF	myoclonus epilepsy with ragged-red fibres
MHD	monohydroxyderivative

min	minute/s
MMR	measles, mumps and rubella
MRI	Magnetic Resonance Imaging
ms	millisecond
MW	molecular weight
nm	nanometre
OCP	oral contraceptive pill
od	once daily
NCSE	non-convulsive status epilepticus
NCYSE	National Centre for Young People with Epilepsy
NICE	National Institute for Clinical Excellence
NSE	National Society for Epilepsy
NTD	neural tube defect
OR	odds ratio
PCT	Primary Care Trust
PE	phenytoin equivalent
PET	positron emission tomography
PME	progressive myodonic epilepsies
PML	progressive multifocal leucoencephalopathy
POP	progesterone-only pill
PDS	paroxysmal depolarization shifts
PPR	photoparoxysmal responses
RCN	Royal College of Nurses
REM	rapid eye movement
RID	relative infant dose
Rx	prescription
SD	standard deviation(s)
sec	second(s)
SIGN	Scottish Intercollegiate Guidelines Network
SJS	Stevens–Johnson syndrome
SLS	Selected List Scheme
SMEB	severe myoclonic epilepsy borderline
SMEI	severe myoclonic epilepsy in infancy
SMR	standardized mortality ratio
SPC	summary of product characteristics
SPECT	single proton emission tomography
SSRI	selective serotonin re-uptake inhibitor
SUDEP	sudden unexpected death in epilepsy
TEN	toxic epidermal necrosis
TIA	transient ischaemic attack
UGT	uridine glucuronyl transferase

UK	United Kingdom
UMN	upper motor neuron
VNS	vagus nerve stimulation
WAIS	Wechsler Adult Intelligence scale
WHO	World Health Organization
WMS	Wechsler Memory Scale

Detailed contents

What is epilepsy?

Introduction

- Epilepsy is a tendency to suffer recurrent epileptic seizures (📖 see Chapter 3a, pp.61–73 for detailed descriptions of epileptic seizures).
- Pragmatically, epilepsy can be defined as having two or more unprovoked epileptic seizures occurring within a time frame of 2 years. The term '**unprovoked**' refers to the absence of acute conditions that can produce seizures in patients who do not normally have seizures (conditions such as hypoglycemia, alcohol withdrawal, hypercalcemia, encephalitis, electroconvulsive therapy, etc.; 📖 see epileptic seizures without epilepsy, pp.156–157).
- In a small proportion of patients with epilepsy, seizures can be triggered by specific stimuli that do not trigger seizures in the general population (e.g. flashing lights, visual patterns, reading). This is called reflex epilepsy.
- Epilepsy is one of the most common serious neurological conditions.
- Epilepsy can affect any age group from any socio-economic background.

The epilepsies

- The term 'epilepsy' includes many different disorders. Hence, there is currently a trend towards using the term 'the epilepsies'.
- The epilepsies identify patients who experience recurrent unprovoked seizures with a vast range of underlying aetiologies.
- The epilepsies can be subdivided into 'syndromes'. An epilepsy syndrome is a cluster of signs and symptoms that occur together with a frequency higher than chance due to a common cause. They define a unique epilepsy condition associated with specific clinical history, seizure types, EEG findings, and prognosis.
- There are approximately 30 different syndromes and around 40 different seizure types.[1]

Incidence

- The incidence is the number of newly diagnosed cases of a condition within a period of time (usually 1 year).
- In the UK, the annual incidence is approximately 46 per 100,000 or 0.46 cases per 1000 population.
- Approximately 27,400 new cases are diagnosed per year or 75 new cases each day in the UK.
- It is estimated that the incidence of epilepsy in developing countries is approximately 100 per 100,000 people per year (estimates vary from 49.3–190).

Prevalence

- The prevalence of a disorder is the proportion of a population with the disorder at a given time.
- The overall prevalence of epilepsy is around 1 in 131 people (approximately one tenth of the prevalance of diabetes)
- Approximately 300,000 people in the UK have epilepsy.[1]
- It is estimated that the total number of people under the age of 18 years with a diagnosis of epilepsy is approximately 42,000 or 1 in 242.
- The highest prevalence is among those above the age of 65 years. The total is approximately 105,000 or 1 in 91.[1]
- Epilepsy prevalence is 25% higher in the most socially deprived areas compared to the least socially deprived.[3]
- The World Health Organization (WHO) has estimated that around 50 million people in the world have epilepsy at any one time and the life time prevalence is approximately 100 million people.[4]

References

1. Joint Epilepsy Council (2006). *Epilepsy Prevalence, Incidence and Other Statistics.* JEC, Leeds. Available at www.jointepilepsycouncil.org.uk

2. MacDonald BK, Cockerell OC, Sander JW, *et al.* (2000). The incidence and lifetime prevalence of neurological disorders in a prospective community based study in the UK. *Brain,* **123**, 665–76.

3. Purcell B, Gaitatziz A, Sander JW, *et al.* (2002). Epilepsy prevalence and prescribing patterns in England and Wales. *Health Statistics Quarterly,* **15**, 23–30.

4. Scott RA, Lhatoo SD, Sander JWAS (2001). The treatment of epilepsy in developing countries: where do we go from here? *Bulletin of the World Health Organization* **79**.

Useful contact

www.ilae-epilepsy.org—website of The International League Against Epilepsy(ILAE).

Prognosis

Remission

The prognosis of epilepsy has traditionally been considered poor. However, between 70–80% of patients become seizure free with medical treatment. The prognosis largely depends on the specific epilepsy syndrome and its aetiology. A question often asked in clinical practice and in the literature is if the prognosis of epilepsy is the same regardless of whether it is treated or untreated with drugs. In other words, whether medical treatment alters the natural evolution of epilepsy.

Definitions

- *Terminal remission:* a seizure free period of 5 years or more lasting to the time of the most recent follow up.
- *Chronic epilepsy:* epilepsy still active 5 years after onset.
- *Prognosis*: the probability of entering terminal remission once a pattern of recurrent epileptic seizures has been established.

Prognosis after a single seizure

The risk of suffering recurrent seizures after having a single seizure is unclear. Estimates vary between 27–81%. Hospital-based studies show lower values than community-based or studies that include patients after 24 hours of the first seizure. This may be due to the fact that the risk of having a second seizure after a first seizure decreases with time.

Risk factors for recurrence after a first seizure

Family history: debatable, perhaps for idiopathic epilepsies.

Etiology: recurrence 12 months after a first seizure was 100% if congenital neurological deficits were present, 75% after acquired central nervous system (CNS) lesions and 40% if associated with an acute precipitant.[1]

Neurological abnormalities: increased risk if neurological examination is abnormal, but only in symptomatic epilepsies.

EEG abnormalities: increased risk, particularly for idiopathic epilepsies.

Head injury: The risk of epilepsy is about 2% if associated with mild trauma (amnesia or loss of consciousness (LOC) <30 min and no cranial fracture); 2–5% if moderate trauma (non-depressed skull fracture, 30 min <amnesia or LOC <24 hours); 12–15% after severe head injury (intracranial bleeding, brain contusions, dural tear, anmesia or LOC > 24 hours); 50% after missile or penetrating injury. Early seizures (within a week of injury) are not epilepsy but increase the likelihood of having epilepsy later.

Intracranial infection: any intracranial infection increases the risk of epilepsy. Postnatal meningitis, brain abscess, and encephalitis increase the risk 3-fold.

Seizure type: partial (focal) non-convulsive seizures are more likely to recur than convulsive seizures. Nocturnal seizures are also likely to recur.

Early medical treatment: appears to reduce the risk of recurrent seizures:[2]
- After 24 months: 26% risk if treated versus 51% if untreated.
- After 12 months: 50% risk if treated versus 67% if untreated.
- After 36 months: 57% risk if treated versus 78% if untreated.

Natural history of treated epilepsy

Newly diagnosed epilepsy can be defined as having two or more unprovoked seizures. It is unclear whether medication should be started after a single unprovoked seizure. After a second unprovoked seizure medication should be started. Under these circumstances:

- The probability of remission within the first year is 65–80%.
- The likelihood of remission is lower for complex partial than for secondarily generalized seizures (remission rates 16–43% versus 48–53%).
- The likelihood of remission is lower in the presence of multiple seizure types, neurological deficits, behavioural, or psychiatric disturbances.
- No particular antiepileptic drug appears to be better in population studies, but individual patients and syndromes may respond better to some antiepileptic drugs.
- Remission rates increase with time: 42% after 1 year, 65% after 10 years, 76% after 15 years.[3]

Once epilepsy becomes chronic, 20-30% of patients do not enter remission (confirmed by hospital based and community studies); only 20% of patients have seizure free periods; and only a few eventually become seizure free on antiepileptic drugs(AEDs).

The majority of patients on AED treatment eventually become seizure free and drug withdrawal is contemplated. The overall risk of seizure relapse after drug withdrawal is 11–41%. The risk of recurrence with withdrawal is lower in children than in adults. The risk of relapse after AED withdrawal is higher in the presence of long history of seizures, more than one seizure type, structural brain lesions, neurological signs, learning difficulties, history of remissions and relapses, juvenile myoclonic epilepsy, acute symptomatic seizures, and EEG abnormalities.

Natural history of untreated epilepsy

Most of what we know about the natural history of epilepsy is from treated patients. This raises two questions that have not been satisfactorily addressed in the literature:

- Is there remission without treatment?
- What is the effect of early treatment on prognosis?

Spontaneous remission without treatment

The prevalence of epilepsy in developed and developing countries seems to be similar, suggesting that remission rates are similar. Measured remission rates in developed and developing world are also similar (40–50%). Since epilepsy in the developed world is usually treated and in the developing world is largely untreated, these findings raise the question of whether medical treatment affects prognosis.

Effects of early treatment on prognosis

Around 50% of treated patients remit in the second 6 months after a previous untreated 6 month period in Kenya, Ecuador, and Malawi. This is similar to that reported with treated epilepsy, suggesting that early treatment may not improve remission rates. However, this does not exclude an effect on prognosis in subgroups (📖 see Risk factors for recurrence after a first seizure).

Prognosis of specific syndromes

The prognosis in epilepsy largely depends on the underlying syndrome (📖 see Chapter 3b, pp.75–130). The prognoses of a few syndromes are summarized here as examples:

- *Benign familial (idiopathic) neonatal convulsions* ('5th day fits'): only 10% have epilepsy later in life.
- *Neonatal convulsions* (occurring within the first 4 weeks of life): these affect 0.5% of infants. 30% die within the year; 25% suffer seizures into adulthood or have learning difficulties or spasticity; only 40% fully recover. Poor prognostic factors are prematurity, early onset seizures (first 2 days), focal brain lesion or malformation, intracranial bleeding, inborn errors of metabolism, abnormal EEG. The prognosis is better if no aetiology is found.
- *Idiopathic generalized epilepsies*: these make up one third of all epilepsies under 20 and generally have good a prognosis:
  - *Childhood absence epilepsy*: 80% become seizure free. Poorer prognosis if tonic–clonic convulsions or other seizure types occur.
  - *Juvenile absence epilepsy*: slightly worse outcome than in childhood absence epilepsy.
  - *Juvenile myoclonic epilepsy*: good response to treatment, but seizures recur if treatment stops; often requires lifetime treatment.
  - *Epilespy with generalized tonic–clonic seizures on awakening*: seizures remit in most; no mental deterioration.
- *Idiopathic focal epilepsies*: generally good prognosis with complete seizure remission. In focal epilepsy with centrotemporal spikes (Rolandic epilepsy), only 2% have lifelong seizures; in other idiopathic focal epilepsies, up to 10% have lifelong seizures.
- *Symptomatic/cryptogenic generalized epilepsies:* neurological and/or cognitive impairment is present in 90% of patients. Prognosis depends on the underlying syndrome but is generally poor:
  - *Infantile spasms* (West syndrome): one in five die and 90% of survivors suffer learning difficulties and chronic epilepsy.
  - *Lennox-Gastaut syndrome*: 60% of patients suffer status epilepticus (convulsive or non-convulsive). Seizure remission occurs in 10%.
  - *Severe myoclonic epilepsy in infancy*: onset in first year of life, generalized tonic–clonic and myoclonic seizures. 16% of patients die within 10 years of onset, all survivors have uncontrolled seizures, and 90% severe learning difficulties.
- *Symptomatic/cryptogenic focal (partial) epilepsies:* prognosis depends on the underlying lesion. Poorer seizure prognosis in congenital lesions (malformations, tuberous sclerosis, Sturge–Weber syndrome). Surgery can be a treatment option. Excellent response to surgery in mesial temporal sclerosis.
- *Epilepsia partialis continua (Kojewnikow's syndrome):*
  - *Rasmussen's encephalitis*: progressive, neurological deficits and mental impairment, antiepileptic drugs are generally not effective, surgical treatment should be considered.
  - *Dysplastic lesions, tumours, vascular malformations*: outcome depending on cause.

- *Epilepsy with continuous spike-and-wave during slow wave sleep:* usually this is a type of symptomatic generalized epilepsy. There is an identifiable cause in 20-30% (meningitis, birth injury, cytomegalovirus infection). It is associated with developmental arrest and behavioural difficulties. The EEG abnormality is age dependent, and seizures remit in many patients but learning and behaviour difficulties tend to persist.
- *Landau-Kleffner syndrome* (acquired epileptic aphasia): 80% of patients enjoy seizure remission, and 60% have persistent learning (particularly language) difficulties.

References

1. Hart YM, Sander JW, Johnson AL, et al. (1990). National General Practice Study of Epilepsy: recurrence after a first seizure. *Lancet*, **336**, 1271–4.

2. First Seizure Trial Group (1993). Randomized clinical trial on the efficacy of antiepileptic drugs in reducing the risk of relapse after a first unprovoked tonic-clonic seizure. First Seizure Trial Group (FIR.S.T. Group). *Neurology*, **43**, 478–83.

3. Annegers JF, Hauser WA, Elveback LR (1979). Remission of seizures and relapse in patients with epilepsy. *Epilepsia*, **20**, 729–37.

Mortality

Introduction

- There are methodological problems in the study of mortality in epilepsy. These relate to differences in definitions, selection bias in cohorts under study, incomplete data particularly in population-based studies, and inconsistent death certification.
- The prevalence of epilepsy depends on incidence, remission, and mortality. An excess mortality is observed in cohorts of patients with epilepsy. Most of the mortality in the first years after diagnosis is related to underlying disease causing the epilepsy. Throughout, there is also a small excess mortality related to the epilepsy itself. This excess is in part preventable. It includes deaths due to accidents, drowning, status epilepticus and sudden death in epilepsy (SUDEP). Deaths related to complications of the treatment of epilepsy can also occur but are very rare. Finally, suicides due to associated psychiatric morbidity are increased in a subgroup of people with epilepsy.
  📖 See Box 1.1.

Standardized mortality ratio (SMR)

Mortality rates are measured using the SMR. The rate observed in a given cohort is compared to that expected, based on known death rates in the general population standardized for age and sex. SMR in epilepsy is 2–3 compared to the general population, but is much higher in selected cohorts; particularly those with intractable epilepsy, or epilepsy associated with other handicap or disease.

Proportionate mortality

This term refers to the proportion of deaths within a given cohort due to a particular cause. Proportions differ depending on the cohort under study. Causes of death usually include cerebrovascular and cardiac disease, neoplasms including brain tumours, pneumonia, suicide, accidents, SUDEP, and other seizure-related deaths.

Box 1.1 Causes of death in epilepsy (these categories may overlap):

- Unrelated to epilepsy
- Death from underlying/associated disease.
- Epilepsy-related:
  • Seizure-related
  • Status epilepticus.
  • Trauma, burns, or drowning consequent to a seizure.
  • Majority of sudden unexpected deaths in epilepsy.
  • Deaths in a seizure with secondary cause identified e.g. clear severe aspiration or airway obstruction by food.
  • Deaths provoked by habitual seizures due to co-existing cardio-respiratory disease.
  • Deaths as a consequence of medical or surgical treatment of epilepsy.
  • Suicides.

Status epilepticus

Mortality associated with status epilepticus is of the order of 20%. Although status epilepticus is more common in children, the mortality rate is higher in adults. In tertiary centres, death is reported largely due to the underlying condition rather than the status per se. Nevertheless, status epilepticus from any cause, particularly if convulsive, should be considered a life-threatening medical emergency requiring prompt treatment.

Accidental deaths—drowning, trauma, and burns

The risk of injury relates to seizure frequency as well as seizure type (seizures associated with falls, carry the highest risk). Epileptic seizures are also a cause of vehicle driver collapse. Drowning is exposure dependent. 📖 See Box 1.2.

> **Box 1.2 Some measures to prevent accidental injury and death in epilepsy**
>
> - Avoid potentially dangerous situations in the event of a seizure, including:
>   - Unprotected heights.
>   - Unprotected waterfronts.
>   - Proximity to fires/heat.
>   - Proximity to dangerous machinery.
>   - Driving.
> - Use sit-down showers with thermostat-controlled water-temperature rather than baths.
> - Follow driving regulations.
> - Take care as a pedestrian and cyclist avoiding traffic.
> - Take care with cooking, hot water, and with home appliances.
> - In severe epilepsy with frequent drop attacks, consider helmet or wheelchair use.

Sudden unexpected ('unexplained') death in epilepsy (SUDEP)

Otherwise well patients with epilepsy sometimes die unexpectedly without a cause for death found at post-mortem examination, although pulmonary congestion is frequently noted, and sometimes congestion in other organs. The majority of deaths are unwitnessed; most often the person is found dead in bed. Often there is evidence suggestive of an epileptic seizure. There is some dispute over definitions with a few investigators excluding death in a documented seizure. A pragmatic workable definition for SUDEP is: sudden, unexpected, witnessed or unwitnessed, non-traumatic, and non-drowning death in epilepsy, with or without evidence for a seizure and excluding documented status epilepticus, where post-mortem examination does not reveal a structural or toxicological cause for death. This definition does not address sudden death in epilepsy with concomitant disease, a category which also needs study.

Where information is incomplete or autopsy is not available the level of uncertainty may be indicated as follows: definite SUDEP (sudden death in benign circumstances with no other known cause and autopsy performed), probable (as before but without autopsy), possible, and not SUDEP.

Incidence rates in different cohorts are listed in Box 1.3. The most likely cause is cardio-respiratory compromise during or shortly after an epileptic seizure. Some risk factors identified in case control studies are listed in Box 1.4. The most important is a history of generalized tonic–clonic seizures and uncontrolled epilepsy. Individual susceptibility is not fully explained and risk prediction is difficult.

Box 1.3 SUDEP incidence

- New onset epilepsy: < 1:5000 person years.
- Controlled epilepsy MRC AED withdrawal study 2:5000 person years.[1]
- Population based studies minimum 0.35/1000 person years.
- UK death certificates for those aged 15–60 = 350–400 individuals in 1997.
- Multicentre hospital series: large unselected 1.21/1000 person years.
- Cohorts with epilepsy and other disability 1:300 person years.
- Hospital series/Intractable cohorts 1:250 person years (higher in pre-surgical cohorts and those with failed epilepsy surgery).
  For a recent review see[(2)].

Suicides

An excess in suicides is mostly reported in selected cohorts, less in population based surveys, for example, in intractable cohorts with temporal lobe epilepsy, suggesting that the pathophysiology of the underlying conditions plays a role. The excess observed is not simply due to the burden of chronic disease. Patients who undergo temporal lobectomy for the treatment of their epilepsy are also at potential risk. There has also been recent concern about the possible modifying effects on risk of AEDs.

Practical implications

The excess mortality associated with epilepsy has practical implications to management both in relation to information provision, treatment decisions, as well as service provision. It also has medico-legal implications. Guidelines generally advocate more information provision to patients regarding risks associated with epilepsy—including SUDEP—than is reportedly commonly practised. While this may be subject to debate, and particularly where the individual is faced with treatment or social choices, an awareness of the risks associated with epilepsy is a prerequisite to informed choice (Box 1.5).

Box 1.4 Some risk factors for SUDEP shown in different case control studies[2]

Seizures [2]

- History of generalized tonic clonic seizures.
- Tonic clonic seizure in past 3 months.
- Tonic clonic seizure in past year.
- More frequent seizures.

Circumstances

- Prone body position at death.
- Bedroom shared by supervising individual (protective).
- Listening devices (protective).

Treatment

- Never treated.
- On two AEDs compared to none or one.
- History of treatment with >4 AEDs ever compared to 1 to 2.
- Polytherapy.
- Frequent medication changes.
- Carbamazepine level greater than usual quoted range; on carbamazepine.
- Increased variation in AED levels in sequential hair samples.

Other

- Full scale IQ <70 compared to >79.
- Younger age of onset of epilepsy.

Box 1.5 Prevention of epilepsy-related deaths

- Prevention of injury and drowning.
- Prevention of seizures.
- Reduction in seizure severity.
- Detection and treatment of psychiatric co-morbidity.
- Choice of treatment appropriate for severity of epilepsy.
- Adequate response to convulsive seizures to minimize cardio-respiratory compromise and risk of injury.

References

1. MRC AED Withdrawal Study Group (1991). Randomised study of AED withdrawal in patients in remission. *Lancet*, **337**, 1175–80.
2. Tomson T, Nashef L, Ruolin P (2008). *Lancet Neurology* **7**(11):1021–31.

Mechanisms of epilepsy

Basic functional anatomy

Cerebral cortex

Most seizures are thought to result from a malfunction of the cerebral cortex and its interaction with subcortical structures. The *cerebral cortex* is a layer of grey matter that surrounds both cerebral hemispheres (therefore the name cerebral cortex, i.e. cerebral bark). It folds in a complicated fashion, defining on the cerebral surface the *sulci* (depressions of the surface of the brain, *sulcus* is singular) and the *gyri* (bulging regions of the brain surface, *gyrus* is singular) (Fig. 2.1). There are four main lobes: frontal, temporal, parietal, and occipital. In addition, there are two deep depressions called **fissures:** the *rolandic* or *central* fissure between frontal and parietal lobes, and the *sylvian* fissures between frontal and temporal lobes. We will use the term cortex to refer to the cerebral cortex in order to distinguish it from the other main brain cortex, the cerebellar cortex, which does not appear to be directly involved in the generation of epileptic seizures.

The cortex is the structure responsible for the most complex brain functions (the so called 'higher brain functions'): perception, voluntary movement, the production and understanding of language, memory, motivation.

Normal functions of the cortex can be altered during epileptic seizures, To a large degree, the nervous system's function is hierarchical. The cortex is the most dominant structure, responsible for higher functions. the remaining brain structures (primarily the thalamus, brain stem and cerebellum) are sometimes termed the *subcortical structures*.

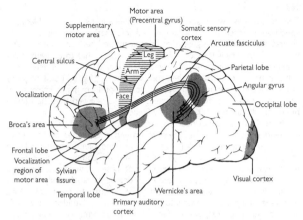

Fig. 2.1 Lateral view of the human left cerebral hemisphere, highlighting the main areas involved in movement control and language. The main lobes, sulci, and gyri are also shown. (Reproduced with permission from Kandel ER and Schwartz JH (eds.) (1985). *Principles of Neural Science*, 2nd edn. Elsevier, New York.)

Neurons and glia

The cortex has two main types of cells—neurons and glia. Neurons specialize in processing information. This information is mainly coded as chemical and electrical signals that are transmitted between neurons. The function of glial cells is much debated, but probably has to do with maintaining the appropriate cellular environment, including immune defence.

Neurons are cells with rather complex shapes (Fig. 2.2) and are very interconnected (one neuron receives information from many neurons and also sends signals to many other neurons). It is believed that the human brain contains around 1,000,000,000,000 neurons.

Although the shape of neurons varies, most neurons have three basic elements (Figs. 2.2 and 2.3). They have a round or triangular central structure called the *neuronal body* (or *cell body* or *soma*, plural is *somata*). From the body, there are usually many ramifications with complex shapes, which make most neurons look like a tree. Most of these ramifications, are called *dendrites*. Dendrites are specialized in picking up signals (usually chemical signals) from other neurons and converting them into electrical signals that travel along the dendrite into the neuronal body. Dendrites and body are thought to be responsible for processing information coming from other neurons. Apart from dendrites, there is usually one other ramification called the *axon*. The initial portion of the axon, closest to the cell body, is usually wider than the rest of the axon, and is called *axon hillock*. Under normal conditions, the axon hillock is thought to initiate self-propagating electrical signals (action potentials). The axon conveys processed electrical signals to other neurons as bursts of action potentials. Electrical signals travel along the axon and are directly responsible for releasing the chemicals necessary to communicate information to the next neurons. A neuron may have many dendrites, but usually a single axon.

Information is transferred from one neuron to another via chemical compounds (called *neurotransmitters* and *neuromodulators*). Information is then converted into electrical signals in the neuron, travels along each neuron as electrical signals, and is processed within each neuron as electrical signals. Information is then converted back into chemical signals before it is transferred to the next neuron.

The anatomical structure that transfers information from one neuron to another is called the *synapse*. Synapses usually, but not always, involve the axon of one neuron and the dendrite of another neuron. Therefore, synapses convert information from electrical form into chemical form in the sending neuron, and back to electrical in the receiving neuron. In most synapses, neurons are not physically in contact with each other. There is a very small space between the two neurons (the *synaptic cleft*) (Fig. 2.4). There is debate about the role or extrasynaptic transmission of information in the human brain.

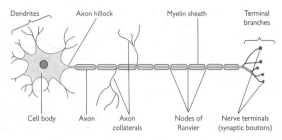

Fig. 2.2 A diagrammatic representation of a CNS neuron. (Reproduced with permission from Pocock G and Richards CD (2006). *Human Physiology*, 3rd edn, Oxford University Press, Oxford.)

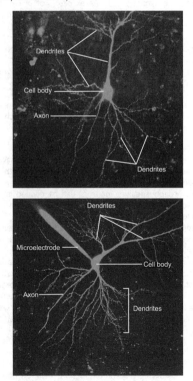

Fig. 2.3 Two neurons stained with a green fluorescent dye (Oregon green BAPTA 1). The lower panel shows the microelectrode used to introduce the dye into the cell. Note the extensive branching of the dendrites and the single axon. (Reproduced with permission from Pocock G and Richards CD (2006). Human Physiology, 3rd edn, Oxford University Press, Oxford.)

Anatomy and physiology of the synapse

As explained in the previous section, the synapse is the region where two neurons become very close, in contact or nearly in contact with each other. It is via synapses that neurons communicate with each other. With the standard (optical) microscope, synapses look like a little pimple on the surface of the neuron (called *synaptic boutons* or *synaptic processes*, Fig. 2.3). However, when seen with the electron microscope, membranes from the two communicating neurons come nearly into contact, only separated by a distance of around 20nm (the *synaptic cleft*). The membrane from the neuron providing information is called the *presynaptic membrane*, and the membrane from the neuron receiving information is called the *postsynaptic membrane* (Fig. 2.4).

When electrical signals (in the form of action potentials) reach the presynaptic membrane, a specific chemical compound (neurotransmitter) is released into the synaptic cleft via *exocitosis* of presynaptic vesicles. *Calcium* is necessary for this process. The postsynaptic membrane has certain proteins (*receptors*) that can specifically couple with a neurotransmitter. When receptors couple with neurotransmitters, pores for specific ions are opened in the postsynaptic membrane (permeability across the membrane for such ions is increased), a process that triggers changes in electrical voltage across the membrane (the *postsynaptic potential*). In this way, *electrical phenomena* in the presynaptic membrane give rise to electrical changes in the postsynaptic membrane via a chemical process.

Some synapses are thought to be only electrical, with pre- and postsynaptic membrane in direct contact. In the human brain, such synapses are thought to be a minority and their role is uncertain.

Cortical neurons

Cortical neurons are not all alike, and many classifications have been made based upon the size and form of neuronal bodies, the length and distribution of their dendritic trees, and the destination and degree of branching of their axons. Broadly speaking, neurons can be divided into two major classes: *pyramidal cells* and *interneuron cells*. The principal neuron types and their connections are shown in Fig. 2.5.

Pyramidal cells are so called because their bodies are shaped like pyramids. Their axons are long and go to other areas of the cortex and brain or to the spinal cord. They are *excitatory*.

Interneurons have a body that is round or oval. Their bodies are small and dendrites may spring from them in all directions (stellate cells, i.e. resembling a star). Their axons typically do not leave the cortex and make synapses with nearby neurons. This is why they are called interneurons. They are mainly *inhibitory*. Several types of interneurons have been described: stellate cells, granule cells, basket cells, chandelier (axo-axonic) cells, double-bouquet cells. The axons of chandelier cells synapse directly with the axonic hillock of pyramidal cells, where action potentials initiate, thus exerting the most powerful inhibitory action.

Regions of the brain with plenty of neuronal bodies and dendrites appear grey, and are called *grey matter*. Regions with few neuronal bodies, tend to have plenty of axons, look whiter and are called *white matter*. The cerebral cortex is grey matter.

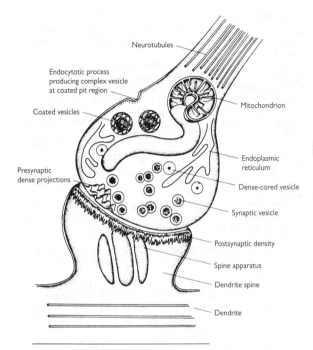

Fig. 2.4 Diagramatic version of and axon terminal (top) forming a synapse on a dendrite spine (bottom). The structures shown are not to scale. Endocytosis produces complex vesicles consisting of a hexagonal basketwork of fibres (cytonet), which form part of the inner surface of the nerve terminal membrane at regions called 'coated pits'. (Reproduced with permission from Bradford HF (1986). *Chemical Neurobiology. An Introduction to Neurochemistry.* WH Freeman and Company, New York.)

Layers of cortex

Cortical cells are not randomly distributed. Different types of cells and axons tend to lay along the cortex with a distribution that, in most regions, makes up six layers:

- Layer I, molecular or plexiform: with few neuronal bodies.
- Layer II or external granular layer: with small pyramidal cells.
- Layer III or pyramidal cell layer: with small pyramidal bodies.
- Layer IV or granular cell layer or internal granular layer: rich in stellate (granular) cells and axons from pyramidal cells.
- Layer V or ganglion cell or giant pyramidal layer: with large bodies of pyramidal cells
- Layer VI or fusiform or multiform cell layer: with cells of different size and shape.

These layers run parallel to the surface of the cortex. Layer I is external (in contact with the meninges) and layer VI is internal (in contact with the white matter).

External axons leave or enter the cortex through the underlying white matter, in the direction perpendicular to the brain cortex. Axons leaving the cortex are called *efferent*, and come from cell bodies in the overlying cortex. Axons entering the cortex, from cell bodies in thalamus or other remote cortex, are called *afferent*. Afferent axons from cortex in the contralateral hemisphere mainly cross the midline through the *corpus callosum* (callosal fibres).

Layers rich in pyramidal cells are predominantly output layers, whereas those rich in granular-stellate cells are mainly input layers, where afferent axons from thalamus and other structures terminate. For instance, layer IV is expanded in thickness in the primary visual cortex, whereas layer V is expanded in the primary motor cortex.

Surround inhibition

When information reaches a cortical region, the axons of interneurons tend to release the inhibitory neurotransmitter gamma-aminobutyric acid (GABA). This creates a small region of inhibition around an active area, called *surround* or *lateral inhibition*. Such inhibition limits the extent of active cortex, often to a rather small area which, when visualized across the cortex, appears as a column of cortex. Such small columns are thought to be the functional units of the cortex. Due to surround inhibition, processed information leaves the cortex mainly through the long axons of pyramidal cells.

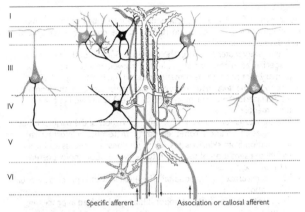

Fig. 2.5 The principal neuron types and their interconnections. The two large pyramidal cells (white) in layers III and V receive multiple synaptic connections from the interneurons (stellate cells, stippled) in layer IV. Basket cell (black) inhibition is directed to the body of cortical neurons. Most input to the cortex arrives from specific thalamic nuclei (specific afferents) and is directed mostly to layer IV. Association and callosal input (association and callosal afferents) is mainly directed to more superficial layers. (Reproduced with permission from Kandel ER and Schwartz JH (eds.) (1985). *Principles of Neural Science*, 2nd edn. Elsevier, New York; adapted from Szentágothai (1969).)

Regions of cortex

As shown in Fig. 2.1, the cortex is divided into lobes (frontal, temporal, parietal, occipital, limbic). Some regions of the cortex are specialized in processing certain tasks:

- The *primary motor cortex* (in the posterior portion of the frontal lobes) is specialized in commanding voluntary movements to muscles. The primary motor cortex is sometimes called the *motor strip*.
- The *supplementary motor cortex* (in the medial aspect of the frontal lobes, anterior to the primary motor cortex) is involved in planning movements.
- The *somatosensory cortex* (in the anterior region of the parietal lobes) processes information from the body (somatosensory information)—information from skin, muscles, joints, tendons. It is necessary for us to feel the sensation of touch and to be aware of our body posture without visual cues.
- The *visual cortex* (in the occipital lobes) is involved in processing visual information.
- The *auditory cortex* (in the temporal lobes) is involved in processing sound.
- The sensory speech area (usually in the left temporal lobe), also called *Wernicke's area*, is responsible for interpreting language (both spoken and written).
- The *motor speech area* (usually in the left frontal lobe), also called *Broca's area*, is responsible for generating speech.
- The *amygdala* and other parts of the *limbic system* are involved in processing emotions.
- The *hippocampus* is involved in processing memories.

The areas other than those mentioned above are generically designated 'association areas'. The functions of association areas are not as clear cut as those of the areas just listed. Generally, the parietal lobe (particularly on the right side) is involved in processing spatial information and body self image. The frontal lobe is involved in thinking, motivation, volition and making decisions.

Motor, somatosensory and visual cortices have a topographic organization (somatotopic representation)—i.e. each area of the cortex process information from (or for) specific areas of the body or visual fields (Fig. 2.6). Auditory cortex shows a tonotopic organization, i.e. certain areas process specific tones. Motor, somatosensory, and visual processing is crossed, i.e. each hemisphere moves and feels the opposite side of the body, and sees the contralateral visual field. Auditory processing is bilateral—each hemisphere receives information from both ears. Consequently, removing or damaging cortex unilaterally can generate severe contralateral motor, somatosensory, or visual deficits, but not major auditory deficits. Some parts of the body have more cortical representation than others in the somatosensory and motor cortices. In particular, hand and face appear to engage a disproportionate area of cortex. It is common practice to draw a subject next to the cortex with the size of body parts proportional to the cortical areas representing them. This creates a distorted figure called *Penfield homunculus* (Fig. 2.6).

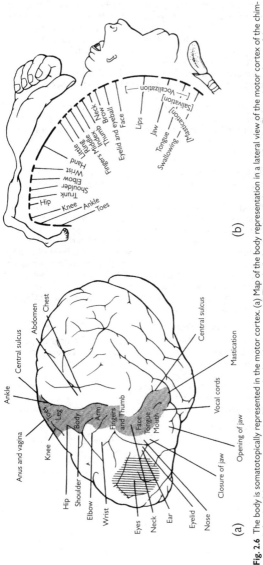

Fig. 2.6 The body is somatotopically represented in the motor cortex. (a) Map of the body representation in a lateral view of the motor cortex of the chimpanzee (left side of the picture is anterior brain and right side is posterior). The shaded area indicates the precentral gyrus. Electrical stimulation of the region highlighted by vertical lines produces eye movements. (b) Body representation in the human motor cortex and corresponding homunculus on a coronal (transversal) section of one hemisphere at the level of the precentral gyrus. (Reproduced with permission from Kandel ER and Schwartz JH (1985). *Principles of Neural Science*, 2nd edn. Elsevier, New York; (a) adapted from Sherrington (1906); (b) adapted from Penfield W and Rasmussen T (1950).)

Hemisphere specialization (asymmetries)

Although both hemispheres can independently process information and make decisions, there is a certain degree of specialization between them— the right hemisphere tends to be better at processing spatial information (e.g.reading maps, solving spatial puzzles) whereas the left hemisphere processes speech in most (not all) subjects. Memory tends to be processed by both hemispheres.

The hemisphere that processes speech is called the dominant hemisphere for speech. The laterality of speech dominance depends on handedness:

- Among right handed people, 96% of subjects have the dominant hemisphere on the left.
- Among left handed people, 70% have the dominant hemisphere on the left, 15% on the right and 15% have speech processing on both sides (codominant).

Function and anatomy of the hippocampus

The main functions of the hippocampus seem to be processing short-term memory and processing spatial information with regard to the position of the subject within its environment. The hippocampus is particularly important in epileptology because it is the source of a high proportion of focal seizures and the most common source of temporal lobe epilepsy. In addition, it has a relatively simple anatomy and internal synaptic connections, which makes it ideal to study the basic mechanisms of synaptic transmission, the mechanisms of epileptogenesis, and the mechanisms of memory. Its basic anatomy is shown in Fig. 2.7. The main input comes from the entorhinal cortex, which itself receives information from wide association cortical areas and subcortical structures (thalamus and amygdala). The main output is the fimbria and fornix.

Connections of the cortex

The cortex receives massive input from subcortical structures, particularly from the thalamus, which is the main subcortical centre involved in processing sensory information. Each cortical area receives and sends information from and to other association areas. The main output of the cortex is the pyramidal tract, composed of axons from the motor area, which convey motor orders to the spinal tracts. Association areas from contralateral hemispheres communicate through the corpus callosum.

Subcortical structures affect cortical excitability

The thalamus and brainstem are connected to the cortex and appear to control global cortical excitability and sleep cycles.

Situation of CA1 abd CA3 in rats and humans

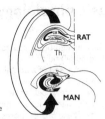

Small arrows show the hippocampal sulcus.
ca1 Regio superior
ca3 Regio inferior
Th Thalamus
The large arrow indicated the inversion of arrangements in the
hippocampus in these two species.

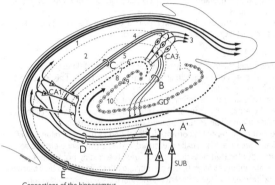

Connections of the hippocampus

Diagram of principal pathways. A B C D E are parts of neuronal chains forming the principal pathways.
A': These perforant fibres join the apical dendrites of the pyramidal neurons directly.

Cornu ammonis:
1 Alveus
2 Stratum pyramidale
3 Axon of pyramidal neurons
4 Schaffer collateral
5 Stratum radiatum and lacunosum
6 Stratum moleculare
7 Hippocampal sulcus

Gyrus dentatus:
8 Stratum moleculare
9 Stratum granulosum
10 Polymorphic layer

GD Gyrus dentatus
CA3, CA1 Fields of the cornu ammonis
SUB Subiculum

Fig. 2.7 Connections of the hippocampus. (Reproduced with permission from
Henri M and Duvernoy JF (1988). *The Human Hippocampus. An Atlas of Applied
Anatomy.* Bergmann Verlag, Munchen.)

Basic physiology

The membrane

- The cell membrane separates intracellular and extracellular (interstitial) fluids.
- It is composed of a double layer of lipids (fat) with sparsely scattered proteins.
- Some proteins behave as pores, which can be open or closed and allow specific charged ions to move between intracellular and extracellular fluids. These protein pores are called *ion channels* (Fig. 2.8)
- Each type of ion channel is generally permeable to one type of ion or to a few types.
- For each ion, the density of ion channels open in the membrane defines the permeability of the membrane to that ion.

The cell at rest

- In every cell there is a voltage difference (potential difference, 📖 see Box 2.1) between intracellular and extracellular fluids. This is called the *membrane potential.*
- In neurons at rest, the intracellular fluid is 60–70mV more negative than the extracellular fluid. The voltage difference between inside and outside the neuron at rest is called the *resting potential.*
- The resting potential is commonly described as having a value of −60 to −70mV because it is usually measured with the reference electrode (0 voltage) located outside the cell. Since the resting potential is generally different from 0, the membrane at rest is said to be polarized.
- In addition to voltage differences, there are also differences in ion concentrations between inside and outside the cell.
- Outside, Na^+, Ca^{2+} and Cl^- exist in much higher concentrations. On the inside, the concentration of K^+ and non-permeable anions (mainly proteins) is much higher (Fig. 2.9).
- Differences in ion concentration, and in electrical potential, existing between inside and outside the cell are also called gradients. Therefore, there is usually a voltage (electrical) gradient and a concentration (chemical) gradient between inside and outside the cell.
- For each ion, the electrical and concentration gradients behave as forces that will move ions between inside and outside the cell, depending on the ion charge and membrane permeability to that ion. According to voltage gradients, positively charged ions tend to move towards negative regions, and negatively charged ions tend to move towards positive regions. In addition, according to concentration gradients, ions tend to move from regions with higher concentrations to regions of lower concentration.
  - For instance, at rest, Na^+ ions will tend to be pushed into the cell because of the concentration gradient (concentration higher outside) and because of the electrical gradient (inside more negative, attracts positively charged external Na^+).
  - On the other hand, K^+ ions tend to be pushed inside by the electrical gradient (inside negativity attracts positively charged K^+) and outside by the concentration gradient (higher concentration inside than outside).

- The passage of charged ions across the membrane behaves as an electrical current (ionic current). Since the electrical resistance of the membrane is relatively high, large voltage changes can be generated by relatively small ionic currents. ($V = I.R$, Ohm's Law) This means that ion concentrations inside and outside the cell tend to change little with voltage changes, unless massive neuronal firing occurs.

Box 2.1 Synonyms

The following terms refer to the same concept:
- Voltage difference
- Potential difference
- Electrical field
- Electrical force
- Voltage gradient
- Potential gradient
- Electrical gradient

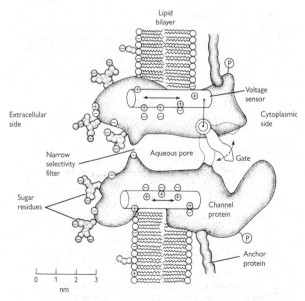

Fig. 2.8 Working hypothesis for a channel. The channel is drawn as a transmembrane macromolecule with a hole through the centre. The external surface (left) of the molecule is glycosylated. The functional regions (selectivity filter, gate, and sensor) are deducted from voltage-clamp experiments and are only beginning to be charted by structural studies. We have yet to learn how they actually look. (Reproduced with permission from Hille B (1992). *Ionic Channels of Excitable Membranes*, 2nd edn. Sinauer Associates, Sunderland, Massachusetts.)

Equilibrium potential

- For each ion, and for a given membrane permeability, there will be a membrane potential at which the forces due to electrical and concentration gradients have similar values and push ions in opposite direction. This is the *equilibrium potential*.
- At the equilibrium potential there will be no net movement of ions across the membrane (since the number of ions that leave the cell due to one gradient will be equal to the number of ions that enter the cell due to the other gradient).
- For each ion type, its equilibrium potential depends on its intracellular and extracellular concentrations, its charge and its membrane permeability. For each value of these variables, the value of the equilibrium potential is given by *Nernst equation*.
- For the usual conditions of mammalians cells, the values for equilibrium potentials are:
  - For Na^+ = +40mV.
  - For K^+ = −100mV.
  - For Cl^- = −75mV.
  - For Ca^{2+} = +250mV.
- Since the value of the equilibrium potential is different for different ions, when there is more than one ion involved an overall equilibrium potential cannot exist, because an equilibrium potential for one ion would be a non-equilibrium potential for another ion. The membrane potential will settle closest to the equilibrium potential of the ion of highest permeability.

Excitable cells and postsynaptic potentials

- For each cell, the value of the resting potential is fairly constant in time.
- In excitable cells (muscle cells, neurons, and a few others), the membrane potential can change as a response to external stimulation. Such stimulation can be the result of the application of electrical current across the membrane, or of the release of specific chemicals (neurotransmitters) into the extracellular fluid.
- In the postsynaptic membrane, changes in the membrane potential seen as a direct response to the release of neurotransmitters are called postsynaptic potentials.
- Postsynaptic potentials can be generated by changes in permeability to specific ions. This occurs due to opening of ion channels as a response to activation of specific membrane receptors by neurotransmitters.
- Neurotransmitters that increase permeability to specific ions tend to drive the membrane potential closer to the equilibrium potentials for these ions.
- Thus, neurotransmitters that increase permeability to Na^+ and/or Ca^{2+} tend to drive the membrane potential closer to the equilibrium potentials for these ions. Since their equilibrium potentials are positive, the membrane potential will become less negative than at rest (and therefore the membrane will become less polarized). This is called *depolarization* (Fig. 2.10).

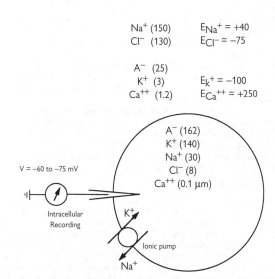

Fig. 2.9 Distribution of ions across neuronal membranes (concentrations in mM) and their equilibrium potentials (expressed as mV). At rest, the cell membrane is permeable to K^+, Na^+, and Cl^-, and exhibits a voltage difference (inside versus outside) of approximately −60 to −70 mV, as seen by an intracellular recording electrode. E = equilibrium potential. (Reproduced with permission from Shepherd GM (1990). *The Synaptic Organization of the Brain*, 3rd edn. Oxford University Press, Oxford.)

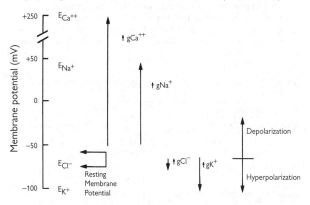

Fig. 2.10 Effect of increasing membrane conductance (or permeability, denoted as g) to Ca^{2+}, Na^+, Cl^-, or K^+. Increases in gCa^{2+} or gNa^+ bring the membrane potential toward more positive values (depolarization), whereas increases in gCl^- or gK^+ bring it toward more negative values (hyperpolarization). E = equilibrium potential. (Reproduced with permission from Shepherd GM (1990). *The Synaptic Organization of the Brain*, 3rd edn. Oxford University Press, Oxford.)

- On the contrary, neurotransmitters that increase permeability to K^+ and/or Cl^- tend to make the membrane potential more negative (and therefore the membrane will become more polarized). This is called *hyperpolarization*.
- Postsynaptic depolarization potentials drive the membrane potential closer to the threshold for action potentials (see below). Therefore, they increase the likelihood of neuronal firing and are called *excitatory postsynaptic potentials (EPSP)*.
- Postsynaptic potentials consisting of hyperpolarization drive the membrane potential away from the threshold for action potentials. Therefore, they decrease the likelihood of neuronal firing and are called *inhibitory postsynaptic potentials (IPSP)*.
- Postsynaptic potentials can add up (Fig. 2.11) and travel along the membrane with a progressive decrement.

Action potentials

In neurons, when the membrane is depolarized to a particular value of membrane potential (called *threshold*), an action potential will occur (Fig. 2.12). Threshold value is variable but is normally between −60 and −50 mV. An action potential is a complex electrical event, which is commonly initiated by a sudden increase in permeability to Na^+. Increases in permeability to K^+ occur later in the action potential (Fig. 2.13). Action potentials are self-propagating (travel along the membrane with no decrement), and are responsible for triggering the release of neurotransmitters when they reach the presynaptic terminal in the axon (Table 2.1). Action potentials are the final electrical events that are responsible for the release of neurotransmitters and therefore for communication of information to the 'next' neuron. Due to their shape, action potentials are sometimes called spikes (different from EEG spikes). A neuron is said to '*fire*' when it generates one action potential or a run of action potentials. The term *adaptation* refers to the decrease in the frequency of action potentials that can be seen during sustained stimulation. Action potentials are usually immediately followed by a relatively long period of hyperpolarization (*after-hyperpolarization*).

Table 2.1 Differences between postsynaptic potentials and action potentials

Postsynaptic potentials	Action potentials
Normally initiated near synapses	Normally initiated at axon hillock
Propagate with decrement (passive propagation)	Propagate without decrement (self-propagating)
Temporal and spatial summation	No summation (refractory period)
Amplitude proportional to stimulus	All-or-nothing

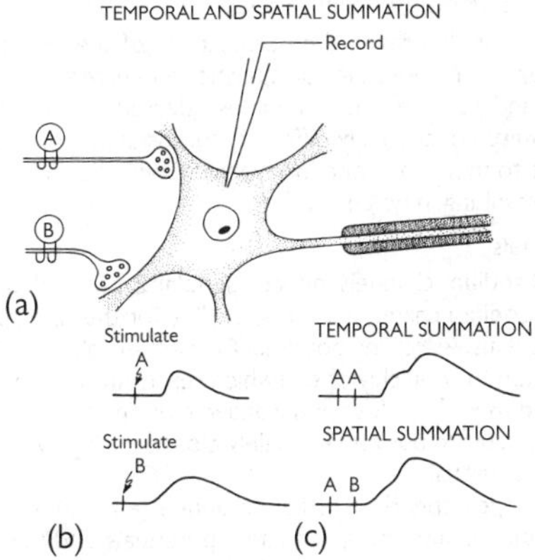

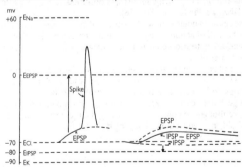

TEMPORAL AND SPATIAL SUMMATION

Fig. 2.11 Temporal and spatial summation of synaptic inputs to a central neuron. (a) The experimental arrangement in which a neuron is impaled by an intracellular recording electrode, and stimulating electrodes. A and B activate two separate inputs that make synaptic contact near each other. (b) Stimulaton of either synaptic input alone evokes an EPSP. (c) The amplitude of the EPSP can be increased either by stimulating the same synaptic contact twice at a short interval (temporal summation) or by stimulating one contact shortly after the other (spatial summation). (Reproduced with permission from Patton DH, Fuchs AF, Hille B, et al. 1989). *Textbook of Physiology*, Vol 1, 21st edn. WB Saunders Company, Philadelphia© 1989, with permission of Elsevier.)

Fig. 2.12 Diagram summarizing the mode of action of postsynaptic excitation and inhibition at chemically operated synapses in the central nervous system in terms of ionic hypothesis. Equilibrium potentials for Na^+, K^+, and Cl^-, and for EPSP and IPSP are shown as dotted lines. At left, EPSP is seen driving membrane potential in depolarizing direction, and at threshold eliciting an action potential in the cell. To right, IPSP and EPSP are shown alone (dotted lines) and when they interact (net effect, continuous line). EPSP is now so depressed by simultaneous IPSP that the membrane potential does not reach cell threshold. Interaction of synaptic influences of opposite signs is the essence of integrative action of single neurons. (Reproduced from Eccles JC, (1963). *Modes of communications between nerve cells. Australian Academy of Science Yearbook*, Waite & Bull with kind permission of the Australian Academy of Science (also published in Montcastle, VB, (1974). Medical Physiology, Vol 1, 13th edn. The CV Mosby Company, Saint Louis).

Membrane channels and currents

Since ion channels determine the permeability of the membrane to specific ions, they are responsible for specific ion currents. For this reason, ion channels and currents are sometimes referred under the same name, although they are conceptually different (for instance, some channels may be permeable to more than one ion type; and one channel might be active but blocked, resulting in no current).

Sodium channels

- Opening of sodium channels induces depolarization. Voltage dependent sodium channels are responsible for the rising phase of action potentials. At resting potential they are mainly closed, with depolarization they quickly open (which results in sodium influx into the cell) and then they close and inactivate during the repolarizing phase. They activate but remain mainly closed during hyperpolarization and resting potential.

- Blocking voltage dependent sodium channels (e.g. with tetradotoxin) prevents initiation and spread of action potentials, and this is thought to be the main mechanism of action of many anticonvulsant drugs (📖 see Neurochemistry of antiepileptic drug action, pp.252–256). The duration of the inactivated state of sodium channels contributes to the cell refractory period and, consequently, determines the maximal firing frequency of the neuron. Therefore, drugs that block voltage dependent sodium channels can block repetitive firing and decrease the threshold for seizures.

- Conversely, late sodium channel openings can result in prolonged depolarization and perhaps seizures, as observed during paroxysmal depolarizing shifts (📖 see Fig 2.16).

- The sodium channels that quickly open and close (*transient*) during the initial half of action potentials were the first to be described. They are blocked by tetradotoxin and their current is called I_{Na} (I stands for current intensity).

- Other sodium channels have been described. There are sodium channels that remain open for much longer, resulting in non-inactivating *persistent* sodium currents (I_{NaP}). They are also blocked by tetradotoxin. Since persistent currents activate at voltage levels below threshold, they are thought to contribute to driving the membrane towards threshold and contribute to initiating transient I_{Na}.

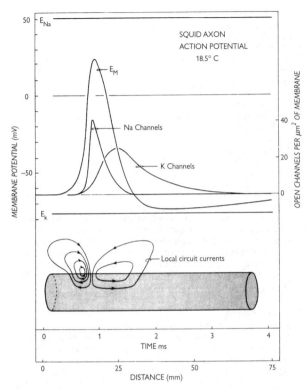

Fig. 2.13 Opening and closing of Na$^+$ and K$^+$ channels during propagated action potential (E$_M$), calculated from Hodgkin–Huxley model. Because the action potential is a non-decrementing wave, the diagram shows the time course of events at one point on the axon or the spatial distribution of event at one time as the action potential propagates from right to left. The absolute calibration in terms of channels per µm^2 is only approximate. The lower diagram shows the local circuit current flowing during the action potential in an axon with greatly exaggerated diameter. (Reproduced with permission from Patton DH, Fuchs AF, Hille B, *et al.* (1989). *Textbook of Physiology*, vol. 1, 21st edn. WB Saunders Company, Philadelphia; adapted after Hodgkin AL and Huxley AF (1952). *J Physiol* (Lond), **117**, 500–44.)

Calcium channels

Opening calcium channels induces depolarization. Brain voltage dependent calcium channels are subclassified into L, P/Q, N, and T channels. L, P/Q and N channels require significant membrane depolarization to become active. T channels can be activated by small depolarization or hyperpolarization. Calcium currents resulting from opening calcium channels are often called $I_{Ca(L)}$, $I_{Ca(P)}$, $I_{Ca(N)}$, or $I_{Ca(T)}$.

- *L channels* are postsynaptic and are responsible for calcium influx during depolarization. They inactivate slowly. Calcium influx can be necessary for gene regulation and for long-term potentiation (see below). Blockade of L-calcium current can be anti- or pro-convulsant, by inhibiting synaptic potentiation, but also inhibiting afterhyperpolarization.
- *N and P/Q receptors* are located in synaptic boutons and mediate calcium entry necessary for neurotransmitter release into the synaptic cleft. They are regulated by G proteins, and therefore modulated by G-protein linked receptors such as $GABA_B$. Inhibiting these calcium currents reduces synaptic release of $GABA_B$.
- *T channels* are activated by hyperpolarization or by small depolarizations, and quickly inactivate. They contribute to the generation of spike-and-wave discharges in absence seizures. Hyperpolarization of thalamo-cortical neurons results in activation of T calcium channels which can be opened by subsequent repolarization, resulting in calcium entry, consequent depolarization, more action potentials and recurrent EEG discharges. Ethosuximide is thought to act as a potent anti-absence drug by blocking T-type calcium channels.

Potassium channels

There are many types of potassium channels. Opening potassium channels generally results in hyperpolarization. *Persistent potassium currents* ($I_{K,leak}$) are responsible for maintaining the membrane resting potential. Voltage-dependent potassium currents can dramatically alter neuronal excitability. *Voltage dependent potassium currents* can influence the resting potential (directly affecting excitability) and are responsible for neuronal repolarization after action potentials. Repolarization rate determines the duration of action potentials, which can influence neurotransmitter release and the propensity for repetitive firing (refractory period).

Voltage-dependent potassium channels are subclassified into:

- *A-type channels* (I_A): they rapidly activate and inactivate. They activate by depolarization of the membrane positive to −60 mV, delaying the onset of action potentials.
- *Delayed rectifier channels* (I_K): they are responsible for some currents that activate during the second half of action potentials. They open during depolarization and do not significantly inactivate.
- *Muscarine-sensitive potassium currents* (I_M): activated by depolarization above −65 mV, and does not inactivate. It is blocked by stimulation of muscarinic cholinergic receptors. Because these are slow and small currents they do not affect the form of the action potentials, but might contribute to adaptation of spike frequency.
- *Inward-rectifying channels* (Kir): the channels open at the resting potential and close during depolarization because they are blocked by

internal ions. Inward rectification refers to the ability of an ion channel to allow greater influx than efflux of ions. In the case of Kir channels, inward rectification is caused by cytoplasmic ions such as polyamines and Mg^{2+}, which plug the conduction pathway on depolarization and thereby impede the outward flow of K^+. Some channels are linked to G-proteins and are therefore activated by G-protein related receptors such as $GABA_B$ receptors. Others open with rises in intracellular ATP.

- In addition to voltage-dependent potassium channels, there are potassium channels that are opened by intracellular calcium (calcium activated potassium channels or $I_{K,Ca}$). They mediate after-hyperpolarization. There are potassium channels activated by intracellular cyclic nucleotides, mainly in retinal photoreceptors. Two calcium activated potassium currents have been described: I_C and I_{AHP}. I_C is sensitive to intracellular calcium and is also voltage dependent, increasing with depolarization. It controls the frequency of action potentials by causing marked hyperpolarization after each action potential. I_{AHP} is slower and generates prolonged after-hyperpolarization (for which it is named), and it is thought to be responsible for frequency adaptation during repetitive firing.

Sodium-potassium currents or hyperpolarizing inward rectification (I_h)

These channels are permeable to potassium and sodium, and depolarize the membrane from a hyperpolarized potential. They activate during hyperpolarization and inactivate during depolarization. They consist of inward cation currents activated by hyperpolarization. Because they are potassium currents that bring the membrane potential towards more positive values (toward resting potential), they are also called I_Q ('queer') or I_f ('funny'). They can depolarize thalamo-cortical neurons, thus inactivating T-type calcium currents. Consequently, they may contribute to terminating thalamo-cortical oscillations responsible for spike-wave activity during absence seizures. Because I_h resists attempts to depolarize the cell, it keeps the resting membrane positive to the equilibrium potential for potassium, close to threshold.

Generation of the electroencephalogram (EEG)

- If relatively large electrodes are placed on the scalp, on the surface of the cortex, or in the cortex, on-going oscillations of electrical potential can be recorded. Such record is called the EEG. The EEG is generated by the addition of all electrical currents simultaneously occurring in the region around the electrodes as a result of ionic currents due to neuronal function.
- In practice, it is believed that most of the EEG signal arises from postsynaptic potentials. Action potentials are thought to be too brief (around 1ms) to add up to generate significant EEG signal.
- For the use and interpretation of the EEG, ▢ see Role of the Encephalogram (EEG), pp.166–175.

Basic neurochemistry

Cortical excitability

- Cortical excitability is determined by a fine balance between excitation and inhibition.
- The main excitatory neurotransmitters in the cortex are aminoacids such as glutamate or aspartate. Apart from acting as neurotransmitters, glutamate and aspartate form part of the structure of many proteins.
- The main cortical inhibitory neurotransmitter is gamma-aminobutyricacid (GABA).
- Glutamate is the main neurotransmitter released by subcortical and intercortical axons that synapse with pyramidal cells.
- GABA is the main neurotransmitter released by cortical interneurons.

Receptors

The receptors to neurotransmitters can be grouped into *ionotropic receptors* (i.e. those where receptor activation is directly coupled to a membrane ion channel) and *metabotropic receptors* (i.e. those where receptor activation is coupled to an intracellular biochemical cascade which may eventually lead to opening or closing of membrane ion channels, amongst other effects). Receptors are usually identified and defined in terms of the chemical compounds that block their actions.

Glutamate receptors

Glutamate is considered the principal excitatory amino acid in the CNS. Postsynaptic glutamate receptors are classified into ionotropic and metabotropic.

Ionotropic receptors (Figs. 2.14 and 2.15)

- Ionotropic receptors to glutamate are classified according to their affinity for three exogenous compounds: *AMPA* (alpha-amino-3-hydroxy-5-methyl-4-isoxazolepropionic acid), *kainate* and *N-methyl-D-aspartate (NMDA)*. Activation of these receptors is associated with EPSP. AMPA receptors were called *quisqualate* receptors in the past. AMPA and kainate receptors are often called *non-NMDA receptors*. AMPA, kainate and NMDA receptors are ionotropic. Most fast excitatory synaptic transmission in the brain is mediated via AMPA and NMDA receptors.
- *Non-NMDA receptors:* EPSPs induced by activation with *AMPA* and *kainate* are due to an increase in permeability to Na^+ and K^+, with a reversal potential around 0 mV. They are fast EPSPs occurring with a short delay after arrival of the action potential to the presynaptic terminal. Non-NMDA receptors consist of at least 4 subunits:
  - AMPA receptors contain subunits GluR1 to GluR4. AMPA receptors lacking GluR2 subunit are permeable to calcium ions.
  - Kainate receptors have subunits GluR5 to GluR7, and KA1 to KA2.
- *NMDA receptors:* EPSPs induced by activation of NMDA receptors result from a *voltage dependent current* due to an increase in permeability to Na^+, K^+ and Ca^{2+}. EPSPs induced by NMDA receptors occur later and have a slower time course than those induced by non-NMDA receptors. The voltage dependence of NMDA-receptor mediated currents is due to blocking of NMDA receptor channels by

magnesium ions (Mg^{2+}). At the resting membrane potential (−75 mV), NMDA receptor channels are blocked by Mg^{2+}. As the membrane depolarizes, Mg^{2+} block becomes weaker or disappears. This can occur during repetitive neuronal activation. NMDA receptor channels can be blocked by *2-amino-5-phophovalerate* (APV).

Activation of NMDA receptors leads to an influx of Ca^{2+} into the post-synaptic cell. This can enhance several cellular biochemical mechanisms resulting in an increased response to excitation (*potentiation*). In rodents, potentiation can last for hours or days (*long-term potentiation*). Long-term potentiation is thought to be the physiological basis of encoding memory in the nervous system and, in particular, in the hippocampus.

Sustained activation of NMDA receptors is thought to result in cell death (*excitotoxicity*). This may be a mechanism by which status epilepticus can lead to brain damage. Neuroscientists have attempted to find specific NMDA receptor blockers to protect against brain damage. NMDA receptors are composed of multiple NR1 subunits, at least one NR2 subunit (NR2A, NR2B, NR2C, or NR2D) and sometimes an NR3 subunit.

Metabotropic receptors
- Metabotropic receptors are also excitatory and their activation induces EPSPs.
- Glutamate metabotropic receptors couple to G-proteins and are classified into three groups:
  - *Group I:* mainly postsynaptic, where they enhance postsynaptic entrance of calcium, calcium release from intracellular endoplasmic reticulum and induce depolarization through inhibition of potassium currents. It is debated whether they play a role in neurodegeneration. Their antagonists have neuroprotective and antiepileptic potential. Group I receptors are subclassified into mGluR1 to mGluR5. They couple to the stimulation of phosphoinositide metabolism through the Gq family of G proteins. The generation of inositol trisphosphate from phosphatidylinositolbiphosphate leads to an increase in intracellular Ca^{2+} by enhancing Ca^{2+} release from the endoplasmic reticulum.
  - *Group II and group III:* group II receptors are subclassified into mGlu2 and mGlu3, whereas group III receptors are subclassified into mGlu4 to mGlu8. They couple to the Gi/o family of G proteins and inhibit adenylyl cyclase. They inhibit GABA and glutamate release.
- AP-4 is a selective agonist at mGluR4 and mGluR6 receptors. Agonists at these receptors could be useful as anticonvulsants through blocking the release of endogenous glutamate.
- 3-5-dihydroxyphenylglycine is an agonist at the mGluR1 and mGluR5 receptors.
- 4-carboxyphenylglycine selectively blocks the mGluR1 receptor.
- The mGluR1 and mGluR5 receptors may play a role in synaptic plasticity and enhance the action of NMDA receptors. Selective mGluR1 and mGluR5 agonists could be useful in the treatment of memory disorders.

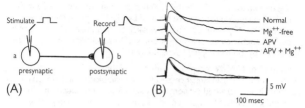

Fig. 2.14 Synaptic potentials mediated by the release of glutamate. (A) Schematic diagram of experimental protocol in which the actions and pharmacology of monosynaptic connections between cultured cortical pyramidal cells is investigated. Intracellular recordings are used to stimulate a generator cell (a) which is monosynaptically connected to a follower cell (b). (B) Activation of an action potential in the generator cell (a) causes a monosynaptic EPSP in the follower cell (b) through the stimulation of AMPA and kainate receptors (top trace). Removal of Mg^{2+} from the medium bathing the cultures enhances the late components of this EPSP (second trace; Mg^{2+}-free). Addition of the NMDA receptor antagonist APV abolishes this late component, indicating that it was due to the activation of NMDA receptors (third trace; APV). Returning Mg^{2+} to the bathing medium now has no additional effect on the EPSP (fourth trace; $APV+Mg^{2+}$). At the bottom of (B) the traces are superimposed for comparison. The data illustrate that the release of glutamate can activate AMPA/kainate and NMDA receptors, and that the NMDA, but not the AMPA/kainate, ionic channel can be blocked by Mg^{2+} ions. (C) Schematic summary diagram illustrating that glutamate release from the presynaptic terminal at a low frequency ('normal synaptic transmission') acts on both NMDA and AMPA/kainate type of receptors. Na+ and K+ flow through the AMPA/kainate channel, but not through the NMDA receptor channel owing to Mg^{2+} block. (D) Depolarization of the membrane potential, or activation of the glutaminergic inputs at a high frequency, relieves the Mg^{2+} block of the NMDA channel, thereby allowing Na+, K+, and, importantly, Ca^{2+} to flow through the channel. Depolarization due to the synaptic potential now also activated other voltage-dependent channels, such as those that conduct Ca^{2+}. (Reproduced with permission from Shepherd GM (1990). *The Synaptic Organization of the Brain*, 3rd edn. Oxford University Press, Oxford. (A) from Huettner JE and Baughman RW (1988). *J Neurosci* **8**, 160–75, with permissions; (C) and (D), data from Nicoll RA (1988). *Science*, **241**, 545–51.)

GABA receptors (Fig. 2.15)

There are two major types of GABA receptors: $GABA_A$ and $GABA_B$. It is interesting to note that glutamate is a metabolic precursor of GABA: glutamic acid decarboxylase (GAD) converts glutamate into GABA.

- *$GABA_A$ receptors (ionotropic):* activation of $GABA_A$ receptors induces fast IPSPs due to an increase in permeability to chloride (Cl^-), with a reversal potential at around −75 mV. $GABA_A$-induced IPSPs have a fast rising phase and a slower decay. They are relatively short, lasting only for a few tens of ms. Many fast IPSPs in the nervous system are thought to be due to activation of $GABA_A$ receptors. There is no second-messenger system involved. Fast ISPSs are directly triggered by $GABA_A$ binding to a receptor located on the ion channel. $GABA_A$ receptors are blocked by bicuculline, picrotoxin or strychnine. Benzodiazepines and barbiturates can also bind $GABA_A$ receptors and enhance the actions of $GABA_A$. Benzodiazepines increase the frequency of channel openings whereas barbiturates increase the duration of channel openings.

- *$GABA_B$ receptors (metabotropic):* activation of $GABA_B$ receptors induces slow IPSPs due to an increase in permeability to potassium (K^+). $GABA_B$-induced IPSPs are mediated by a second-messenger system (G-proteins). Release of GABA is under the control of presynaptic $GABA_B$ receptors. $GABA_B$ receptors are blocked by phaclofen.

Summary of receptors involved in epileptogenesis

Glutamatergic synapses—excitatory

- Ionotropic receptors:
  - AMPA.
  - Kainate.
  - NMDA.
- Metabotropic receptors.

GABAergic synapses—inhibitory

- $GABA_A$ (ionotropic).
- $GABA_B$ (metabotropic).

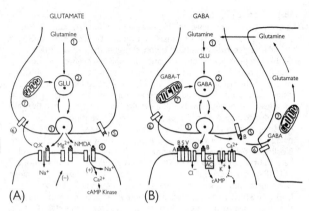

Fig. 2.15 Molecular mechanisms of amino acid synapses. (A) Glutaminergic synapses: (1) synthesis of glutamate (GLU) from glutamine; (2) transport and storage; (3) release of GLU by exocytosis; (4) binding of GLU to quisqualate (Q), kainate (K), and NMDA receptors. The Q and K receptors gate Na^+ and K^+ flux; the NMDA receptor also allows Ca^{2+} entry when the membrane potential is depolarized (+). When the membrane potential is hyperpolarized (-), Mg^{2+} blocks NMDA receptors. The release of GLU may be regulated by presynaptic receptors (?5). Once GLU is released, it is removed from the synaptic cleft by reuptake (6) and processed intracellularly (7). B. GABAergic synapse: (1) synthesis of GABA from glutamine; (2) transport and storage of GABA; (3) release of GABA by exocitosis; (4) binding to a $GABA_A$ receptor which can be blocked by bicuculline (B), picrotoxin, or strychnine (S) and can also be modified by benzodiazepines, such as valium (V); $GABA_B$ receptors, by contrast, are linked via a G-protein to K^+ and Ca^{2+} channels which are blocked by GABA; (5) release of GABA is under the control of presynaptic $GABA_B$ receptors; GABA is removed from the synaptic cleft by uptake into terminals or glia (6); (7) processing of GABA back to glutamine. (Reproduced with permission from Shepherd GM (1990). *The Synaptic Organization of the Brain*, 3rd edn. Oxford University Press, Oxford.)

Mechanisms of epileptogenesis

(By Dr Antonio Valentín)

Epileptogenesis (the generation of epileptic seizures) can be explained by a number of mechanisms. It is believed that epileptic seizures result from synchronous *repetitive firing (bursts)* of action potentials in many cortical neurons. Basically, seizures can result from *increase excitability* or *decreased inhibition* (both increasing the likelihood of cell firing) and from *hyper-synchronicity* of neuronal firing. The basic mechanisms of epileptogenesis can be studied *in vitro* (in individual cells or in tissue slices) or *in vivo* (in the complete animal).

In vitro experiments have elucidated some mechanisms that might be involved in the generation of interictal EEG spikes. The mechanisms of focal seizures are less well developed.

Cellular and network mechanisms of epileptogenesis

Bursts of action potentials often occur during a long depolarization. Prolonged depolarizations can occur spontaneously in a neuronal network, or can be induced by artificially injecting current into a neuron (e.g. during current clamp experiments). When studying brain tissue slices, prolonged depolarizations with superimposed trains of action potentials (*paroxysmal depolarization shifts* or *PDS*) can occur, either spontaneously or as a result of neuronal stimulation (Fig. 2.16). PDS have the following characteristics:

- PDS are large depolarizations of the neuronal membrane (20–40 mV), similar to a giant EPSP.
- PDS drive the membrane potential above threshold, making neurons fire rapid bursts of action potentials.
- PDS are generated by voltage-sensitive sodium currents induced by activation glutamate receptors, and by voltage-sensitive calcium channels which can generate slow action potentials.

There are some theoretical and experimental factors, which are necessary for the generation of PDS:

- Existence of a synaptic network with strong excitatory (pyramidal) neurons that are able to drive the membrane potential above threshold.
- Large population of connected neurons, probably >1000 neurons.

PDS are thought to be the equivalent event in cortical slices to interictal EEG spikes seen *in vivo*.

In some epilepsies, particularly in idiopathic epilepsies, seizures might result from changes in the intrinsic properties of voltage-dependent ion channels (potassium, sodium channels) and synaptic receptors (mainly GABA or nicotinic receptors).

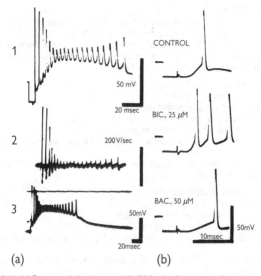

Fig. 2.16 (a) Paroxysmal depolarizing shift (PDS) of a CA3 neuron. The PDS is evoked by stimulation of mossy fibres after bicuculline. High- and low gain DC recordings with different time-scales in lines 1 and 3, the electrically differentiated record of the signal in line 2. Starting with the first action potential, the spike repolarization is stepwise reduced and the membrane is strongly depolarized for nearly 60ms, until the membrane repolarizes very slowly (A3). (b) Suppression of bicuculline-induced multiple discharges by baclofen. After adding bicuculine to the perfusate, the gyrus dentatus cells responded with multiple spikes to a stimulation of the perforant pathway (B2). Adding baclofen (50μM) to the same solution blocks the multiple spikes (D3). (Reproduced with permission from Wieser HG, Speckmann E-J, Engel J (1987). *The Epileptic Focus.* John Libbey, London–Paris; adapted from Misgeld U, Klee MR, Zeise ML (1982). In *Physiology and Pharmacology of Epileptic Phenomena*, Klee MR, Lux HD, and Speckman EJ (eds.), pp.131–9. Raven Press: New York.)

The most common acute experimental procedure used to understand the basic mechanisms of epileptogenesis is the hippocampal slice, mainly obtained from rat brain. In essence, transversal slices of the hippocampus are cut in an attempt to gain direct access to neuronal tissue while preserving local connections within the slice.

Advantages of slice technique

- Simple preparation of slices.
- Control of the experimental conditions
- No physiological movements—pulse, breathing, etc.
- Good access and visualization of tissue.
- Easy to modify the extracellular medium—adding drugs or changing ionic concentrations.
- Connections in the hippocampus are maintained in the slice preparation— tri-synaptic circuit.

Disadvantages of slices technique

- Neurons without their normal afferents.
- Neurons without their normal efferents.
- Some damage to the tissue is unavoidable.
- Slices can lose their normal electrophysiological characteristics with time.
- Excitability can change with anoxia provoked during manipulation of the slices.

Basically two types of experimental designs can be performed in hippocampal slices:

- *Extracellular recordings:* to stimulate extracellularly an area of the hippocampus (e.g. gyrus dentatus, CA3, CA1) and record extracellular responses from a connected region. For instance, stimulating CA3 and recording from the striatum radiatum of CA1, where axons from CA3 synapse with dendrites from CA1 (📖 see Fig. 2.7, p.25).
- *Intracellular recordings:* to record the effects of stimulation, neurotransmitters or changes in extracellular fluid composition on intracellularly recorded membrane potential or currents via voltage or current clamp techniques.

Mechanisms of generating hyperexcitable networks

Most hypotheses on how cortex becomes hyperexcitable are based on changes in the balance between excitation and inhibition, leading to overall hyperexcitability. However, as neurons are part of networks with profuse interconnections, other mechanisms such as hypersynchrony can be involved in the generation of seizures. Some of the suggested mechanisms involved in the epileptogenesis are:

Loss of inhibition

Loss of inhibition can be due to two possible mechanisms:

- Destruction of inhibitory cells.
  - Although loss of GABAergic inhibitory interneurons may contribute to epileptogenesis, several studies have provided evidence that inhibition is not depressed in epileptogenic regions and may actually be enhanced.

- Some studies suggest that in epilepsy there is selective loss of inhibitory neurons which project to dendrites of granule cells, and that there is preservation of perisomatic inhibitory cells, which are responsible for the synchronization of large cell populations.
- Deafferentation of inhibitory cells—e.g. destruction of the excitatory neurons of the hilus.

Excitatory axonal sprouting

Axonal sprouting—of which the best known example involves the mossy fibres—can produce increased synaptic connectivity with the following characteristics:

- Axonal sprouts from relatively mature neurons tend to synapse locally rather than travelling long distances.
- New synapses are mainly excitatory.
- Some axons synapse onto inhibitory interneurons, resulting in strengthening of recurrent inhibition.

Hypersynchrony

Some factors are important for the generation of hypersynchrony between different areas of the hippocampal slice:

- *Inhibition block:* in normal conditions there are hardly any spontaneous field potentials in the hippocampus. If IPSPs are blocked (e.g. with bicuculline), spontaneous multipeaked field potentials appear in CA1, CA2, and CA3, suggesting a degree of neuronal synchronicity.
- *Neuronal connectivity:* neurons from areas CA3 and CA2 show 'bursting activity' even when isolated, but the neurons from CA1 require input from CA3/CA2 for burst firing.
- *Inhibition block plus neuronal connectivity:* if inhibition is intact, CA3 cannot drive spontaneous activity in CA1.
- *Non-synaptic mechanisms:* electrical field effects may induce rapid synchronization of action potentials.
- *Electrical synapses:* electrotonic (gap) junctions can lead to rapid synchronization and reduce seizure threshold.

Changes in extracellular ionic concentrations

Increases in extracellular K^+ concentration (e.g., because of prolonged cell firing during seizures) will increase neuronal hyperexcitability.

Thalamocortical circuits

In generalized seizures, the question arises as to the mechanisms by which most of the cortex synchronizes at once. There is ample anatomical and physiological evidence suggesting that non-specific thalamic nuclei and reticular formation play an important role in controlling cortical excitability and, in particular, in the generation of seizures in generalized epilepsies. It was initially thought that a midbrain or thalamic disturbance was the origin of generalized seizures—*centrencephalic hypothesis*. However, further evidence from the amytal test and other sources suggested that generalized seizures arise from a disturbance in the interaction between cortex and midbrain, possibly associated with a globally hyperexcitable cortex—*corticoreticular theory*.

Absence epilepsy is a type of generalized epilepsy where there is a detailed model of the basic mechanisms originating generalized seizures. They arise from the thalamocortical system, and appear to depend on the properties of both cortex and thalamus.

Thalamic neurons have 'oscillating' currents that can trigger action potentials after repolarization and after-hyperpolarization:

- *Calcium I_T current:* low threshold calcium spikes (calcium action potentials when the neuron is only slightly depolarized)
- *Potassium I_H or I_Q currents:* depolarization after hyperpolarization of the cell.

The thalamus is reciprocally connected with the cortex. For every one fibre from thalamus to cortex, there are about 40 fibres from cortex to thalamus. Synchronization between thalamus and cortex during typical absences with 3Hz spike and wave activity depends on synchronization of the thalamus by rhythmic activity of networks.

Conclusion

Some of the basic mechanisms of epileptogenesis in some forms of epilepsy have been carefully studied. Nevertheless, many important aspects remain an active area of research. Identifying specific physiological mechanisms can provide useful insight into new treatments.

Experimental models of epilepsy

Experimental models of epilepsy and seizures—on animals or tissue slices—are used to investigate the mechanisms responsible for epilepsy, to screen for new antiepileptic drugs, and to establish the mechanisms of action of antiepileptic drugs. Models carried out on live animals are called *in vivo*, whereas those models obtained in tissue slices or cells are called *in vitro*.

In vivo models of focal (partial) seizures

The following *in vivo* techniques have been used as models of focal seizures:

- Cortical application of antagonists of inhibitory amino acid receptors (penicillin, bicuculline, picrotoxin, strychnine): spike-like discharges develop within minutes.
- Cortical application of metals (aluminium, cobalt, tungsten, zinc, iron): it takes 4 –9 weeks to develop focal seizures.
- Cortical application of convulsants:
  - Pentylenetetrazol.
  - Tetanus toxin.
  - Kainic acid: a glutamate receptor agonist.
  - Pilocarpine: a muscarinic agonist.
  - GHB (gamma-hydroxybutyrate).
  - THIP (4,5,6,7-tetrahydroxyisoxazolo-4,5,c-pyridine-3-ol): a $GABA_A$ receptor antagonist.
  - AY-9944: inhibits the reduction for 7-dehydrocholesterol to cholesterol.
  - Flurothyl.
  - Homocysteine.
- Cooling of a cortical region: focal cryogenic stimulation.
- Focal electrical stimulation:
  - *Acute effects:* stimulation of the cortex with runs of electrical pulses (at a frequency above 5Hz) induces focal seizure like EEG patterns (called afterdischarges) around the stimulated area. If stimulation continues, an overt clinical seizure can occur.
  - *Chronic effects (kindling model):* in non-epileptic animals, daily repeated subconvulsive electrical stimulation with runs of electrical pulses initially do not induce seizures. After a few weeks stimulation can induce seizures. If daily stimulation continues, spontaneous focal seizures can occur, ultimately unrelated to stimuli. Limbic structures (amygdala, hippocampus) of the rat appear to be particularly susceptible to kindling.

In vivo models of generalized seizures

The following *in vivo* techniques have been used as models of generalized seizures:

- Systemic injection (intravenous) of drugs:
  - *Convulsive seizures:* pentylenetetrazol, bicuculline, kainic acid, pilocarpine, flurothyl, homocysteine.
  - *Absence-like seizures*: penicillin, gamma-hydroxybutyrate (GHB), THIP (4,5,6,7-tetrahydroxyisoxazolo-4,5,c-pyridine-3-ol), AY-9944.

- Electroshock: trains of electrical currents at 50–60Hz applied through corneal electrodes for 200ms induce seizures in mice and rats. Two parameters are commonly measured: the stimulus intensity needed to induce 5sec of continuous clonus (minimal) and the stimulus needed to induce tonic–clonic seizures (maximal electroshock [MES]). This model has been particularly useful in testing anticonvulsant properties of compounds to identify new antiepileptic drugs.
- Environmental trauma: hypoxia, hyperbaric conditions, overhydration (hypo-osmolarity).
- Genetic models (📖 see pp.50–51).

In vitro models of epilepsy

The following *in vitro* models have been developed:
- Dissociated cell cultures.
- Tissue slices from normal mammalian hippocampus and neocortex.
- Tissue slices from animals previously injected with an epileptogenic agent—usually tetanus toxin.
- Slice culture.
- Isolated brain (guinea pig).
- Reptilian (turtle) preparation: slices or hemispheres.

In addition to exposing brain tissue to the convulsant agents, *in vitro* models permit manipulation of the composition of the extracellular fluid. Events resembling interictal and ictal discharges can be seen with low magnesium, low calcium, high potassium, and in the presence of blockers of potassium channels such as 4-aminopyridine.

Models of status epilepticus

- *Systemic administration of convulsants in vivo:* bicuculline, allylclycine, 4-deoxypyridoxine, kainic acid, flurothyl, pilocarpine, pilocarpine after lithium pretreatment, pentylenetetrazol, pentylenetetrazol/phenytoin, soman (a cholinesterase inhibitor).
- *Cortical application of convulsants in vivo:* alumina gel/4-deoxypyridoxine, cobalt/homosysteine, bicuculline injected into area tempestas, domoic acid, kainic acid in amygdala or hippocampus, withdrawal of GABAergic drugs.
- *Electrical stimulation in vivo:* long lasting stimulation, kindling stimuli administered over several months.
- *In vitro models:* as models for seizures. In particular, conditions with low magnesium, low calcium, high potassium, or with 4-aminopyridine.

Genetics and epilepsy

Key points

- Genetic factors contribute to the aetiology of at least 40% of people with epilepsy.
- Epilepsy may be one of many clinical features in a number of inherited diseases. This is addressed as appropriate in other sections.
- Epilepsy is inherited as a simple Mendelian trait in no more than 1–2%.
- In most, idiopathic epilepsy inheritance is complex.
- Genetic idiopathic epilepsy is more likely to present early in life, namely in childhood and young adulthood. However, genetic contributions in later presentations are harder to ascertain.
- There is overlap between epilepsies that are primarily genetic and those that are acquired.
- Causative genetic mutations have been found in Mendelian pedigrees with idiopathic epilepsy.
- *De novo* mutations have also been found in a few syndromes occurring sporadically, such as severe myoclonic epilepsy in infancy.
- Most but not all mutations identified so far in idiopathic epilepsy are in ion channel or receptor genes.
- There are many genetic animal models of epilepsy.

Genetic animal models of epilepsy

- These include animals with seizures occurring either spontaneously or in response to stimuli—audiogenic, photic, or sensory. In some, the epilepsy is associated with other deficits such as ataxia or poor survival.
- There are models of idiopathic epilepsy and models of epilepsy associated with cortical malformations.
- The genetic mutation may be known particularly where the epilepsy segregates as a Mendelian trait.
- Examples of epileptic animals include dogs usually with generalized tonic clonic seizures, chicken, photosensitive baboons (*Papio papio*), mice, rats, and gerbils.
- Some animal models show spike-wave absences. The tottering, lethargic, and stargazer mice, for example, have recessively inherited voltage gated calcium sub-unit gene mutations and display spike/wave absences, motor seizures, and ataxia.

Idiopathic epilepsy in humans

- Most idiopathic epilepsies are complexly inherited.
- Identifying susceptibility traits is difficult and will require large-scale genome-wide association studies using efficient molecular technology.
- Genetic defects have been identified in less common Mendelian pedigrees.
- It is possible, indeed likely, that the same genes will turn out to be relevant in complexly-inherited epilepsies, although this remains to be shown.
- Examples of genes where mutations have been shown to cause epilepsy are listed in Box 2.2. Some of these are inherited mutations and others are sporadic.

- Familial studies have shown that the same causative genetic defect can be associated with varying phenotypes in the same pedigree, presumably because of the interaction with other genes or with environmental factors. A good example is that of the syndrome of generalized epilepsy with febrile seizures plus, or GEFS+ (🕮 see also Chapter 3b, p.98). This is an autosomal dominant familial syndrome with reduced penetrance and more than one phenotype observed within each pedigree. Affected individuals usually experience febrile seizures, which may persist beyond 6 years. Afebrile seizures occur in a proportion. Afebrile seizures are usually generalized and include absences, myoclonic seizures, and atonic seizures. Most affected individuals have relatively benign epilepsy but more severe phenotypes—such as myoclonic-astatic epilepsy and severe myoclonic epilepsy of infancy—may occur. Some pedigrees have prominent absences, less commonly focal seizures. A small proportion of patients develop intractable focal epilepsy with hippocampal sclerosis.
- Not only can the same genetic defect be associated with different phenotypes in the same pedigree, but some syndromes have been shown to be due to different genes/genetic defects (🕮 see Box 2.2), although these may be related.

Box 2.2 Some genetic mutations in idiopathic human epilepsy

Potassium, chloride, sodium channel, and GABA genes:
- Benign familial neonatal convulsions—KCNQ2, KCNQ3
- Benign familial neonatal infantile convulsions—SCN2A
- Benign familial infantile convulsions—SCN2A
- Generalized epilepsy with febrile seizures plus—SCN1B, SCN1A, SCN2A, GABRG2
- Absence epilepsy and febrile seizures—GABRG2
- Severe myoclonic epilepsy of infancy—SCN1A
- Autosomal dominant juvenile myoclonic epilepsy—GABRA1
- Autosomal dominant febrile seizures—SCN1A, GABRG2
- Autosomal dominant idiopathic generalized epilepsy—CLCN2

Acetylcholine receptor
Autosomal dominant nocturnal frontal lobe epilepsy—CHRNA4, CHRNB2

Other
- Juvenile myoclonic epilepsy—EFHC1 (Myoclonin1, encodes protein with a Ca(2+)-sensing EF-hand motif)
- Autosomal dominant focal epilepsy with auditory features—LGI1 (leucine-rich, glioma inactivated gene 1)

Causes of human epilepsy

Epilepsy can run in families with no particular cause other than a genetic predisposition to suffer epileptic seizures. This type of epilepsy is called *primary* or *idiopathic epilepsy*. There is no evidence of brain damage in this type of epilepsy. These epilepsies are likely to be due to subtle genetic mutations.

On the other hand, epilepsy can be caused by virtually any insult (damage) to the cortex, whether it occurs *in utero*, at birth, after birth or as a consequence of genetic abnormalities associated with brain damage. This type of epilepsy is called *secondary* or *symptomatic epilepsy*.

Causes of symptomatic epilepsy are multiple and include:

- Pre- or perinatal hypoxia.
- Porencephaly, a sequel of a perinatal middle-cerebral artery infarct.
- Cerebral hypoxia in adult life.
- Head (brain) injury: particularly if associated with loss of consciousness or amnesia >24 hours, intracranial haematoma, or following penetrative injuries (33–53% of patients having cerebral missile injuries develop epilepsy).
- Neurosurgery.
- Intracranial tumours: 📖 see Epilepsy after cerebral tumours, hamartomas, and neurosurgery, pp.486-488
- Cerebrovascular disease: 📖 see Cerebrovascular disease, p.490.
- CNS infections: encephalitis, meningitis, abscess, tuberculoma, parasitosis.
- Alzheimer disease: seizures occur late in the disease in 15% of patients.
- Genetic disorders associated with brain damage: Down's syndrome.
- Metabolic disorders: Unverricht–Lundborg disease, Lafora disease, neuronal ceroliopofuscinosis, type III Gaucher disease, gangliosidosis, mitochondrial disease, sialidosis, etc.
- Hippocampal sclerosis.
- Developmental abnormalities: focal cortical dysplasia, cortical malformations, hemimegaloencephaly, etc. 📖 see Abnormalities of cortical development, pp.478-484.

Pathology of epilepsy

- The terms *neuropathological abnormalities*, *neuropathology*, *structural abnormalities and pathology* refer to the abnormalities that can be seen on visual inspection of the brain or during microscopic examination. Many neuropathological abnormalities (but not all) can also be identified with modern neuroimaging techniques.
- Idiopathic epilepsies may not show structural abnormalities. Routine neuroimaging in these epilepsies is normal. No clear detectable neuropathological abnormalities are thought to be present in idiopathic epilepsies.
- Symptomatic epilepsies are due to some form of brain damage, which leaves a structural abnormality. Presumed symptomatic (cryptogenic) epilepsies are also thought to be due to brain damage, although no evidence of a structural abnormality can be found, presumably due to the limited sensitivity of present diagnostic methods.
- Most of what we know of neuropathology of epilepsy derives from brain specimens removed during surgery for the treatment of epilepsy, e.g. in patients with symptomatic focal epilepsy.

Neuropathological abnormalities associated with epilepsy

Lesions originating during intrauterine life

These lesions are developmental abnormalities, generally of unknown cause. Suggested causes include genetic conditions, placental abnormalities, anoxia, malnutrition, radiation, chemicals, and viral infection. They can be divided into *disorders of neuronal migration* (heterotopias, polymicrogyria, megalencephaly, focal cortical dysplasia, tuberous sclerosis, hamartomas, meningoangiomatosis) and *disorders of vascular organization* (cavernous haemangioma, arteriovenous malformation and Sturge–Weber syndrome). There is some debate about whether some conditions of the latter group can originate after intrauterine life.

Heterotopias: neurons are abnormally present in the subcortical white matter forming lamina or nodules (laminar or nodular heterotopia). Laminar heterotopias tend to occur within the centrum semiovale (the core of the hemispheric white matter). Nodular heterotopia tends to occur around the angles of the lateral ventricles. Heterotopias are often bilateral and may or may not be associated with learning difficulties.

Polymicrogyria: this is characterized by the presence of many small abnormally formed gyri with the so-called cobblestone appearance. Polymicrogyria can be localized, widespread, or bilateral and appears to have a predilection for the opercula of the insula. The affected cortex may show fused cortex (unlayered polymicrogyria) or rarely has only four layers (four-layered polymicrogyria). Polymicrogyria is most frequently caused by intrauterine ischaemia but rarely it can be seen in neonates infected with cytomegalovirus and even familiar cases are known.

Megalencephaly: the brain is abnormally large due to thickening and disorganization of the cerebral cortex. It can be bilateral or unilateral (hemimegalencephaly). Heterotopias are often present. Hydrocephalus or storage diseases should be excluded.

Focal cortical dysplasia (FCD)(Fig. 2.17): in this condition normal lamination of the cortex is lost, as is the demarcation between grey and white matter. There are abnormally large (dysmorphic) neurons scattered throughout the cortex and may extend in small clusters into the subjacent white matter. FCD may present with or without balloon cells (abundant glassy cytoplasm and dysplaced nuclei). The findings resemble cortical tubers in tuberous sclerosis. Interesting, the first seizure in patients with focal cortical dysplasia can occur with a long delay after birth, between 2–31 years of age.

Tuberous sclerosis: cortical tubers resemble those described in focal cortical dysplasia. However, lesions are often multiple, and characterized by cortical nodularity and calcification. Patients may have learning difficulties and may have subependymal nodules from which subependymal giant cell astrocytoma may develop. In most instances, cutaneous lesions (sebaceous nevi) and hamartomatous visceral tumours (angiomyolipoma, rhabdomyoma, and perivascular epithelioid cell tumour) are also present. There are *formes frustes*, where learning difficulties and/or cutaneous manifestations are absent.

Hamartomas: these contain clusters of neurons arranged in a disorganized manner and do not expand. They often show calcification. They tend to occur in the amygdala, fusiform gyrus, and less frequently in the hippocampus. Hypothalamic hamartomas can be associated with gelastic (laughing) seizures, precocious puberty, and learning difficulties.

Meningioangiomatosis: in this condition, cerebral cortex is replaced by meningovascular tissue which does not grow (in contrast to meningiomas). Not to be confused with multiple meningiomas sometimes seen in neurofibromatosis 2 disease.

Cavernous haemangiomas: they are static lesions composed of endothelial lined distended vascular channels with frequently thrombosed vessels, thick collagenuous walls surrounded by gliotic brain and haemosiderin deposition due to previous bleeding. Calcification is common. They show predilection for peri-central location, often inducing focal motor seizures.

Arteriovenous malformations: these are responsible for shunting of arterial blood into altered venous channels, inducing local alterations of cerebral flow. Gliosis and haemosiderin deposition is also seen around the lesion.

Sturge–Weber syndrome (encephalofacial angiomatosis): in this condition these is a triad of seizures, facial nevus flammeus and intracerebral calcification with occipital predilection. Intracranial lesions include calcified cortex with pial venous angioma.

Lesions originating at childbirth

Prematurity, and perinatal hypoxia can generate cerebral lesions, often leading to epilepsy.

- *Perinatal arterial occlusion* can generate cerebral infarcts and later epilepsy. Infarcts can be massive and, when affecting the middle cerebral artery, can induce massive necrosis and loss of most parietal lobe (porencephaly). The cause of perinatal arterial occlusion is unclear (embolism from the placenta, thrombus generated in fetal placental veins or heart).
- *Neonatal hypoxia* can be associated with *ulegyria* (mushroom-like gyri, affecting mainly the depths of the sulci rather than the crowns of gyri).

Lesions resulting from febrile convulsions

Children <2 years have relatively high susceptibility to suffer epileptic seizures during febrile illness. Prolonged and recurrent febrile convulsions
may lead to neuronal damage affecting hippocampus, amygdala, and medial
temporal lobe, possibly causing mesial temporal sclerosis. Genetic susceptibility is likely.

Lesions resulting from inflammation or infection

Brain inflammation and infection—meningitis, encephalitis—often resolve
leaving multiple patchy infarcts, necrosis, cerebral abscess, granulation, or
scar tissue. Astrocytic and microglial infiltration can be seen during the
active phase or in chronic encephalitis such as Rasmussen's. Parasites can
be seen in parasitic infestations.

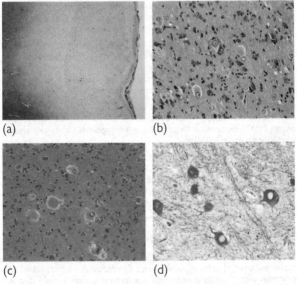

Fig. 2.17 Focal cortical dysplasia, type IIB. (a) The cortex is focally distended and the
demarcation is lost between grey and white matter (Luxol fast blue). (b–c) Presence
of dysmorphic neurons and balloon cells (H&E). (d) Immunohistochemistry for
neurofilament demonstrates dysmorphic neurons with disoriented neuronal
processes. Figure kindly provided by Dr Istvan Bodi.

Head injury

Residual lesions of trauma usually include multiple wedge-shaped scars—particularly over orbital frontal and lateral temporal gyri—mainly composed of collagenuous fibrosis intermingled with glial proliferation with destruction of cortical layers. Haemosiderin deposition is frequent in the wall of the cystic lesions.

Stroke in adults

Infarcts typically leave wedge-shaped or cystic scars. Epilepsy, however, occurs relatively infrequently after stroke (estimated at 10% more frequently after severe or haemorrhagic strokes.

Anoxic enchephalopathy

Anoxic encephalopathy is increasingly encountered as a result of cardiopulmonary resuscitation. It is often associated with persistent myoclonic jerks and sometimes generalized convulsive seizures. It is associated with laminar cortical necrosis with accentuation of sulci depth. Arterial watershed distribution can sometimes be seen or can be superimposed with more widespread abnormalities. Similar findings can be seen after profound hypoglycaemia.

Tumours

- Any brain tumour may lead to seizures due to space occupation. However, the low-grade tumours which are more commonly associated with chronic epilepsy are:
- *Low grade astrocytoma*: prominent fibrillary background, hyperchromatic angular nuclei, rare mitoses, hypercellularity, and minimal pleomorphism. Although benign, these tumours are infiltrative, often distorting the junction between grey and white matter.
- *Oligodendroglioma*: most affect white matter and overlying grey matter, and are sometimes cystic. The tumour cells form characteristic perinuclear halos, giving fried egg appearances, without prominent fibrillary background. Calcification is often prominent.
- *Ganglioglioma*: most commonly found in temporal lobes. The tumour is often cystic and is composed of dysplastic neurons and astrocytic tumour cells. Tumours are often reticulin rich, with prominent calcification and perivascular lymphocytes.
- *Pleomorphic xanthoastrocytoma*: usually located superficially, next to the meninges. The tumour is moderately cellular, without necrosis or mitosis, rich in reticulin, with multinucleate giant cells and lipid-laden xanthomatous cells. Infiltration by lymphocytes and plasma cells is common.
- *Dysembryoplastic neuroepithelial tumour (DNET)*: superficial cortical lesions most commonly in temporal or frontal lobes, usually arranged in solitary or multiple nodules. The oligodendroglial-like immature neurocytes produce myxoid background and include scattered floating neurons. Sometimes they are associated with cortical dysplasia.

Inborn errors of metabolism—endogenous metabolic encephalopathies or storage disease

Genetically-determined absence of specific enzymes can be responsible for neuronal accumulation of non-metabolized compounds. In some, the biochemical mechanism has been established (Tay–Sachs disease,

GM2 gangliosidosis, hexosaminidase deficiency) whereas others are sometimes classified as neurodegenerative disease. For detailed descriptions of neuropathological abnormalities in these conditions see Scaravilli.[1]

Metabolic encephalopathies

Mitochondrial diseases may lead to multiple subcortical infarcts, usually not respecting arterial territories. Muscle biopsy may reveal ragged red fibres. The most common mitochondrial conditions are known as MERRF (myoclonic epilepsy with ragged-red fibres) and MELAS (mitochondrial myopathy, encephalopathy, lactic acidosis, and stroke-like episodes). Secondary mitochondrial DNA defects also occur because of mutations in the nuclear gene, POLG (DNA polymerase gamma) on which maintenance of mitochondrial DNA is critically dependent.

Mesial temporal sclerosis (Fig. 2.18)

This is the most common cause of symptomatic focal epilepsy. Neuropathological findings include loss of pyramidal neurons, predominantly in the CA1 of the hippocampus, associated with astrocytic gliosis and atrophy. Neuronal loss and gliosis may be observed in the amygdala and parahippocampal gyrus. In some cases, there is mild atrophy of most temporal cortex. Mild cases might be restricted to the end folium of the hippocampus (end folium sclerosis).

Iatrogenic lesions

For instance chronic treatment with phenytoin can induce gingival hyperplasia, lymphadenopathy (most commonly involving cervical nodes) and cerebellar atrophy.

Neuropathological abnormalities found in temporal lobe epilepsy

- Mesial temporal sclerosis.
- Tumours: astrocytomas and other glioneuronal tumours, oligodendrogliomas, dysembryoplastic neuroepithelial tumours.
- Vascular malformations: arteriovenous malformations, cavernous angiomas.
- Developmental lesions: focal cortical dysplasia, hamartomas.
- Post-traumatic lesions.
- Others: developmental cysts, fibroglial scars, infection, inflammation, infarct.

Neuropathological abnormalities found in frontal lobe epilepsy

Lesions are similar to those seen in the temporal lobes except for mesial temporal sclerosis:

- Post-traumatic lesions.
- Tumours: gliomas, particularly low-grade astrocytomas, oligodendrogliomas. Dysembryoplastic neuroepithelial tumours are much less common than in the temporal lobe.
- Vascular malformations: arteriovenous malformations, cavernous angiomas.
- Developmental lesions: focal cortical dysplasia (particularly peri-central cortex).

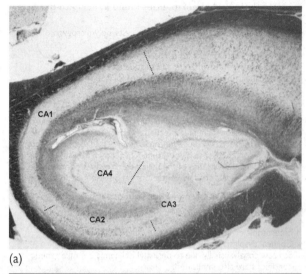

(a)

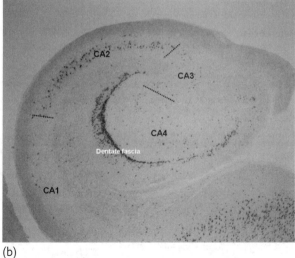

(b)

Fig. 2.18 Hippocampal sclerosis. Subtotal neuronal loss in the CA1 segment of the hippocampus. The neuronal loss is moderate in the CA3-4 segments and the neurons of CA2 segment are relatively preserved. (a) Luxol fast blue; (b) Neu-N immunohistochemistry). Figure kindly provided by Dr Istvan Bodi.

Neuropathological abnormalities found in occipito-parietal epilepsy

- Peri-natal injury: atrophy, porencephalic cysts, polymicrogyria, schizencephaly, ulegyria.
- Developmental lesions: focal cortical dysplasia.
- Tumours: low-grade astrocytomas, oligodendrogliomas.
- Vascular malformations: arteriovenous malformation, cavernous angiomas, Sturge–Weber syndrome, stroke in MELAS.

Disorders that affect most of cerebral hemispheres

- Unilateral: perinatal vascular lesions, porencephaly, ulegyria, syndrome of hemiconvulsion–hemiplegia–epilepsy (HHE), Rasmussen's encephalitis, Sturge–Weber syndrome, hemimegalencephaly, extensive unilateral cortical dysplasia, focal subcortical heterotopia.
- Bilateral: bilateral varieties of the unilateral disorders, perinatal anoxia, metabolic storage disorders, mitochondrial disease megalencephaly.

Disorders of neuronal migration and organization

- Lissencephaly, agyria, pachygyria.
- Heterotopia: subependymal, focal, subcortical, or diffuse (band heterotopia or double cortex).
- Cortical dysplasia.
- Schizencephaly: usually due to perinatal ischaemia but rare genetic conditions are also implicated.
- Megalencephaly.
- Tuberous sclerosis (Bourneville's disease).

References

1. Scaravilli F (ed.) (1998). *Neuropathology of Epilepsy. World* Scientific, Singapore.

Key reading

1. Laidlaw J, Richens A, and Chadwick D (eds.) (1993). *A Textbook of Epilepsy*, 4th edn. Churchill Livingstone, London.

2. Dichter MA, Schwartzkroin PA, Heinemann U, et al. (1997). The Neurobiology of Epilepsy. In *Epilepsy: A Comprehensive Textbook.*, Engel Jr and Pedley TA (eds), pp.231–512. Lippincott-Raven Publishers, Philadelphia.

3. Delgado-Escueta AV, Wilson WA, Olsen RW, et al. (1999). *Jasper's Basic Mechanisms of the Epilepsies. Advances in Neurology, vol 79*. Lippincott Williams & Wilkins, Philadelphia.

Types of epileptic seizures

International classifications

Two classifications are often used in the diagnosis, management and study of epilepsy:
- Classification of epileptic seizures.
- Classification of the epilepsies (epileptic syndromes).

The term epileptic seizure refers to a specific event, which is a symptom of epilepsy. Each seizure is characterized by a duration, and by the specific feelings, perceptions, or actions that the patient has or performs during the seizure as a result of abnormal neuronal activity.

The term epilepsy (or epileptic syndrome) refers to a disease characterized by a chronic propensity to suffer epileptic seizures. Like most chronic conditions, each syndrome is characterized by an age of onset, a constellation of symptoms and signs, a prognosis, presence or absence of genetic predisposition, a specific cause(s), and response to treatment. Seizures are only one element among the constellations of symptoms and signs that characterize each epileptic syndrome.

Generally, a subject will have *one epileptic syndrome* but can have *one or more seizure types*.

Both classifications, of seizures and epilepsies, are necessary. An epileptic syndrome can present several seizure types, and a particular seizure type can be seen in several epileptic syndromes. *There is a relationship but no one-to-one correspondence between seizure type and epileptic syndrome.*

Many classifications of seizures and epilepsies have been developed since epilepsy was first described in Babylonian tablets. Currently the most widely used classifications are those periodically proposed by the International League Against Epilepsy (ILAE). In this chapter, seizure classification, will be discussed. Classifications of syndromes will be discussed in Chapter 3b.

Classification of seizures

Seizures have traditionally been classified into two main groups: focal and generalized (📖 see Box 3a.1 for a list of useful terms):
- *Focal seizures:* these start in a localized region of the cerebral cortex of one hemisphere, in other words, they arise from a cortical focus. Focal seizures have also been called partial or local seizures.
- *Generalized seizures*: these arise simultaneously from both cerebral hemispheres, usually from most cerebral cortex at once.

Partial seizures are true seizures (focal seizures), although the term 'partial seizure' has sometimes been misunderstood as not referring to genuine seizures (only partially being a seizure).

Box 3a.1 Useful terms in relation to seizures

Ictal: occurring during a seizure.

Post–ictal: occurring shortly after a seizure (within minutes or sometimes hours), while the patient is not fully recovered from a seizure.

Inter–ictal: occurring while the patient is not having a seizure (between seizures).

Clonus or clonic movements or clonic convulsions: repetitive and rhythmic brisk contractions of muscle groups which generate fast movement of one or several parts of the body in one direction, usually followed by more gradual muscle relaxation that brings the body parts involved back to the original position before the next brisk contractions occur. Contractions usually occur at around 3Hz. They can be focal (involving one limb or body parts on one side of the body) or generalized (involving all limbs or limbs on both sides).

Rhythmic: a movement or EEG waveform that repeats at regular intervals.

Dystonia or tonic or dystonic posture: sustained contraction of muscles for several seconds which result in slow movements of one or several body parts that often end up rigid in a sustained posture, usually in a rather unnatural position. This can be focal or generalized

Fencing posture: bilateral symmetrical dystonic posture where one arm is extended and the other one is flexed. Often seen in seizures involving the supplementary motor cortex.

Head version: rotation of the head.

Forced head version: slow gradual head rotation where the head ends up in an extreme unnatural position looking to one side over the shoulder. It is due to a tonic contraction of neck muscles. Sometimes there are superimposed small head clonic movements. Forced version is claimed to have lateralizing value (the face looks away from the side of the seizure focus).

Adversive head version: head rotation where the face looks away from the side of the seizure focus.

Myoclonus, myoclonia, or myoclonic jerk: isolated sudden jerk of a body part due to a brisk contraction of a number of muscles lasting for <200ms.

Aphasia: inability to speak or understand speech because of dysfunction of the speech areas.

Dysphasia: impaired communication involving language without dysfunction of the relevant primary motor or sensory pathways, manifested by impaired comprehension, anomia or difficulty in naming, paraphasic errors, or a combination of these.

For a more detailed description of terms see ILAE Commission report.[1]

Focal seizures

Symptoms and manifestations of focal seizures depend on the area where they originate.

Focal seizures have been classified according to a number of criteria:
- According to severity: whether consciousness is lost or whether they lead to convulsions.
- According to the site of initiation: in the four main lobes (temporal, frontal, parietal, or occipital lobe seizures), or in more specific structures (limbic seizures, medial temporal seizures, medial frontal seizures, insular seizures, etc).

For many years impairment of consciousness has been considered an important feature to classify focal seizures (it was considered a cardinal classification criteria for the 1981 ILAE seizure classification, but not in recent propasals).

For practical purposes, consciousness is defined as the ability to appropriately respond to questions or requests, and to remember events happening during the seizure.

Impairment of consciousness is considered an important feature to evaluate seizure severity for the following reasons:
- Since each hemisphere is able to maintain consciousness independently, impairment of consciousness means that the seizure has spread to both hemispheres.
- Seizures where consciousness is lost should be considered more severe because patients are more prone to accidents which can be serious or fatal.
- Loss of consciousness can lead to more severe convulsive seizures that can be associated with falls, carpet burns, bruises, fractures, respiratory arrest, and convulsive status epilepticus.

During focal seizures consciousness can be either:
- Preserved throughout.
- Can be lost from the start, or
- Might be initially preserved and then lost, depending on the functional relevance of the cortex initiating the seizure.

Focal seizures without impairment of consciousness
- These are focal seizures starting close to or within a functionally relevant area—visual, olfactory, auditory, somatosensory, primary motor or speech areas, hippocampus, amygdala.
- Seizures without impairment of consciousness were called *simple partial seizures* in the 1981 ILAE seizure classification.
- Traditionally, the term *aura* or *warning* has been used to describe the subjective experience preceding loss of consciousness, or sometimes occurring on their own. Auras and warnings are very localized focal seizures that have not yet spread far enough to affect consciousness.

- Focal seizures with preserved consciousness can show the following manifestations depending on the areas involved:

Motor signs
- In seizures involving the primary motor cortex: unilateral clonic movements or tonic posturing occur most commonly affecting one hand or one side of the face, since these are the body parts with largest cortical representation. Occasionally, motor seizures may propagate to neighbouring cortical areas, sequentially affecting neighbouring body parts (for instance, starting in the hand, then involving the forearm, arm, same side of the face). This phenomenon is called a 'Jacksonian march' (after Hughlings Jackson who first described it).
- In seizures involving the prefrontal cortex: adversive head turning (towards the side opposite the hemisphere originating the seizure), fencing posture.
- In seizures involving speech areas: aphasia, dysphasia.

Sensory symptoms
Simple sensations or illusions depend on the sensory areas involved:
- In seizures involving the somatosensory cortex: tingling, numbness, less frequently pain or burning sensation occur. These sensations most commonly affect one hand or one side of the face, since these are the body parts with the largest cortical representation.
- In seizures involving the visual cortex: flashing lights, simple geometrical figures such as circles and sometimes more complex figures are reported. They are seen in the visual field contralateral to the hemisphere affected.
- In seizures involving the auditory cortex: hearing sounds, melodies, or sentences.
- In seizures involving the olfactory or gustatory cortex: perceiving smells (often putrid or burnt) or taste (often metallic).
- In seizures involving the insula and parietal lobes: vertiginous sensation.

Autonomic symptoms and signs
- Epigastric sensation: the commonest epileptic aura.
- Pallor.
- Flushing.
- Sweating.
- Pupillary dilatation.
- Piloerection.
- Changes in heart rate: tachycardia, bradicardia, asystole.
- Changes in respiratory rate.
- Erection.
- Urination.
- Defaecation.

Psychic symptoms
- Memory disturbances: flashbacks, déjà vu (sensation as if a new experience has been experienced before), jamais vu (sense of a familiar experience seeming novel or unfamiliar), panoramic vision (rapid recollection of episodes from the patient's past experience).
- Affective symptoms: fear, terror, anger, rage, extreme pleasure, or displeasure, depression.

- Cognitive disturbances: forced thinking, dreamy states, distortion of time, sensations of unreality, detachment, and depersonalization.
- Illusions: this term refers to an alteration of an actual perception. Illusions in seizures include distortions of object size (micropsia, macrosia), distortions of distance, distortions of sounds (microacusia, macroacusia), altered perception of size or weight of a limb.
- Structured hallucinations: this term refers to the experience of perceptions not corresponding to external stimuli. Hallucinations seen during seizures include hearing music or seeing scenes which are not real.

Focal seizures with impairment of consciousness

If focal seizures propagate to both hemispheres, consciousness will be impaired or lost. The patient will be unresponsive or only partially responsive and have no recollection of what is happening. After the seizure, some patients might not be aware that they had a seizure.

Consciousness can be lost from the beginning of the seizure (if it arises from a cortical area that is not very functionally relevant, and symptoms only occur after spreading to both hemispheres), or consciousness may be preserved initially (showing the symptoms and signs described in the previous section) to be impaired if or when the seizure becomes bilateral.

Manifestations of seizures with impaired consciousness:
- Patient might stare and appear distant.
- Patient might appear distant and carry out normal but apparently purposeless movements called 'automatisms'—for instance, lip smacking, walking, saying stereotyped sentences, looking around, fidgeting, fiddling or fumbling with things, clapping, bicycling movements, etc.
- Patient might suffer convulsions: these seizures are often called 'tonic–clonic' seizures, secondarily generalized seizures, or 'grand mal' seizures. Convulsions usually start with some or all limbs and head becoming rigid for a few seconds (tonic phase) often associated with uttering grunting noises or a scream ('the epileptic cry'). This is usually followed by repetitive contractions of all limbs and head (clonic phase) at about 3Hz, where the body parts jerk fast in one direction and more slowly recover the initial position before jerking again. Convulsions can be preceded by forced head rotation (slow and extreme rotation of the head, usually away from seizure focus). Convulsive movements can start earlier or be more pronounced on the body side contralateral to seizure focus. Convulsive seizures can be followed by paralysis or paresis (weakness) contralateral to the seizure focus (*Todd's paralysis*). The patient might be incontinent or bite his/her tongue (particularly the side of the tongue) during convulsive seizures.

The first two groups (patient staring and/or showing automatisms) are grouped under 'complex partial' seizures in the 1981 ILAE Classification.

Automatisms have been classified into two categories:
- *De novo automatisms:* actions that appear with the seizure. They can be *spontaneous* (such as chewing, swallowing, lip smacking, walking, running, saying stereotyped sentences, looking around, fidgeting, fiddling or fumbling with things, clapping, carrying out bicycling movements in the air, taking clothes off), or they may be actions carried out *as*

a response to an external stimulus occurring during the seizure (pushing off an approaching observer, drinking from a nearby cup, withdrawing a limb held by an observer, etc.).
- *Preservative automatisms:* continuation of any complex activity initiated prior to loss of consciousness such as continue eating with a spoon, chewing, carry on walking, carry on sewing, etc.

Cautionary note!

The terms complex partial seizures, temporal lobe seizures, and psycho-motor seizures are often used as synonyms. This is not correct. Although the most frequent source of complex partial seizures is the temporal lobe, it is not the only one, as complex partial seizures can arise from any lobe. The term psychomotor seizure is now obsolete.

Brief complex partial seizures can resemble absence seizures, 📖 see Box 3a.2, p.69.

Gelastic seizures: gelastic seizures are those that include laughter as one of their clinical manifestations. Laughter is usually a short manifestation (<30sec). Laughter can be a manifestation of several seizure types such as partial seizures with motor symptoms, myoclonic seizures, axial tonic seizures, spasms, generalized convulsive seizures, and petit mal absences. Gelastic seizures have been observed mainly in association with hypotha-lamic hamartomas, but also in temporal and frontal lobe lesions as well as in metabolic conditions (Niemann–Pick disease type C).

Hemiclonic seizures: consisting of clonic movements involving only one side (right or left). They can involve one side of the face and/or limbs.

Classification of focal seizures according to the site of origin
Seizures can be classified according to the site of initiation. The site of onset can be suggested in many focal seizures with preserved conscious-ness by the motor manifestations or from the symptoms experienced by the patient (📖 see above Focal seizures without impairment of con-sciousness, pp.64–66). For instance, flashing lights in the right visual field most likely arise from the left occipital lobe.

Temporal lobe seizures tend to be associated with an epigastric sensa-tion, memory disturbances (most commonly déjà vu), staring, oroalimen-tary automatisms,(manual automatisms, fidgeting, fumbling with objects) unilateral dystonia, and sometimes convulsions. If unilateral, automatisms tend to be ipsilateral to seizure onset and dystonia contralateral. They last for about 1min and are followed by postictal confusion and gradual recovery.

Frontal lobe seizures are usually brief, with prominent bizarre motor and gestural automatisms (limb thrashing, kicking, grimacing), sometimes asymmetrical tonic postures, often occurring in clusters during sleep and with little post-ictal confusion unless there is secondary generalization.

Occipital lobe seizures tend to start with visual symptoms and/or blinking.

Focal seizures from any location can have impairment of consciousness and/or convulsions.

Generalized seizures

Generalized seizures are those arising simultaneously from both cerebral hemispheres, usually from most of the cerebral cortex at once. Consequently, generalized seizures have the following characteristics:

- Consciousness is lost from outset.
- There is no early stage where consciousness is preserved: there is no specific aura or warning to the seizures, although patients often refer to non-specific brief warnings such as cephalic sensations.
- There are no consistent focal features either clinically or on the ictal EEG: convulsions and muscle contractions do not consistently start on one side, there are no warnings, there is no consistent head rotation to one side, and there are not consistent earlier EEG changes one hemisphere compared to the other over.

There are several types of generalized seizures.

Generalized tonic–clonic seizures: tonic–clonic seizures similar to those described under focal seizures with impairment of conciousness (p.66) but with no consistent focal components (movements are symmetrical from the start and if there is head rotation, it does not occur consistently to the same side).

Clonic seizures: they are similar to tonic–clonic seizures but without an initial tonic phase. There are no focal features.

Tonic seizures: the patient's limbs and neck suddenly go rigid for a few seconds and, if standing, the patient might fall backwards or forwards. As the limbs become rigid, the legs extend and the arms slowly flex or extend, or first flex and then extend, in a rather symmetrical fashion.

Atonic seizures: brief attacks consisting of a sudden loss of muscle tone causing the patient to suddenly nod the head or fall to the floor. Atonic seizures have previously been named 'akinetic' or 'astatic' seizures.

The term *'drop attack'* is applied to seizures where patients suddenly fall to the ground and frequently injure themselves. They are usually *tonic* or *atonic seizures*. Patients are often *at risk from injury, especially to head and face,* and may require protective helmets to be worn while standing or sitting.

Spasms: spasms consist of brief massive contractions of axial muscles that can provoke flexion or extension of the trunk. Each spasm last for a fraction of a second, but spasms can occur in clusters of 5–50, several clusters occurring each day, often on awakening. They may be symmetrical or asymmetrical, with lateral deviation of the eyes or head, or involving only one side of the body. The child often cries after each spasm. They tend to occur between the age of 3–12 months. They tend to be associated with learning difficulties, developmental delay and hypsarrhythmia on the EEG (West syndrome). Spasms have been sub-classified into flexor spasms, extensor spasms, or flexor–extensor spasms (neck and arms flex, but legs extend). Flexor spasms have also been called 'salaam convulsions' or 'salaam attacks'.

Absence (petit mal) seizures: they are characterized by a period of unresponsiveness lasting for several seconds with or without a variety of associated phenomena—staring, cessation of ongoing activities and speech, eyelid flutter, mild automatisms, mild clonic movements, decreased postural tone without fall (mild atonic components), mild tonic components, mild autonomic components (incontinence, pupil dilatation, pallor, flushing, tachycardia, blood pressure changes). Automatisms are mild, usually consisting of small peri-oral movements or finger fiddling and are more likely in prolonged episodes. Simple absences are those with only impairment of consciousness. Absence seizures have been subclassified into typical and atypical:

- *Typical absences:* show generalized spike-and-wave activity at 2.5–3.5 Hz. Spikes are rather sharp.
- *Atypical absences:* show generalized spike-and-wave activity at <2.5 Hz. Spikes are usually more blunt than in typical absences.

Myoclonic absence seizures are associated with bilateral rhythmic clonic jerks or brief tonic contractions. Jerks mainly involve muscles of the shoulders, arms, and legs. Facial muscles are less commonly involved. When facial myoclonias occur, they are more evident around the chin and mouth, whereas eyelid twitching is typically absent or rare. The jerks and tonic contractions may be symmetrical or predominant on one side, causing turning of the head and body.

Eyelid myoclonia with absences: seizures consist of a brief episode of marked jerking of the eyelids with upwards deviation of the eyes, associated with a generalized discharge of spike-wave occurring on eye closure. All patients are photosensitive. Absence seizures are induced by changes in light associated with eyelid jerking or closure, which can be voluntary, involuntary, or reflex. The majority of the seizures are induced immediately after closure of the eyes in the presence of uninterrupted light. Eye closure in total darkness is ineffective. Intermittent photic stimulation potentiates the effect of eye closure and is capable of inducing seizures when eyes are open or closed. Eyelid myclonia without prominent absences may occur particularly in adult patients.

Box 3a.2 Caution!

Since staring and automatisms can be seen in absence and in complex partial seizures, it can be difficult to distinguish between them on clinical grounds (the ictal EEG is distinctly different):

- Absence seizures are brief, usually lasting for <10sec and rarely >45sec, whereas complex partial seizure often last for >1min.
- Absence seizures have a sudden onset, without warning, whereas complex partial seizures may or may not have a warning.
- In absence seizures, recovery of consciousness is also sudden, without post-ictal confusion, whereas complex partial seizures are often followed by a variable period of confusion sometimes lasting for several minutes.

Generalized myoclonic seizures (jerks) or myoclonias: generalized myoclonic seizures consist of an isolated, sudden, fast, brief (<200ms) and symmetrical muscle contraction, usually involving the arms and neck. Hands and arms suddenly flex upwards while head and neck usually flex down, for a few hundreds of milliseconds. Sometimes there are 2–3 superimposed contractions within a few hundreds of milliseconds. Neverthelss, myoclonias are essentially isolated events. Repetitive rhythmic contractions, usually several per second, lasting for several seconds, should be considered 'clonus' or 'clonic convulsions' (📖 see Generalized tonic–clonic seizures, p.68).

Negative myoclonus: sudden and abrupt interruption of muscular activity. The EMG shows a brief (< 500ms) silent period, not preceded by enhancement of EMG activity (i.e. myoclonus). Epileptic negative myoclonus is time-locked to a spike on the EEG, without evidence of a previous myoclonia. Clinically, negative myoclonus appears as a shock-like involuntary jerky movement due to a sudden brief interruption of muscular activity and can resemble real (positive) myoclonus.

Reflex seizures: reflex seizures are those triggered by stimuli. Stimuli that can trigger seizures include visual stimuli (flashing lights, particularly at around 18–20 Hz; and geometrical patterns, particularly stripes), thinking, music, eating, praxis, somatosensory stimulation, proprioceptive stimuli, reading, hot water, and startle.

Variations of myoclonic seizures

- Myoclonic seizures may not always be *truly* generalized (they might not affect all muscles).
- Sometimes they are bilateral and symmetrical but do not affect all muscles. For instance, they may affect only both shoulders. Such symmetrical but not generalized myoclonic jerks are sometimes called *segmental myoclonus*.
- Some patients have multiple, nearly continuous, small myoclonic jerks, affecting only a few muscles at a time, often unilaterally, affecting different muscles one after another. Eventually most muscles will jerk, but not simultaneously. This is sometimes called *migratory myoclonus, multifocal myoclonus, fragmentary myoclonus* or *polymyoclonus*.
- Myoclonic jerks can occur immediately preceding, during, or at the end of an atonic seizure (*myoclonic–astatic seizures*).
- Myoclonic seizures (movements) may occur in conditions other that epilepsy. They can arise from the brainstem (*subcortical myoclonus*) or from the spinal cord (*spinal myclonus*).
- Myoclonic seizures should be distinguished from spasms and tonic seizures (Fig.3a.1)
- Normal myoclonus occurs in sleep 📖 see Chapter 3c, pp.173–175.

EEG manifestations of seizures

EEG changes occurring during seizures can be very important to establish if seizures are focal or generalized, as well as to identify certain seizure types, since EEG changes can be specific. The EEG changes that can be seen during different seizure types are described in the section on Ictal EEG recording.

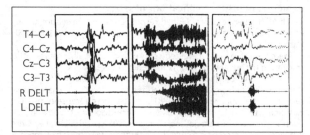

Fig. 3a.1 Polygraphic recording of a myclonic seizure, a tonic seizure, and a spasm. The top four channels correspond to EEG recordings and the bottom two chanels correspond to right and left deltoid muscle activity (electromyogram or EMG). Note that the myoclonic jerk (left) consist of a brief burst of muscle activity lasting for <200ms followed by a tail of less intense activity, whereas the spasm (right) has a more gradual build up and decay of EMG activity lasting for 1–2sec and showing a characteristic rhomboidal morphology. The tonic seizure (centre) shows more sustained EMG activity lasting for several seconds. (Reproduced from Vigevano *et al* (2001). Neurophysiology of spasms. *Brain and Development*, **23**, 467–72,© 2001, with permission from Elsevier.)

Evolution of ILAE classifications of seizures

The ILAE has periodically published recommendations on seizure classifications over the last 50 years. Table 3a.1 broadly compares 1981 and 2001 classifications.

The classification of generalized seizures has essentially changed little, apart from the addition of spasms and reflex seizures.

However the classification of focal seizures has changed more substantially. The 2001 proposal re-coined the term 'focal' to replace partial seizures. In addition, whereas in 1981 non-convulsive focal seizures were classified into simple (with preservation of consciousness) and complex (with impairment of consciousness), in the 2001 classification they were largely grouped according to whether symptoms were motor or sensory. As a result, the meaning of 'focal motor seizure' has changed. Traditionally, the term 'focal motor seizure' referred specifically to seizures consisting of focal convulsions thought to arise from selective involvement of the motor strip, usually showing clonic convulsions involving hand or face. In the 2001 classification, the term 'focal motor seizure' has a wider meaning, referring to focal seizures with any movement, including automatisms.

In some respects, the 1981 classification is more useful. The distinction between simple and complex focal seizures makes physiological, clinical, and electroenecephalographic sense because loss of consciousness implies bilateral involvement and a higher degree of clinical severity. The 1981 classification is still routinely used in clinical practice, and will be used throughout some sections of this book, for instance in the section 📖 Ictal EEG recordings, pp.173–175 and What to do during a seizure, pp.228–232.

In addition, the 1981 classification does not really attempt to classify reflex seizures or status epilepticus (apart from epilepsia partialis continua). In contrast, the 2001 classification includes a detailed classification of reflex seizures and status epilepticus (the so called 'continuous seizure types', 📖 see Diagnosis of status epilepticus, pp.198–205).

References

1. Blume WT, Lüders HO, Mizrahi E, *et al.* (2001). Glossary of descriptive terminology for ictal semiology: report of the ILAE task force on classification and terminology. *Epilepsia*, **42**, 1212–18. Available at: 🖳 www.ilae–epilepsy.org/Visitors/Centre/ctf/glossary.cfm#1.0

Key reading

1. Commission on Classification and Terminology on the International League Against Epilepsy (1981). Proposal for Revised Clinical and Electroencephalographic Classification of Epileptic Seizures. *Epilepsia*, **22**, 489–501.

2. Engel, J Jr. (2001) ILAE Commission Report. A Proposed Diagnostic Scheme for People with Epileptic Seizures and with Epilepsy: Report of the ILAE Task Force on Classification and Terminology. *Epilepsia*, **42**, 796–803.

3. Lüders HO and Noachtar S (eds.) (2000). *Epileptic seizures. Pathophysiology and Clinical Semiology.* Churchill Livingstone, New York.

Table 3a.1 Approximate equivalence of the self-limited seizure types described in the two most recent ILAE seizure classifications

Generalized seizures	
ILAE Classification (1981)	**ILAE Classification (2001)**
Tonic–clonic seizures	Tonic–clonic seizures
Clonic seizures	Clonic seizures: With tonic features Without tonic features
Absence seizures: with impairment of consciousness only with mild clonic components with atonic components with tonic components with automatisms	Typical absence seizures Atypical absence seizures Myoclonic absence seizures
Tonic seizures	Tonic seizures
Not defined	Spasms
Myoclonic seizures	Myoclonic seizures Myoclonic atonic seizures Negative myoclonus
Not defined	Eyelid myoclonia: With absences Without absences
Atonic seizures	Atonic seizures
Not defined	Reflex seizures in generalized epilepsy syndromes
Focal (partial, local) seizures	
ILAE Classification (1981)	**ILAE Classification (2001)**
Simple partial seizures (with no impairment of consciousness)	Focal sensory seizures: With elementary sensory symptoms With experiential sensory symptoms
Complex partial seizures (with impairment of consciousness)	Focal motor seizures With elementary clonic motor signs With asymmetrical tonic motor seizures (e.g., supplementary motor seizures) With typical (temporal lobe) automatisms (e.g., mesial temporal lobe seizures) With hyperkinetic automatisms With focal negative myoclonus With inhibitory motor seizures Gelastic seizures Hemiclonic seizures
Secondarily generalized seizures	Secondarily generalized seizures
Not defined	Reflex seizures in focal epilepsy seizures

From seizures to syndromes

What type of epilepsy do I have?

We have seen that epileptic seizures are discrete, usually brief, events that can take several forms.

Epilepsy is defined as a long lasting (chronic) propensity to suffer epileptic seizures. Normally, the patient must have suffered more than one seizure to establish that he/she suffers from epilepsy. Once established, epilepsy is not necessarily a life-long condition, with remission occurring in a significant proportion of patients.

Such susceptibility to suffer epileptic seizures (epilepsy) can be caused by a variety of circumstances, which can be grouped into two:

- *First*, nearly any type of brain damage or brain lesions can cause epilepsy: stroke, scarring after head injury, brain tumours, anoxia, metabolic disorders, brain infections, etc. The epilepsies caused by such conditions that are associated with some form of brain damage are called '*symptomatic*' epilepsies (they are a symptom of the underlying condition that caused brain damage). Previously, such epilepsies were called '*secondary*' epilepsies (they were secondary to some brain insult causing damage).

- *Second*, epilepsy can occur without any evidence of brain damage. It appears that some families or individuals can have a particularly low threshold to suffer epileptic seizures without having any underlying disease, in the same way that some families or individuals can be particularly tall or particularly short without having any underlying disorder. Such epilepsies occurring without evidence of brain damage are called '*idiopathic*' epilepsies. Previously, such epilepsies were called '*primary*' epilepsies. The cause of idiopathic epilepsies is supposed to be genetic, but too subtle to cause obvious brain damage. There is no brain damage in these epilepsies and patients generally tend to have normal development, normal intelligence, normal memory, normal neurological function, normal imaging, and normal EEG background. Nevertheless, if the epilepsy is severe or has early onset, it can have an adverse impact on development or function.

General features of idiopathic epilepsies

- Normal development, except in early onset severe syndromes.
- Age of onset in infancy, childhood, or early adulthood.
- Normal intelligence and normal memory.
- Normal background on the EEG.
- Normal neuroimaging.
- Family history is often present, but not always.

General features of symptomatic epilepsies

- Normal or abnormal development.
- Age of onset at any time, depending on the onset of the brain insult.
- Learning difficulties or subtle deficits in brain function (for instance, low verbal IQ) or normal brain function, depending on the extent and location of the underlying brain damage.
- Abnormal or normal background on the EEG.
- Normal or abnormal neuroimaging.
- Weak or no family history of epilepsy.

A common conceptual mistake—what is 'secondarily' generalized epilepsy?

Convulsive seizures can be generalized or secondarily generalized. Secondarily generalized seizures are convulsive seizures that start focally and later (secondarily) become generalized—although sometimes the seizure can spread so fast that the focal onset may not be clinically or electroencephalographically apparent.

On the other hand, the epilepsies can be primary (idiopathic) or secondary (symptomatic).

Therefore, the following terms *are correct* (although obsolete to some):
- Secondarily generalized seizure.
- Secondary epilepsy.
- Secondary generalized epilepsy.

Though the term 'secondarily generalized epilepsy' is commonly used, it is wrong and best avoided!

In addition to establishing whether an epilepsy is idiopathic or symptomatic, it is important to determine if the seizures are focal or generalized (📖 see Chapter 3a Types of epileptic seizures, pp.61–73). Epilepsies with focal seizures are called *focal epilepsies* and result from a focal functional abnormality (restricted to one region of one hemisphere). In contrast, epilepsies presenting generalized seizures are called *generalized epilepsies* and usually result from a functional abnormality affecting most cortex on both hemispheres. Generalized seizures occur either because there is diffuse brain damage (symptomatic generalized epilepsies), or because there is a generalized increase in cortical excitability due to abnormal interactions between cortex and thalamus (idiopathic generalized epilepsies).

Focal epilepsies have previously had a variety of names: local, partial, and localization-related epilepsies.

If brain damage in symptomatic epilepsies is very localized, its impact on brain function might be undetectable, subtle, or might only become evident on performance of neuropsychological tests. For instance, a right-handed patient with left mesial temporal sclerosis might show normal speech during everyday activities and perhaps complain of difficulties in remembering some names. On neuropsychological testing, their verbal memory or IQ might be much lower than their non-verbal memory or performance IQ.

In contrast, early massive diffuse brain damage (for instance, after perinatal hypoxia) usually manifests as developmental delay and learning difficulties or disability.

Therefore, epilepsy can be classified into four types according to whether they are symptomatic, idiopathic, focal, or generalized:
- Idiopathic focal epilepsies: susceptibility to focal seizures without brain damage.
- Idiopathic generalized epilepsies: susceptibility to generalized seizures without brain damage.

- Symptomatic focal epilepsies: susceptibility to focal seizures caused by focal brain damage or lesions.
- Symptomatic generalized epilepsies: susceptibility to generalized seizures caused by diffuse (generalized) brain damage.

Examples of epilepsy classification

- A patient having seizures caused by a brain tumour will be suffering from symptomatic focal epilepsy.
- A patient having seizures caused by right mesial temporal sclerosis will be suffering from symptomatic focal epilepsy.
- A patient having multiple angiomas on both hemispheres with seizures arising only from an angioma located on the left frontal lobe will be suffering from symptomatic focal epilepsy.
- A patient with focal cortical disyplasia on MRI who has never had a seizure is not suffering from epilepsy of any type.
- Patients with multiple seizure types and learning difficulties as a result of a metabolic brain storage disease with an autosomal recessive inheritance is likely to be suffering from symptomatic generalized epilepsy.
- The more recent ILAE proposals reconize that some syndromes may be undermined as to whether focal or generalized. Patients with generalized and focal seizures and learning difficulties are usually treated as per a symptomatic generalized epilepsy.
- Patients with infrequent focal seizures of early onset, on the background of normal development and positive family history, are likely to have idiopathic focal epilepsy.
- Patients with generalized seizures, on the background of normal development and normal MRI are likely to have idiopathic generalized epilepsy.

Is this the complete story?

No, it is not. There is often difficulty in classifying patients where there is no direct evidence of structural brain abnormalities. For instance, patients may have learning difficulties, diffusely abnormal EEG background, and delayed milestones with normal neuroimaging and no clear history of a brain injury. Nevertheless, the presence of learning difficulties, diffusely abnormal EEG background, and developmental delay strongly suggest that these patients have suffered some form of diffuse brain pathology. Thus, these patients cannot be classified as idiopathic, or as symptomatic (symptomatic to what? We have not identified an underlying lesion). The International League Against Epilepsy (ILAE) recommends the term 'presumed symptomatic' for these patients (previously called cryptogenic). Conceptually and in terms of management, presumed symptomatic (cryptogenic) epilepsies are identical to symptomatic epilepsies. If it is believed that presumed symptomatic epilepsies are symptomatic epilepsies where our present diagnostic methods are not sensitive enough to find a specific cause. Presumed symptomatic epilepsies can be generalized or focal.

What is the relevance of all this?

Although a patient might have several seizure types, he/she will generally have only one type of epilepsy.

It is important to establish the type of epilepsy that a patient has because different types of epilepsies have different prognosis and management in terms of patient development, natural evolution of the seizures, treatment choices, seizure response to treatment, patient integration in society, and genetic counselling.

Idiopathic epilepsies tend to have good prognosis, with no developmental delay, there is often good response to medical treatment, and seizures in some syndromes may disappear with age. Resective surgical treatment is not indicated, since there is no underlying structural abnormality to remove and patients may grow out of their seizures.

Symptomatic generalized epilepsies have poor outcome, seizures tend to continue throughout life, with poor response to treatment, and resective surgery is not indicated since most of the brain might be structurally abnormal.

Symptomatic focal epilepsies may or may not respond to medical treatment and, if not, they may benefit from resective surgery.

But even within the four broad groups of epilepsies already described, there are several subtypes of epilepsies—the so called, epileptic (epilepsy) syndromes. Although the ILAE recommends the term 'epileptic syndrome', we feel that 'epilepsy syndrome' seems more appropriate. It is important to identify the epilepsy syndrome because different syndromes have different prognoses and response to treatment. Like any medical syndrome, epilepsy syndromes are characterized by a constellation of symptoms and signs that tend to occur together. The criteria used to characterize epilepsy syndromes are shown in the Box 3b.1.

Box 3b.1 Criteria used to identify an epilepsy syndrome

- Age of onset of seizures.
- Seizure type(s).
- Patient development—milestones.
- Patient intelligence and memory function.
- Family history.
- Inte-rictal EEG:
- EEG background abnormalities.
- EEG paroxysmal abnormalities—(inter-ictal epileptiform discharges).
- Ictal EEG—not always available.
- Neuroimaging.
- Aetiology.

Epilepsy syndromes—summary of characteristics

The following pages show a summary of characteristics for some epilepsy syndromes. Some of these are addressed again later in this chapter (pp.131–151).

Benign idiopathic neonatal convulsions or **fifth day fits** or **non-familial benign neonatal convulsions** or **benign neonatal seizures (non-familial)**

Prevalence: rare.

Age of onset of seizures: 1–7 days of life, usually on the 5th day.

Seizure types: focal clonic seizures or subtle neonatal seizures—apnoea, suckling. Seizures are often unilateral but may change sides. They may occur in clusters, leading to prolonged status epilepticus.

Patient development (milestones): normal or minor delay.

Patient intelligence and memory function: usually normal when they grow up.

Family history of epilepsy: no.

Inter-ictal EEG: asynchronous Rolandic bursts of theta rhythms—'théta pointu alternant'.

Ictal EEG: rhythmic localized spikes or slow waves.

Neuroimaging: normal, usually not required.

Aetiology: idiopathic; de novo mutations in KCNQ2 have been reported.

Medical treatment: none, phenobarbitone, phenytoin, benzodiazepines.

Resective surgical treatment: no

Prognosis: excellent, seizures do not usually continue after neonatal period.

Epilepsy type: while this has been classified as idiopathic generalized, the seizures are focal and classification is uncertain.

Benign familial neonatal convulsions *or* benign familial neonatal seizures

Prevalence: rare.

Age of onset of seizures: day 2–3 after birth, but occasionally up to 3 months.

Seizure types: generalized clonic or tonic–clonic seizures.

Patient development (milestones): normal.

Patient intelligence and memory function: normal when patients grow up.

Family history of epilepsy: yes, autosomal dominance inheritance.

Inter-ictal EEG:
- EEG background: normal.
- EEG paroxysmal abnormalities: none, focal or multifocal.

Ictal EEG: brief flattening followed by asymmetrical spike-wave activity for 1–2min.

Neuroimaging: normal.

Aetiology: idiopathic. Associated with mutations in KCNQ2 and KCNQ3.

Medical treatment: none, phenobarbital, valproate.

Resective surgical treatment: no.

Prognosis: generally good, seizures cease by age 6 months but 10% develop other syndromes (usually well controlled) later in life.

Epilepsy type: idiopathic, unclear if generalized (ILAE) or focal.

The following related syndromes have been described:
- Benign familial neonatal-infantile seizures present later and may be due to mutations in SCN2A.
- Benign familial infantile seizures occur later than the above but there is overlap. Loci have been reported.

Early myoclonic encephalopathy (Fig. 3b.1) or neonatal
myoclonic encephalopathy or myoclonic encephalopathy
with neonatal onset or neonatal epileptic encephalopathy
with periodic EEG bursts

Prevalence: rare.

Age of onset of seizures: neonatal period.

Seizure types: polymyoclonus (fragmentary, segmental, erratic myoclonus), generalized myoclonus, evolving to infantile spasms after several months, focal motor seizures.

Patient development (milestones): delayed.

Patient intelligence and memory function: poor.

Family history of epilepsy: often present.

Inter-ictal EEG: the EEG consists of continuous patterns of burst-suppression (bursts of spikes, sharp waves and slow waves alternating with flat periods), sometimes accentuated by sleep.

Ictal EEG: as inter-ictal.

Neuroimaging: normal (particularly initially) or abnormal.

Aetiology: genetic and metabolic disorders, including non-ketotic hyperglycinaemia.

Medical treatment: usually ineffective, but the following among others, have been tried: corticosteroids, valproate, vigabatrin, benzodiazepines.

Resective surgical treatment: no.

Prognosis: poor, 50% die within a year, all neurologically abnormal with severe developmental delay. May transiently evolve to West syndrome.

Epilepsy type: symptomatic or presumed symptomatic generalized.

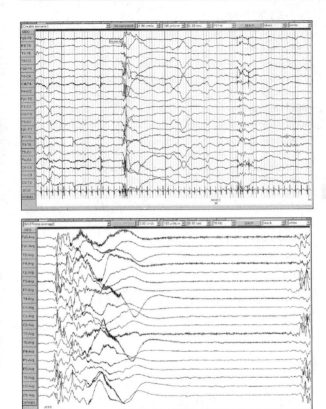

Fig. 3b.1 Suppression-burst pattern in a patient with early myoclonic encephalopathy: 9-day-old neonate presented with generalized and erratic stimulus sensitive myoclonus (upper graph), diagnosed with non-ketotic hyperglycineamia. Generalized discharges occurred in association with myoclonus (lower graph). Figure kindly provided by Dr Sushma Goyal.

Early infantile epileptic encephalopathy *or* **Ohtahara's syndrome (Fig. 3b.2)**

Prevalence: rare.

Age of onset of seizures: first months of life.

Seizure types: brief tonic spasms (main difference with early myoclonic encephalopathy).

Patient development (milestones): delayed.

Patient intelligence and memory function: poor when grown up.

Family history of epilepsy: not usually. some have family history of febrile serizures.

Inter-ictal EEG: burst-suppression (bursts of spikes, sharp waves and slow waves alternating with flat periods), with longer bursts and shorter suppression than in early myoclonic encephalopathy.

Ictal EEG: as inter-ictal.

Neuroimaging: usually abnormal.

Aetiology: major brain malformations.

Medical treatment: as in early myoclonic encephalopathy.

Resective surgical treatment: generally not. Reported in some cases.

Prognosis: poor, as in early myoclonic encephalopathy. Frequent evolution into West syndrome and Lennox-Gastaut syndrome.

Epilepsy type: symptomatic or presumed symptomatic generalized.

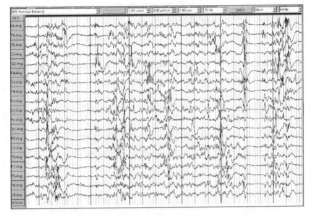

Fig. 3b.2 Early infantile epileptic encephalopathy (Ohtahara's syndrome): neonate with suppression–burst on the EEG who presented with tonic spasms. Figure kindly provided by Dr Sushma Goyal.

Pyridoxine dependency *or* **vitamin B6 dependency**

Prevalence: unknown, probably rare.

Age of onset of seizures: *in utero* to 18 months (peak at 24–72 hours after birth).

Seizure types: multifocal or generalized (myoclonic, tonic, clonic, spasms).

Patient development (milestones): often delayed, particularly if treatment is delayed.

Patient intelligence and memory function: sometimes affected, particularly if treatment is delayed.

Family history of epilepsy: autosomal recessive inheritance.

Inter-ictal EEG: hypsarrhythmic, burst-suppression, multifocal discharges.

Neuroimaging: normal.

Aetiology: genetic (autosomal recessive). Vitamin B6 is a co-factor for glutamic acid decarboxylase, a crucial enzyme for synthesis of GABA. Most commonly caused by mutations in ALDH7A1 gene (antiquitin) which result in α-amino-adipic semialdehyde dehydrogenase (α–AASA dehydrogenase) deficiency. Other inborn errors of metabolism have also been reported.

Medical treatment: vitamin B6.
● In newborn: 50mg/kg/day.
● In older children: 3–30mg/kg/day.

In unclear cases, oral trial for 2 weeks is recommended. In some cases, treatment with pyridoxine is not effective and pyridoxal phosphate is needed.

Any infant <3 years with intractable seizures of unknown cause should have a trial.

Resective surgical treatment: no.

Prognosis: seizure response to intravenous treatment is immediate, although EEG response might take days or weeks. Poor prognosis if treatment is delayed. Even if treated early, children are likely to have developmental delay.

Epilepsy type: unclear, symptomatic generalized?

West's syndrome (Fig. 3b.3) *or* infantile spasms

Syndrome definition:
- Infantile spasms.
- Hypsarrhythmia on EEG (Fig. 3b.4).
- Arrest of psychomotor development.

Prevalence: uncommon.

Age of onset of seizures: 3–12 months.

Seizure types: spasms (flexor, extensor, or flexor-extensor). Sometimes subtle, with head nods. In clusters, especially on awakening.

Patient development (milestones): severely affected.

Patient intelligence and memory function: poor.

Family history of epilepsy: unusual.

Inter-ictal EEG: hypsarrhythmia (severely slowed EEG in the delta and theta ranges plus superimposed frequent multifocal and generalized epileptiform discharges). Hypsarrhythmia is not always present.

Ictal EEG: high amplitude generalized spike and wave followed by EEG flattening with fast rhythms for a few seconds.

Neuroimaging: normal or abnormal, according to aetiology.

Aetiology: perinatal hypoxic ischaemic encephalopathy, malformations (particularly tuberous sclerosis), pre- and postnatal infections, metabolic disorders (phenylketonuria).

Medical treatment: many drugs have been tried, including vigabatrin, valproate, corticosteroids, nitrazepam, immunoglobulins, pyridoxine. Vigabatrin and corticosteroids appear to be particularly effective and are considered first line treatment. There are reports of the successful use of the ketogenic diet which require further evaluation.

Surgical treatment: where brain lesions demonstrated. Callosotomy for drop attacks.

Prognosis: poor. Developmental delay (85%), learning disabilities, and intractable seizures. 50–60% develop other epilepsy syndromes, in particular Lennox–Gastaut syndrome.

Epilepsy type: presumed symptomatic (20–30%) or symptomatic (70–80%) generalized.

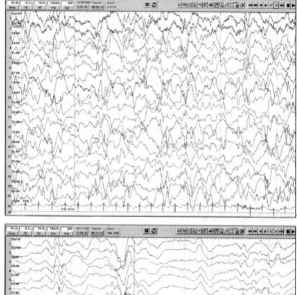

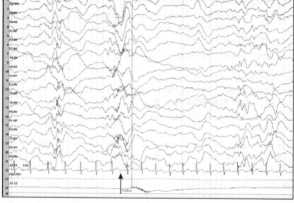

Fig. 3b.3 West syndrome: 5-month-old with a history of neonatal hypoxi ischemic encephalopathy, presented with clusters of spasms lasting up to 10min. He had been smiling and laughing less in the previous 2 weeks. The inter-ictal EEG showed hypsarrhythmia: high amplitude EEG dominated by low frequencies and superimposed multifocal sharp waves (upper graph). Spasms were associated with EEG and EMG changes (arrow in lower graph). Figure kindly provided by Dr Sushma Goyal.

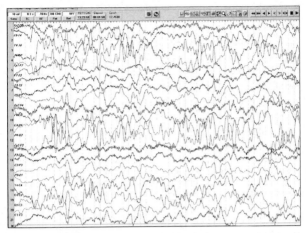

Fig. 3b.4 Asymmetrical or hemi hypsarrythmia: this 3-month-old child presented with infantile spasms. MRI later demonstrated right polymicrogyria with sub-cortical heterotopia. Figure kindly provided by Dr Sushma Goyal.

Benign myoclonic epilepsy in infancy (BMEI) (Fig. 3b.5)

Prevalence: rare.

Age of onset of seizures: 4 months to 3 years.

Seizure types: generalized myoclonic, often while falling asleep. No other seizure types. Febrile seizures in 20% of patients.

Patient development (milestones): normal.

Patient intelligence and memory function: normal.

Family history of epilepsy: present in 30% of patients.

Inter-ictal EEG:
- EEG background: normal.
- EEG paroxysmal abnormalities: generalized spike-wave and polyspikes, particularly during drowsiness and early sleep. Myoclonic attacks and generalized spine-wave discharges can also be precipitated by noise, contact, and photic stimulation. The latter despite the young age at presentation.

Ictal EEG: generalized spike-wave and polyspikes.

Neuroimaging: normal.

Aetiology: idiopathic.

Medical treatment: valproate (best), benzodiazepines.

Resective surgical treatment: no.

Prognosis: good.

Epilepsy type: idiopathic generalized.

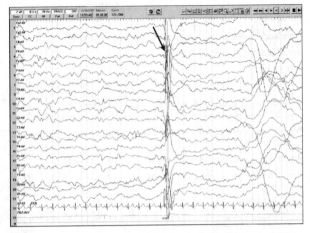

Fig. 3b.5 Benign myoclonic epilepsy of infancy: 3-month-old child presented with myoclonus on with normal development. The EEG showed a normal EEG background with generalized spike-wave discharges accompanying myoclonus (arrow). Figure kindly provided by Dr Sushma Goyal.

Severe myoclonic epilepsy in infancy (SMEI) or Dravet's syndrome or polymorphic epilepsy (Fig. 3b.6)

Prevalence: approximately 6% of epilepsies starting before the age of 3.

Age of onset of seizures: 3–8 months.

Seizure types:
- Initially (before 1 year of age) febrile seizures, usually prolonged and lateralized.
- Second year: generalized or segmental myoclonic seizures.
- 40–60% have additional absence seizures and focal motor seizures.

Patient development (milestones): initially normal, but pyschomotor delay from 2 years.

Patient intelligence and memory function: learning difficulties.

Family history of epilepsy: 15–25% have a family history of epilepsy or fertile seizures.

Inter-ictal EEG:
- EEG background: initially normal during the first year of life, later diffuse and multifocal abnormalities.
- EEG paroxysmal abnormalities: generalized and multifocal epileptiform discharges, often photosensitive.

Ictal EEG: sharp spikes and polyspikes with myoclonic seizures.

Neuroimaging: normal or abnormal (largely diffuse atrophy).

Aetiology: Most often due to a sporadic sodium channel mutation, in SCN1A. Similar mutations have been found in post-vaccine epileptic encephalopathy and in SMEB (a varient of SMEI).

Medical treatment: valproate, benzodiazepines, stiripentol, topiramate, amongst other. Not very effective. Carbemazepine and lamotrigine can have an aggravating effect.

Resective surgical treatment: no.

Prognosis: poor. Intractable seizures, learning difficulties, progressive ataxia.

Epilepsy type: initially considered symptomatic, or presumed symptomatic, with focal and generalized features. Later classified as epileptic encephalopathy. Now being reclassified as idiopathic.

SMEB refers to infants with presentations close to SMEI, but excludes all the features (e.g. myoclonus).

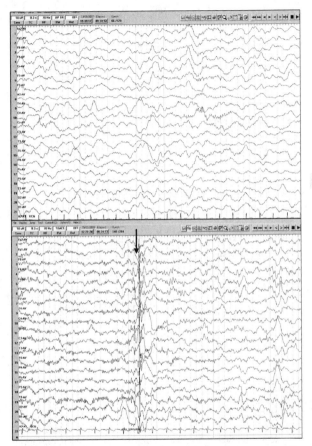

Fig. 3b.6 Severe myoclonic epilepsy of infancy: Patient presented at 5 months with an afebrile generalized seizure. The EEG was normal apart from mild right temporal slowing (upper graph). 11 months later he developed intractable generalized tonic–clonic seizures and myoclonus. *SCN1A* gene mutation was positive. The EEG then showed generalized spike-and-wave discharges (arrow) associated with myoclonus (lower graph). Figure kindly provided by Dr Sushma Goyal.

Lennox–Gastaut syndrome (Fig. 3b.7)

Syndrome definition:
- Seizures: tonic, atonic, atypical absences.
- EEG abnormalities: generalized slow spike-wave while awake and generalized bursts of fast rhythms at 10Hz while asleep.
- Developmental delay, learning disability, neuropsychological and psychiatric disorders.

Prevalence: uncommon.

Age of onset of seizures: 1–8 years.

Seizure types:
- Generalized tonic.
- Atypical absences.
- Atonic.
- Myoclonic.
- Drop attacks—falls during tonic or atonic seizures.

Patient development (milestones): severely delayed. Plateau after epilepsy onset in de novo cases.

Patient intelligence and memory function: poor.

Family history of epilepsy: Low but depends on aetiology.

Inter-ictal EEG:
- *EEG background*: slowed.
- *EEG paroxysmal abnormalities*: multifocal or slow generalized spike-wave discharges while awake. Generalized bursts of fast rhythms at 10Hz while asleep.

Ictal EEG:
- Tonic and atonic seizures: EEG flattening with diffuse fast activity.
- Atypical absences: generalized spike-wave at <2.5Hz.
- Myoclonic: generalized spike or polyspike and wave.

Neuroimaging: normal or abnormal.

Aetiology: unknown, West syndrome, diffuse cerebral atrophy, other forms of widespread brain damage.

Medical treatment: not very effective. The most effective AEDs appear to be valproate, lamotrigine, benzodiazepines, levetiracetam, topiramate, rufinamide, corticosteroids, immunoglobulin. Rufinamide recently introduced.

Surgical treatment: callosotomy for drop attacks. Deep brain stimulation has been used is some centers.

Prognosis: poor. Seizures might eventually remit but learning difficulties persist.

Epilepsy type: symptomatic or presumed symptomatic generalized. Epileptic encephalopathy.

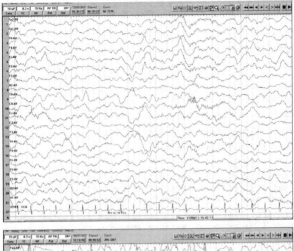

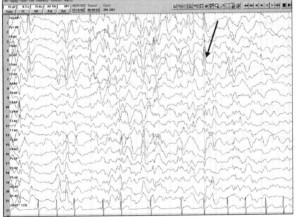

Fig. 3b.7 Lennox–Gastaut syndrome: a 5-year-old child with global developmental delay with tonic seizures. The EEG shows diffuse slowing and bilateral slow spike-wave-discharges (arrow). Figure kindly provided by Dr Sushma Goyal.

Myoclonic-astatic epilepsy *or* **epilepsy with myoclonic-astatic seizures** *or* **Doose syndrome (Fig. 3b.8)**

Prevalence: 1–2% of all childhood epilepsies.

Age of onset of seizures: 2–5 years.

Seizure types: myoclonic-astatic (myoclonic-atonic), myoclonic, astatic (atonic), tonic–clonic, absences occurring in previously healthy subjects. Presence of tonic seizures is an exclusion criterion. Non-convulsive status epilepticus (NCSE) is common.

Patient development (milestones): often delayed after onset of seizures.

Patient intelligence and memory function: 75% normal.

Family history of epilepsy: in 30%.

Inter-ictal EEG:
- EEG background: initially normal, later posterior slowing.
- EEG paroxysmal abnormalities: initially absent, irregular generalized fast spike-wave and polyspike-wave. Most cases are photosensitive.

Ictal EEG: irregular generalized fast spike-wave and polyspike-wave at above 2.5Hz in myoclonic and atonic seizures. Atonia is usually synchronous with a slow wave.

Neuroimaging: normal.

Aetiology: possibly genetic. Some GEFS+(📖 p.98) probands have myoclonic-astatic epilepsy.

Medical treatment: valproate, lamotrigine, ethosuximide, topiramate, and levetiracetam. Ketogenic diet. Narrow spectrum drugs may worsen the condition.

Surgical treatment: callosotomy for drop attacks.

Prognosis: variable.

Epilepsy type: symptomatic/cryptogenic generalized according to 1989 ILAE classification. Idiopathic generalized according to the latest 2001 ILAE classification.

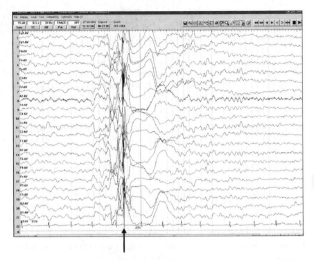

Fig. 3b.8 Myoclonic-astatic epilepsy: 9-year-old child with multiple seizures: GTCS and myoclonus, with falls (arrow). Positive family history. The EEG showed EEG changes associated with myoclonus. Note: the silent period after the jerk. Figure kindly provided by Dr Sushma Goyal.

Epilepsy with febrile seizures plus (EFS+) *or* **generalized epilepsy with febrile seizures plus (GEFS+)** *or* **autosomal dominant epilepsy with febrile seizures plus**

This entity includes several seizure types and syndromes with febrile seizures plus (febrile seizures continuing beyond the age of 6), such as severe myoclonic epilepsy in infancy (SMEI), severe myoclonic epilepsy borderline (SMEB, similar to SMEI but without myoclonias) and myoclonic-astatic epilepsy. Most probands, however, do not have severe epilepsy.

Prevalence: rare.

Age of onset of seizures: varies from first months of life to childhood, depending on the underlying syndrome.

Seizure types:
- Initially febrile seizures plus (febrile seizures which will continue beyond the age of 6).
- Later afebrile generalized seizures (absences, myoclonic, tonic or myoclonic-atonic seizures).
- Focal frontal or temporal seizures in 13% of subjects.

Patient development (milestones): depends on underlying syndrome.

Patient intelligence and memory function: depends on underlying syndrome.

Family history of epilepsy: frequent.

Inter-ictal EEG: depends on underlying syndrome.

Ictal EEG: depends on underlying syndrome and seizure type.

Neuroimaging: usually normal. Hippocampal sclerosis has been reported in a minority.

Aetiology: genetic, heterogeneous autosomal dominant with variable, often reduced penetrance and evidence for likely modifier genetic effects. Mutations found in sodium channel genes (*SCN1A, SCN1B*) and in gamma2 GABA receptor subunit gene (*GABRG2*). Other loci have been reported.

Medical treatment: depends on underlying syndrome.

Resective surgical treatment: not usually.

Prognosis: depends on underlying syndrome.

Epilepsy type: depends on underlying syndrome. Idiopathic.

Progressive myoclonic epilepsies (PME) (Fig. 3b.9)
Prevalence: rare.

Age of onset of seizures: depends on cause, but usually between 8–14 years.

Seizure types: generalized myoclonus, often involving mainly shoulders, arms, and neck. Myoclonus can be spontaneous but it is often exacerbated by a variety of stimuli (light, sound, touch, action, emotional stress). There may be other seizure types. Gelastic seizures in Niemann–Pick disease type C.

Patient development (milestones): delayed. Other neurological deterioration may occur, including cognitive or movement disorders.

Patient intelligence and memory function: poor.

Family history of epilepsy: often but not always. Depends on syndrome.

Inter-ictal EEG:
- EEG background: slowed.
- EEG paroxysmal abnormalities: mutifocal or generalized.

Ictal EEG: sharp spike or polyspike and wave, sometimes followed by EEG flattening for a few seconds.

Neuroimaging: abnormal or normal.

Aetiology: a variety of serious neurodegenerative and genetic metabolic diseases affecting the brain, including storage diseases. The most common causes are Unverricht–Lundborg disease and Lafora body disease. More rarely sialidosis types I and II, myoclonic epilepsy with ragged-red fibres (MERRF), Alper's syndrome (POLG1 mutations), neuronal ceroid lipofuscinoses, dentatorubral-pallidoluysian atrophy, galactosialidosis, mucolipidosis type I, juvenile neuropathic Gaucher's disease type 3, juvenile neuroaxonal dystrophy, Wilson's disease, childhood form of Huntington's disease, Hallervorden–Spatz disease, non-ketotic hyperglycinaemia, Tay–Sachs disease (GM2 gangliosidosis type 1), Sandhoff's disease (GM2 gangliosidosis type 2), sulphite oxidase deficiency, biopterin deficiency.

Medical treatment: limited efficacy. Most drugs tried. Phenytoin in Unverricht–Lundborg disease is contraindicated, valproate in PME due to mitochrondrial disease including POLG1 mutations is also contraindicated. Some metabolic conditions may benefit from abstinence from certain food as early as possible. Depending on syndrome, valproate, levetiracetam, piracetam, clonazepam, topiramate and zonisamide may be effective.

Resective surgical treatment: no.

Prognosis: Very variable, depending on syndrome. Often poor, both in terms of seizures and development. If food sensitive, prognosis might be better if diet started earlier.

Epilepsy type: symptomatic generalized.

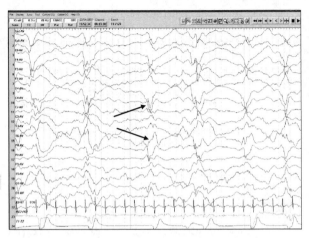

Fig. 3b.9 Progressive myoclonic epilepsy (Alper's syndrome): 3-month-old baby, previously well, presenting with sudden onset of almost continuous myoclonic jerks. Sibling had Alper's disease. The EEG showed myoclonic status epilepticus, with continuous bilateral myoclonus and asymmetrical EEG changes with discharge predominance in the right hemisphere (arrows). Figure kindly provided by Dr Sushma Goyal.

Childhood absence epilepsy *or* absence epilepsy of childhood *or* typical absence epilepsy of childhood *or* pyknolepsy *or* petit-mal epilepsy (Fig. 3b.10)

Prevalence: common. Male:female = 1:2.5 (60–70% are girls).

Age of onset of seizures: 4–10 years; peak at 5–7 years.

Seizure types: typical absences (simple, with clonic components, with atonic components, with tonic components, with automatisms, with autonomic components). Often very frequent, hundreds per day—pyknolepsy. Hyperventilation virtually always induces seizures, which is a useful diagnostic test in clinic and during EEG. Myoclonic absences are not present. Infrequent GTCS can be seen in adolescence or adult life, not preceding or concomitant with the period of active absence seizures.

Patient development (milestones): normal.

Patient intelligence and memory function: normal.

Family history of epilepsy: frequent.

Inter-ictal EEG:
- EEG background: normal.
- EEG paroxysmal abnormalities: generalized spike-and-wave.

Ictal EEG: generalized spike-and-wave at 2.5–3.5Hz.

Neuroimaging: normal.

Aetiology: idiopathic. History of febrile seizures in 15–20% of patients.

Medical treatment: valproate, ethosuximide, lamotrigine amongst others. Seizure exacerbation occurs with narrow spectrum AEDs.

Resective surgical treatment: no.

Prognosis: good. Seizures respond to medical treatment in 70–90%, but 40% develop tonic–clonic seizures in adolescence. There is no developmental delay but there might be subtle cognitive impairment if seizures are very frequent (in around 30% of patients).

Epilepsy type: idiopathic generalized.

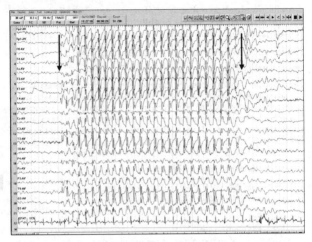

Fig. 3b.10 Childhood absence epilepsy: since age 2½, daily vacant episodes sometimes associated with eyelid flickering and head droop. They occur many days and may have clusters of them, especially when tired. Sometimes appears tired afterwards. 3Hz generalized spike-wave discharges were recorded on the EEG in association with clinical absence seizures (arrows point to onset and offset of absence seizure). Figure kindly provided by Dr Sushma Goyal.

Epilepsy with myoclonic absences or myoclonic absence epilepsy

Prevalence: rare. Male preponderance (69%).

Age of onset of seizures: 1–12 years; peak at 7 years.

Seizure types: typical absences with associated rhythmic generalized myo-clonic jerks involving mainly shoulders, arms and legs, superimposed on a concomitant tonic contraction. Eyelid twitching is absent but perioral myoclonus is frequent.

Patient development (milestones): moderate delay is common.

Patient intelligence and memory function: unimpaired in about 30%.

Family history of epilepsy: in 20%.

Inter-ictal EEG:
- EEG background: normal.
- EEG paroxysmal abnormalities: generalized spike-and-wave.

Ictal EEG: generalized spike-and-wave at 2.5–3.5Hz.

Neuroimaging: normal.

Aetiology: unknown.

Medical treatment: valproate, ethosuximide, valproate + ethosuximide, lamotrigine (or combinations thereof) amongst others.

Resective surgical treatment: no.

Prognosis: treatment less effective to suppress seizures than in typical absence epilepsy of childhood. Developmental delay is common.

Epilepsy type: unclear.

Juvenile absence epilepsy *or* **epilepsy with non-pyknoleptic absences** *or* **epilepsy with spanioleptic absences**

Prevalence: common.

Age of onset of seizures: 7–17 years; peak at 9–13 years.

Seizure types:
- Typical absences, occurring less frequently than in absence epilepsy of childhood.
- Tonic–clonic seizures, often on awakening.
- Myoclonic seizures, less common, overlapping with juvenile myoclonic epilepsy (JME).

Patient development (milestones): normal.

Patient intelligence and memory function: usually unimpaired or mildly impaired.

Family history of epilepsy: present in 10–40%.

Inter-ictal EEG:
- EEG background: normal.
- EEG paroxysmal abnormalities: generalized spike-and-wave.

Ictal EEG: generalized spike-and-wave at 3.5–4Hz.

Neuroimaging: normal.

Aetiology: idiopathic.

Medical treatment: valproate, ethosuximide, lamotrigine (or combinations thereof) amongst others. Seizure exacerbation occurs with narrow spectrum AEDs.

Resective surgical treatment: no.

Prognosis: treatment less effective to suppress seizures than in absence epilepsy of childhood.

Epilepsy type: idiopathic generalized.

Perioral myoclonia with absences—not officially recognized by the ILAE

Prevalence: rare. Mainly females.

Age of onset of seizures: 2–13 years. Median at 10 years.

Seizure types: brief (2–9sec) typical absences with perioral myoclonia (rhythmic contractions that cause protrusion of lips and twitching of the corners of the mouth). Often misdiagnosed as focal motor seizures. Absence seizures can be very frequent or sporadic. All patients suffer generalized tonic–clonic seizures, often starting before or around the time of onset of absence seizures. Absence status epileptics is very common (57%).

Patient development (milestones): normal.

Patient intelligence and memory function: normal.

Family history of epilepsy: reportedly common.

Inter-ictal EEG:
- EEG background: normal.
- EEG paroxysmal abnormalities: generalized spike-and-wave, often abortive and/or asymmetrical. Also focal discharges. No photosensitivity.

Ictal EEG: generalized spike-and-wave at 3–4Hz, often irregular and fragmented.

Neuroimaging: normal.

Aetiology: unknown.

Medical treatment: valproate, ethosuximide, valproate + ethosuximide, lamotrigine, clonazepam or combinations thereof, amongst others.

Resective surgical treatment: no.

Prognosis: seizures are often resistant to medication and lifelong.

Epilepsy type: idiopathic generalized.

Eyelid myoclonia with absences (EMA) *or* **Jeavons syndrome** (Figs. 3b11 and 3b.12)—not officially recognized by the **ILAE** as a syndrome, but recognized as a seizure type.

Syndrome definition
- Eyelid myoclonia with or without absences.
- Eye-closure induces seizures or EEG epileptiform discharges or both.
- Absences without eyelid myoclonia do not occur.
- Photosensitivity.

Prevalence: rare. More in females than males (2:1).

Age of onset of seizures: 2–14 years; peak at 6–8 years.

Seizure types: eyelid myoclonia (jerking of eyelids often associated with jerky upwards deviation of eyeballs and retropulsion of the head). Eyelid myoclonia are brief (3–6sec) and induced by eye closure. Consciousness can be preserved (eyelid myoclonia without absence) or consciousness may be impaired during or following eyelid myoclonia (eyelid myoclonia with absence). GTCS are spontaneous or induced by light. Spontaneous GTCS are rare but can be precipitated by sleep deprivation or alcohol. Myoclonic jerks are rare. Eyelid myoclonia status epilepticus occurs in 20%, either spontaneously or induced by light.

Patient development (milestones): normal.

Patient intelligence and memory function: normal.

Family history of epilepsy: frequent.

Inter-ictal EEG:
- *EEG background:* normal.
- *EEG paroxysmal abnormalities:* generalized discharges as described for ictal recordings.

Ictal EEG: brief (1–6sec, commonly 2–3sec) and frequent generalized spike-and-wave discharges and polyspikes at 3–6Hz occurring immediately (within 0.5–2 sec) after eye closure in an illuminated room. They disappear in total darkness. All patients are photosensitive.

Neuroimaging: normal.

Aetiology: genetic.

Medical treatment: valproate, ethosuximide, lamotrigine, levetiracetam, clonazepam, or combinations of thereof amongst others. Can be refractory though often the eyelid myoclonic is unnoticed by the adult patient. GTCS are infrequent and easier to control.

Resective surgical treatment: no.

Prognosis: lifelong even if seizures are controlled on AEDs. Often refractory in terms of EMA. Photosensitivity may disappear in middle age.

Epilepsy type: reflex photosensitive idiopathic.

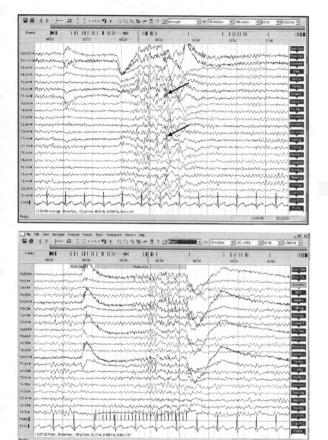

Fig. 3b.11 Eyelid myoclonia with absences: blinking or eye closure induces generalized spike-and-wave activity (arrows, upper graph) and absence seizures with eyelid myoclonus. Patients are photosensitive (lower graph).

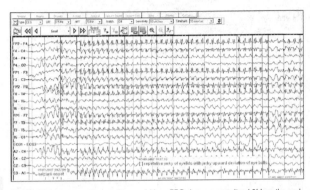

Fig. 3b.12 Jeavons syndrome: 5-year-old boy. EEG shows generalized 3Hz spike-and-wave discharges up to 15sec with repetitive eyelid myoclonus. Figure kindly provided by Dr Sushma Goyal.

Idiopathic generalized epilepsy with phantom absences—not officially recognized by the ILAE

Syndrome definition
- Phantom absences (see below for description).
- GTCS usually starting in adulthood and infrequent, often being the first reported clinical manifestation.
- Absence status epilepticus, in 50% of patients.

Prevalence: rare. Men and women equally affected.

Age of onset of seizures: GTCS start in adulthood, although patients may have suffered unrecognized absence seizures earlier.

Seizure types: phantom absences are absence seizures causing mild impairment of consciousness, unrecognized by the patient or observer, but often associated with delays or error if the patient is asked to count, and occasionally with blinking. GTCS are often the first reported clinical manifestation. Absence status epilepticus in 50% of patients.

Patient development (milestones): normal.

Patient intelligence and memory function: normal.

Family history of epilepsy: frequent.

Inter-ictal EEG:
- *EEG background:* normal.
- *EEG paroxysmal abnormalities:* generalized discharges as described below for ictal recordings. Half of the patients show additional focal discharges. Photosensitivity is exceptional.

Ictal EEG: absence seizures are associated with brief (3–4sec) generalized polyspike and wave discharges at 3–4Hz. Tonic–clonic seizures are generalized.

Neuroimaging: normal.

Aetiology: genetic.

Medical treatment: valproate, ethosuximide, lamotrigine, levetiracetam, clonazepam, or combinations of these amongst others.

Resective surgical treatment: no.

Prognosis: lifelong even if seizures are controlled on AEDs. Patients can have a normal life (except for driving) if only absence seizures occur.

Epilepsy type: idiopathic generalized.

Benign childhood epilepsy with centro-temporal (Rolandic) spikes *or* **Rolandic epilepsy** *or* **Rolandic epilepsy of childhood (Fig. 3b.13)**

Prevalence: the most common epilepsy syndrome in childhood.

Age of onset of seizures: 3–13 years.

Seizure types: focal sensory and/or motor seizures. Sensory aura (unilateral tingling often in mouth or hand) is followed by unilateral focal tonic or clonic seizure usually involving hand or face and larynx. They occur while awake or asleep, but in some patients may occur only from sleep. Consciousness usually preserved, often secondarily generalized convulsions during sleep.

Patient development (milestones): normal.

Patient intelligence and memory function: normal.

Family history of epilepsy: frequent.

Inter-ictal EEG:
- EEG background: normal.
- EEG paroxysmal abnormalities: Rolandic (T3/T4) focal or bilateral independent spike and wave, often increasing in incidence during sleep.

Ictal EEG: repetitive Rolandic spikes which may secondarily generalize.

Neuroimaging: normal.

Aetiology: idiopathic.

Medical treatment: carbamazepine, sultiame, or none.

Resective surgical treatment: no.

Prognosis: usually excellent. Seizures remit spontaneously at puberty.

Epilepsy type: focal idiopathic.

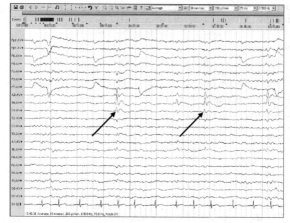

Fig. 3b.13 Benign childhood epilepsy with centro-temporal (rolandic) spikes: 6-year-old boy with normal development and infrequent nocturnal seizures. The EEG shows right centro-sylvian spike-and-wave discharges (arrows), occurring in runs during sleep. Figure kindly provided by Dr Sushma Goyal.

Benign childhood occipital epilepsy *or* benign childhood epilepsy with occipital paroxysms (Fig. 3b.14)
(Panayiotopoulos syndrome and Gastaut-type syndrome)

Prevalence:
- *Panayiotopoulos syndrome:* common, 2–3 per 1000 children, 6–13% of children with non-febrile seizures.
- *Gastaut-type syndrome:* rarer. 2–7% of benign childhood focal epilepsies.

Age of onset of seizures: 1–17 years.

Seizure types: Two forms of this syndrome have been recognized.
- *Panayiotopoulos syndrome:* early onset (1–14 years, peak at 4–5 years), infrequent seizures consisting on autonomic seizures, mainly emetic, eye deviation, ictal syncope, high incidence of autonomic status epilepticus.
- *Gastaut-type syndrome:* late onset (3–15 years, peak at 8 years), seizures with elementary visual hallucinations (flashing lights) and blindness (amaurosis), or both, consciousness usually preserved, sometimes with eye deviation, vomiting, severe post-ictal headache. Sometimes followed by hemiclonic seizures and automatisms.

Patient development (milestones): normal.

Patient intelligence and memory function: normal.

Family history of epilepsy: common for epilepsy and/or migraine.

Inter-ictal EEG:
- EEG background: normal.
- EEG paroxysmal abnormalities: occipital spikes, unilateral or bilateral independent, activated by eye closure (fixation-off).

Ictal EEG: repetitive occipital focal spikes which may secondarily generalize.

Neuroimaging: normal.

Aetiology: idiopathic. Needs to be differentiated from symptomatic occipital epilepsies.

Medical treatment: none if infrequent seizures, carbamazepine otherwise.

Resective surgical treatment: no.

Prognosis: excellent.

Epilepsy type: focal idiopathic epilepsy.

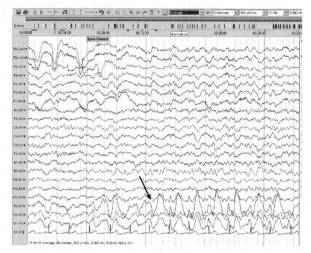

Fig. 3b.14 Benign childhood epilepsy with occipital paroxysms: 5-year-old child with infrequent prolonged nocturnal seizures associated with vomiting. The EEG showed left occipital spike-and-wave discharges (arrow) on eye closure. Figure kindly provided by Dr Sushma Goyal.

Landau–Kleffner syndrome *or* acquired epileptic aphasia (Fig. 3b.15)

Syndrome definition

- Acquired aphasia (aphasia occurring after a period of normal speech development), initially mainly sensory aphasia, with normal hearing (100% of patients).
- Seizures (70% of patients), usually infrequent.
- Behavioural difficulties (70% of patients).
- Continuous status epilepticus during slow wave sleep (common but not required for diagnosis).

Prevalence: rare, possibly underdiagnosed.

Age of onset of seizures: 2–10 years.

Seizure types: infrequent tonic–clonic or focal motor seizures.

Patient development (milestones): poor outlook for remittance of language deficits.

Patient intelligence and memory function: mainly verbal deficits until adolescence.

Family history of epilepsy: in 12%.

Inter-ictal EEG: the awake EEG is normal or shows multifocal discharges particularly with temporal prominence. The sleep EEG shows nearly continuous generalized spike-and-wave activity with posterior temporal predominance, occurring during most sleep (normal sleep phenomena are hardly seen), although full criteria for ESES may not be reached.

Ictal EEG: not well defined, as they are infrequent. Mainly nocturnal. Ususally GTCS or focal motor seizures. Atypical absences, atonic seizures and secondarily generalized seizures can also occur.

Neuroimaging: normal.

Aetiology: unknown. Functional abnormality of speech areas is thought to cause aphasia, seizures, and continuous secondarily generalized discharges during sleep. Behavioural difficulties may be due the chronic lack of normal sleep.

Medical treatment: an initial short trial with corticosteroids is recommended, as it is often effective in controlling continuous spike-wave during sleep and aphasia and behavioural difficulties may improve dramatically. If ineffective, then benzodiazepines, valproate, lamotrigine, or other AEDs.

Surgical treatment: multiple subpial transection over sylvian and perisylvian cortex has been tried with variable success.

Prognosis: good for seizure control, but poor for language recovery. In 40% aphasia remits in adolescence, but might be too late to retrieve psychosocial skills. 50% can lead a relatively normal life. Worse prognosis if earlier onset.

Epilepsy type: undetermined as to whether focal or generalized (1989 ILAE classification). Epileptic encephalopathy (2001 ILAE diagnostic scheme). Epileptic encephalopathy with CSWS including LKS (2006 ILAE classification core group report).

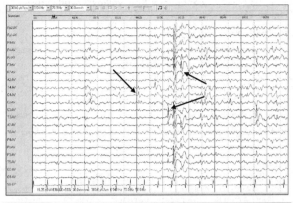

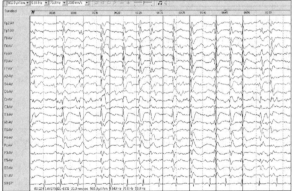

Fig. 3b.15 Landau–Kleffner syndrome: 6-year-old boy presented with a left-sided motor seizure, in addition to deterioration in receptive and expressive language. The awake EEG (upper graph) shows independent left and right centro-temporal discharges, more widespread over the left hemisphere. The sleep EEG (lower graph) showed electrical status epilepticus in sleep—ESES. Figure kindly provided by Dr Sushma Goyal.

Epilepsia partialis continua or **Kojewnikow's syndrome** (Fig. 3b.16)

Prevalence: rare.

Age of onset of seizures: depends on cause, commonly before 10 years of age for Rasmussen's encephailtis.

Seizure types: frequent or continuous focal clonic seizures usually restricted to hand or face, with preserved consciousness (focal motor status epilepticus). Sometimes focal convulsions last for days or weeks.

Patient development (milestones): depending on cause and age of onset.

Patient intelligence and memory function: varying degrees of deficits.

Family history of epilepsy: usually not present.

Inter-ictal EEG:
- EEG background: slow, particularly on the affected side.
- EEG paroxysmal abnormalities: focal, particularly over frontotemporal regions, sometimes rhythmic and linked to the clonic jerks, sometimes not clearly linked with the jerks.

Ictal EEG: as inter-ictal.

Neuroimaging: usually abnormal, although initially may be normal.

Aetiology: two types: type I (secondary to Rasmussen's, tick borne, viral, renal, hepatic or paraneoplastic encephalitis, mitochondrial disorders including POLG1 and other mutations). Type II (secondary to a focal lesion of the motor cortex). Rasmussen's encephalitis is a progressive unilateral encephalitis associated with cortical hemiatrophy. Focal lesions close to the motor cortex can be tumours or vascular lesions.

Medical treatment: drugs usually ineffective, except perhaps corticosteroids. Avoid valproate in mitochondrial (including POLG1 mutations) as this can precipitate liver failure.

Resective surgical treatment: hemispherectomy in Rasmussen's encephalitis, focal resection if due to a focal lesion.

Prognosis: variable, can be poor, depending on cause, often progressive hemiplegia, dysphasia and intellectual decline.

Epilepsy type: focal symptomatic or presumed symptomatic.

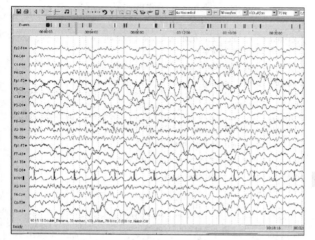

Fig. 3b.16 Rasmussen's encephalitis: girl age 12, who was witnessed to have her first seizure whilst at school. 2 weeks later she developed drooping of the right side of her face, with loss of tone and shaking down the right side of her body. She suffered several episodes of right-sided facial dropping and twitching associated with right arm shaking, lasting for several hours. Imaging was essentially normal. The EEG showed a massive asymmetry of the background activity, with widespread slowing over the left hemisphere and preserved background on the right hemisphere.

Juvenile myoclonic epilepsy (JME) *or* Janz syndrome *or* impulsive petit mal (Fig. 3b.17)

Prevalence: the most common epileptic syndrome with onset in adolescence, often unrecognized.

Age of onset of seizures: 8–24 years, peak between 12–18 years.

Seizure types: myoclonic seizures (most often affecting upper limbs), generalized tonic–clonic and, less frequently, absence seizures. Absence seizures resemble those of JAE. Seizures are more frequent in the mornings. They can be triggered by sleep deprivation, alcohol, abrupt awakening, stress, and in some, photic stimulation.

Patient development (milestones): normal.

Patient intelligence and memory function: normal.

Family history of epilepsy: frequent.

Inter-ictal EEG:
- EEG background: normal.
- EEG paroxysmal abnormalities: generalized polyspike-and-wave, often activated by sleep. 30% are photosensitive. Additional focal sharp waves in 25%.

Ictal EEG: generalized polyspike-and-wave during myoclonic jerks. Generalized fast activity followed by generalized spike-wave during generalized tonic–clonic seizures. Generalized spike-and-wave during absence seizures.

Neuroimaging: normal.

Aetiology: idiopathic. Genetic.

Medical treatment: valproate is broad spectrum and is the most effective, covering all seizure types but is not ideal in women of child-bearing age. The role of new AEDs is still being assessed. Topiramate is broad spectrum. Information on zonisamide, in juvenile myclonic epilepsy is limited. A small dose of lamotrigine added to valproate may be synergistic. Lamotrigine monotherapy is less effective than valproate. It may exacerbate seizures in a proportion, particularly myoclonus. Levetiracetam is licensed for myoclonus in JME. Its effect on GTCS is less predictable. Carbamazepine may make control worse particulary myoclonus and absence seizures. Narrow spectrum antiepileptic drugs should be avoided. An important issue is which medication to choose, as medical treatment is to be continued lifelong.

Resective surgical treatment: no.

Prognosis: good. Excellent response to valproate but propensity to seizures is lifelong in more than 50%, with seizures recurring if therapy withdrawn.

Epilepsy type: idiopathic generalized.

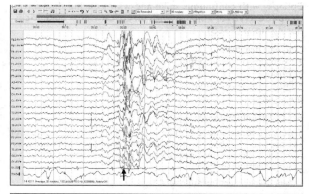

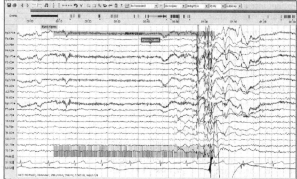

Fig. 3b.17 JME: 15-year-old presented with one generalized tonic–clonic seizure and myoclonic jerks. The EEG shows generalized polyspike-and-wave discharges (arrow on upper graph). Photic stimulation at 25Hz was associated with generalized photparoxysmal responses and myoclonus (lower graph). Figure kindly provided by Dr Sushma Goyal.

Epilepsy with continuous spike-and-waves during slow wave sleep (ECSWS) or epilepsy with electrical status epilepticus during sleep (ESES)

Syndrome definition
- Continuous generalized spikes during >85% of slow sleep.
- Seizures.
- Neuropsychological decline.

Prevalence: rare.

Age of onset of seizures: 4–10 years.

Seizure types: nocturnal focal motor seizures (hemifacial, hemiconvulsive), absence seizures (typical or atypical), absence status, atonic, clonic, generalized tonic–clonic. Tonic seizures are not present or infrequent (unlike in Lennox–Gastaut syndrome).

Patient development (milestones): delayed.

Patient intelligence and memory function: severely affected. Remission of EEG abnormality after 2–7 years, but rarely recover normal function.

Family history of epilepsy: rare (10%).

Inter-ictal EEG: generalized, focal or multifocal discharges while awake. Bilateral or generalized continuous spike-and-wave during sleep at 1.5–2Hz, with frontal emphasis.

Ictal EEG: according to seizure type.

Neuroimaging: abnormal in 30% (unilateral or diffuse cortical atrophy, porenchephaly, developmental malformations).

Aetiology: unknown or widespread brain abnormalities (cortical atrophy, porencephaly, malformations of cortical development).

Medical treatment: valproate + benzodiazepines, ethosuximide, corticosteroids. Carbamazepine might make it worse.

Resective surgical treatment: no.

Prognosis: seizures and EEG abnormalities eventually remit. Neuropsychological deficits improve but rarely completely recover.

Epilepsy type: undetermined as to whether focal or generalized (1989 ILAE classification). Epileptic encephalopathy (2001 ILAE diagnostic scheme and 2006 ILAE classification core group report).

Epilepsy with grand mal (GTCS) on awakening and epilepsy with generalized tonic–clonic seizures only

GTCS on awakening

Prevalence: rare.

Age of onset of seizures: 6–20 years.

Seizure types: GTCS while waking up or when relaxing. Myoclonic and absence seizures are not uncommon.

Patient development (milestones): normal.

Patient intelligence and memory function: normal.

Family history of epilepsy: frequent.

Inter-ictal EEG:
- EEG background: normal.
- EEG paroxysmal abnormalities: occasional generalized discharges.

Ictal EEG: generalized spike-and-wave.

Neuroimaging: normal.

Aetiology: idiopathic.

Medical treatment: broad spectrum AED medication is preferred.

Resective surgical treatment: no.

Prognosis: good. Seizures respond to drugs but relapse if medication withdrawn.

Epilepsy type: idiopathic generalized.

Epilepsy with generalized tonic–clonic seizures only: this is finally recognized as a syndrome, not just a seizure type. It is similar to the above with GTCS being the only seizure type occurring at any time of the day or from sleep (thus, it includes epilepsy with GTCS on awakening). The syndrome is idiopathic generalized, with generalized spike-and-wave on EEG, and responds to broad-spectrum AEDs.

Temporal lobe epilepsy (Fig. 3b.18)

Prevalence: the most common focal epilepsy in adults.

Age of onset of seizures: any age, depending on cause, usually before middle age if starting in adulthood.

Seizure types: temporal lobe seizures (aura of epigatric sensation, taste or déjà vu, vertigo, or hearing melodies or sounds if lateral temporal onset, loss of consciousness, oral automatisms, fiddling, fumbling, walking, automatic speech if non-dominant onset, sometimes contralateral dystonia, post-ictal confusion, post-ictal dysphasia if onset from dominant hemisphere, sometimes secondarily generalized convulsions).

Patient development (milestones): usually normal or mild delay.

Patient intelligence and memory function: normal or mild lateralized deficits if onset in adulthood, particularly affecting memory.

Family history of epilepsy: sometimes.

Inter-ictal EEG:
- EEG background: normal or temporal slowing.
- EEG paroxysmal abnormalities: none or anterior temporal discharges, unilateral or bilateral asynchronous.

Ictal EEG: focal rhythmic sharp waves or spikes, focal slowing and later diffuse slowing, sometimes focal slowing from onset (on scalp).

Neuroimaging: normal or abnormal.

Aetiology: temporal lesion. The most common lesions are mesial temporal sclerosis, temporal tumours, focal cortical dysplasia, or DNET. Mesial temporal sclerosis tends to be unilateral but can be bilateral. The term 'dual temporal pathology' refers to the presence of hippocampal sclerosis and an extra-hippocampal lesion in the same patient. Dual pathology can be observed in as much as 20–30% of temporal lobes resected for surgical treatment. Extrahippocampal lesions tend to be tumours, developmental cysts or trauma. A small proportion are idiopathic and not associated with structural pathology with a good prognosis.

Medical treatment: most AEDs.

Resective surgical treatment: possible for symptomatic cases (temporal lobectomy). 70% become seizure free.

Prognosis: many patients are controlled by drugs. If not, surgery is an option.

Epilepsy type: largely focal symptomatic or presumed symptomatic.

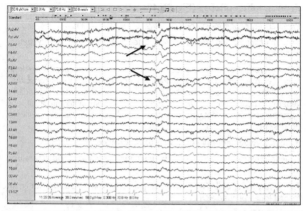

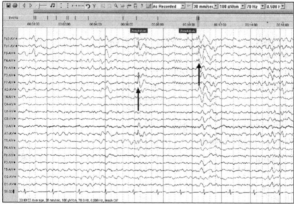

Fig. 3b.18 Temporal lobe epilepsy. Temporal delta waves (arrows, upper graph) and bilateral independent temporal epileptiform discharges (arrows, lower graph) in two patients with temporal lobe epilepsy.

Frontal lobe epilepsy (Fig. 3b.19)

Prevalence: second most common focal epilepsy in adults.

Age of onset of seizures: any age, depending on cause, usually before middle age.

Seizure types: frontal lobe seizures (brief, often during sleep, sometimes many per night, variable aura, sometimes indescribable, loss of consciousness, frantic or bizarre automatisms, dystonia, sometimes secondarily generalized convulsions). Orbital seizures can be similar to temporal lobe seizures. (for more detailed descriptions 📖 see Frontal lobe epilepsy, pp.146–149.

Patient development (milestones): usually normal or mild delay.

Patient intelligence and memory function: normal or mild lateralized deficits.

Family history of epilepsy: sometimes, particularly in autosomal dominant frontal lobe epilepsy(ADFLE).

Inter-ictal EEG:
- EEG background: normal or frontal slowing.
- EEG paroxysmal abnormalities: frontal discharges.

Ictal EEG: frontal or diffuse abnormalities, slowing or discharges may be normal.

Neuroimaging: normal or abnormal.

Aetiology: frontal lesion (head injury, tumour, focal cortical dysplasia, etc). Some are idiopathic (autosomal dominant frontal lobe epilepsy or ADFLE).

Medical treatment: most AEDs

Resective surgical treatment: possible. Only 50% improve.

Prognosis: worse response to medication and surgery than temporal lobe epilepsy, more prone to status epilepticus.

Epilepsy type: focal symptomatic or presumed symptomatic. ADFLE is idiopathic.

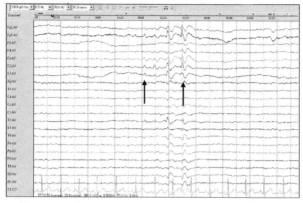

Fig. 3b.19 Frontal lobe epilepsy: Burst of left frontal spike-and-wave in a patient with frontal lobe epilepsy due to focal cortical dysplasia.

Parietal lobe epilepsy (Fig. 3b.20)

Prevalence: rare.

Age of onset of seizures: any age, depending on cause, usually before middle age.

Seizure types: somatosensory aura, vertigo, distortions of space, sometimes loss of consciousness, automatisms, sometimes secondarily generalized convulsions.

Patient development (milestones): usually normal.

Patient intelligence and memory function: normal or mild lateralized deficits.

Family history of epilepsy: sometimes

Inter-ictal EEG:
- EEG background: normal or parieto-central slowing.
- EEG paroxysmal abnormalities: focal parietal or central discharges.

Ictal EEG: focal or diffuse abnormalities, slowing or discharges.

Neuroimaging: normal or abnormal.

Aetiology: parietal lesion (head injury, tumour, focal cortical dysplasia, etc.).

Medical treatment: most AEDs.

Resective surgical treatment: possible.

Prognosis: variable, depending on cause.

Epilepsy type: focal symptomatic or presumed symptomatic.

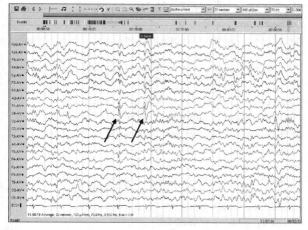

Fig. 3b.20 Right central spikes: the patient had two seizures preceded by feeling unwell and followed by loss of awareness and then whole body shaking for 4–5min. Afterwards he felt tired and had a headache.

Occipital lobe epilepsy (Fig. 3b.21)

Prevalence: rare.

Age of onset of seizures: any age, depending on cause, usually before middle age.

Seizure types: occipital lobe seizures (visual aura such as seeing lights or geometrical figures, sometimes complex hallucinations, blinking, loss of consciousness, automatisms, sometimes secondarily generalized convulsions). Sometimes they may resemble temporal lobe seizures.

Patient development (milestones): usually normal.

Patient intelligence and memory function: normal.

Family history of epilepsy: sometimes.

Inter-ictal EEG:
- EEG background: normal or posterior slowing.
- EEG paroxysmal abnormalities: focal occipital discharges.

Ictal EEG: focal or diffuse abnormalities, slowing or discharges.

Neuroimaging: normal or abnormal.

Aetiology: visual lesion (head injury, tumour, porencephalic cyst, etc.).

Medical treatment: most AEDs.

Resective surgical treatment: possible.

Prognosis: variable, depending on cause.

Epilepsy type: focal symptomatic or presumed symptomatic.

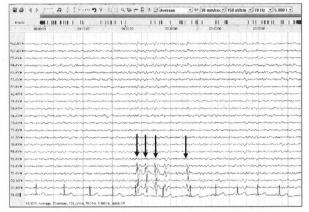

Fig. 3b.21 Occipital lobe epilepsy: burst of left occipital discharges (arrows) in a patient with occipital lobe epilepsy.

Epilepsy syndromes at a glance

- A syndrome may be defined as a cluster of symptoms and signs, which may include evidence from clinical assessment (e.g. history, seizure type), and neurophysiological and neuroradiological investigations.
- Original classification was proposed by ILAE in 1989; and revised in 2001.[1]
- It was revised in view of increasing number of syndromes and some ambiguity in terminology.
- Current classification is based on 5-axis system to aid diagnosis (Box 3b.2).
- When defining the syndrome it is important to determine whether it is focal or generalized.
- The syndrome may then be defined as idiopathic, symptomatic, or presumed symptomatic.
- More specific syndrome diagnosis may then be possible depending on the information available.
- 📖 See Box 3b.3 for an outline of more common syndromes.
- A full classification and description of terminology may be found at:
  ⌁ http://www.ilae-epilepsy.org/Visitors/Centre/ctf/index.cfm

Box 3b.2 ILAE classification 2001

- Axis 1: is it an epileptic seizure?
- Axis 2: what type of epileptic seizure?
- Axis 3: epilepsy syndrome
- Axis 4: underlying aetiology
- Axis 5: are there any additional impairments?

Box 3b.3 Some epilepsy syndromes in childhood

Infancy

- Early myoclonic encephalopathy.
- Early myoclonic epileptic encephalopathy (Ohtahara).
- Migrating partial seizures of infancy.
- West syndrome.
- Severe myoclonic epilepsy of infancy.
- Symptomatic focal epilepsy.

Mid childhood

- Childhood absence epilepsy.
- Benign epilepsy with centrotemporal spikes.
- Panayiotopoulos syndrome.
- Myoclonic astatic epilepsy.
- Landau–Kleffner syndrome/continous spike wave of slow sleep.
- Lennox–Gastaut syndrome.
- Symptomatic focal epilepsy.

Seizures in neonates—younger than 1 month

- Incidence 0.7–2.7/1000 term infants (58–132/1000 preterm).
- Seizures in the neonatal period may take many forms including clonic, myoclonic, and tonic, but more subtle seizures (e.g. suckling, blinking, small finger movements) account for at least 50%.
- Many movements may occur that are not epileptiform in origin, e.g. benign neonatal sleep myoclonus.
- More commonly overt seizures are only a fraction of the true seizure load: electrographic seizures (seizures seen on the EEG) can also occur.
- The most common aetiology in neonatal seizures is *hypoxic ischaemic encephalopathy*, accounting for 30–53%. Other causes include:
  - Cerebral haemorrhage/infarction (15–30%).
  - Cerebral malformations (3–17%).
  - Meningitis (2–14%)
  - Metabolic (8–30%).
  - Maternal drug withdrawal.
- Epilepsy syndromes with onset in the neonatal period account for a very small number (<1%).
- *Benign idiopathic neonatal convulsions* are rare but occur, so called 5th day fits. Typically onset is at age 4–6 days; seizures include clonic seizures with or without apnoea. Although they may require treatment, duration is short (days, weeks, perhaps months). Prognosis for seizure control and development is extremely good.
- *Investigation* of a neonate presenting with seizures should include glucose, electrolytes, lumbar puncture, cranial ultrasound (and further detailed imaging as required), virology, and metabolic screen.
- *Treatment options* in the neonatal period remain limited, and data as to effective medication scant. Phenobarbital and phenytoin remain the drugs of choice when treatment is administered intravenously.
- *All children presenting seizures within the first year of life should have a trial course of pyridoxine*, up to 50/kg per day for up to 2 weeks, looking for pyridoxine dependency. If response is shown, then further assessment including urinalysis and mutation assessment should be sought.

Seizures in infants—age 1 month to 1 year

- It is unusual in infancy to encounter truly generalized seizures.
- Description of episodes is vital to the diagnosis.
- It must be remembered that the differential diagnosis is wide.[1]
- There are certain seizure types—such as spasms—that are specific to this particular age group and likely to be related to brain maturation.
- Unfortunately, apart from febrile seizures, there are few syndromes presenting in this age group with good prognosis with regard to seizure control or developmental outcome.

Febrile seizures

Febrile convulsions are included within the ILAE classification.[2] They are extremely common but in the majority of cases are single and of no major implications.

- Convulsions occur in the presence of fever, at least 38°C.
- Can occur up to 5 years of age but the majority occur below 2 years.
- 70% are what would be defined as simple febrile convulsions (generalized, <10min duration, no recurrence within 24 hours or in the same febrile illness)
- 30% are defined as complex febrile convulsions (focal features, >10min duration, two or more within 24 hours or in the same febrile illness).
- If there is an obvious source of infection and the child rapidly recovers, no investigations are needed. If there is no obvious source, a septic screen should be considered, including lumbar puncture in children <12 months.
- Risk factors for recurrence include age (50% chance recurrence if first seizure <12 months, 20% if >36 months), family history, duration of illness (higher risk if shorter duration of fever), and temperature at time of seizure (higher risk if lower temperature).
- Risk factors for development of epilepsy include abnormal neurological or developmental status prior to the first febrile seizure, family history of afebrile seizures or complex febrile seizures. Some epilepsy syndromes present with febrile seizures as first manifestation (e.g. Dravet's syndrome, GEFS+).
- Most children who have febrile seizures do not require chronic treatment with medicines.
- Management is to cool, and advice about keeping cool should temperature occur. If recurrent (especially if prolonged) supply of rescue medication (benzodiazepine) may be considered with protocol for use. There is no role for prophylactic anticonvulsant medication in the prevention of recurrent febrile seizures.
- The vast majority of children with febrile seizures do not have seizures without fever after age 5 years. Risk factors for later epilepsy include:
  - *Abnormal development* before the febrile seizure.
  - *Complex febrile seizures*: these are defined as seizures that last >10min, more than one seizure in 24 hours, or seizures in which only one side of the body is affected.
  - Seizures without fever in a parent or a brother or sister.

Children with one of these risk factors have a 2.5% chance of later epilepsy. Those with two or three risk factors have a risk of later epilepsy that ranges from 5% (1 in 20) to >10%.

West syndrome

- Initially described as the presence of the following triad:
  - Infantile spasms.
  - Hypsarrhythmia on EEG.
  - Developmental delay.
- Patients present with *infantile spasms* at 3–6 month of age. Infantile spasms typically involve sudden flexion of trunk with abduction of arms in front of the head (*Salaam* or *jackknife attacks*). They may be restricted to head flexion (nodding spasms).
- Flexor generalized myoclonic jerks can also be present.
- Spasms show short duration and occur in clusters, typically on waking.
- Children show developmental plateau at time of presentation.
- The EEG shows an abnormality termed *hypsarrhythmia* which consists of high amplitude chaotic background activity and superimposed multifocal spike and slow waves. The presence of hypsarrhythmia is necessary for the diagnosis of West syndrome.
- This is the most common form of epileptic encephalopathy, where it is presumed that the associated developmental compromise is related to ongoing epileptic activity and is therefore potentially reversible.
- Treatment of infantile spasms is with vigabatrin or steroids according to local protocol.
- There is some evidence that early prompt treatment is related to better developmental outcome.
- Prognosis remains poor:
  - 85% likely to have long-term developmental compromise, and
  - 60% ongoing seizures
- The range of causes is wide, including structural brain malformations, vascular lesions, and metabolic disease. Nevertheless, the underlying diagnosis is obtained in only 60% of patients.
- A very small proportion may be idiopathic and have good outcome, particularly in the presence of:
  - Normal development until the onset of the attacks.
  - Normal neurological and neuroradiological examination.
  - No evidence of a trigger for the spasms.

Severe myoclonic epilepsy of infancy (Dravet's syndrome)

- Described by Charlotte Dravet in 1978.
- This syndrome is usually heralded by prolonged febrile seizures, often lateralized, in the first year of life.
- Prone to recurrent status epilepticus, especially over first 5 years of life.
- During the second year patients develop myoclonic jerks, and other seizure types.
- Plateauing of development seen in second year.
- Early inter-ictal EEG recordings are typically normal although photic stimulation may be positive in up to 40%. Later EEGs show generalized discharges of fast spike wave or polyspike wave complexes, as well as focal or multifocal spikes.

- Also classified as 'epileptic encephalopathy'—possible evidence that control of seizures and reduced status epilepticus result in better developmental outcome.
- Prognosis remains poor however for both seizure control and developmental outcome.
- Up to 70% associated with mutation in *SCN1A* gene, usually sporadic.
- The variety named borderline severe myoclonic epilepsy of infancy (SMEB) refers to patients lacking some of the typical features such as myoclonic seizures.

Epileptic encephalopathies

By definition this is a group of disorders whereby ongoing epilepstic activity and/or seizures are responsible for developmental compromise. Therefore, the premise is the effects are potentially reversible. In the 2001 ILAE classification, the epileptic encephalopathies are listed as a specific group of syndromes. In this group of syndromes, developmental progress is initially normal but plateaus or regresses with the onset of the epilepsy. It appears likely that the aetiology to such developmental problems is likely to be multifactorial, of which the epilepsy will play a part. Further, the possibility of an epileptic encephalopathy remains in any of the early onset childhood epilepsis where epileptic activity may be interfering with cognitive function.

Epilepsis classed as Epileptic Encephalopathies (ILAE 2001)

- Early myoclonic encephalopathy (EME).
- Ohtahara Syndrome.
- West Syndrome.
- Dravet Syndrome (Severe Myoclonic Epilepsy of Infancy) (SMEI).
- Lennox Gastaut Syndrome (LGS, p.137).
- Myoclonic status in nonprogressive encephalopathies.
- Landau Kleffner Syndrome (LKS, p.138).
- Epilepsy with continuous spike waves during slow sleep (CSWS, p.138).

What and when to investigate when seizures present in infants and early childhood?

- All children presenting with epileptic seizures should undergo an EEG.
- All children presenting with seizures <2 years should undergo MRI of the brain.
- Seizure disorders presenting in the first year of life are more likely to be a manifestation of underlying genetic or metabolic disorder than at a later age. Children presenting in this age group should therefore undergo full investigation including liver function tests, copper, caeruloplasmin, plasma amino acids, urinary amino acids and organic acids, calcium, urate, and karyotype.
- Requirements for other investigations will depend on the associated features at presentation and clinical course.

- The key to a decision about further investigation will depend on clinical assessment. Often there is ongoing discussion as to whether a child may have shown neurological regression. Assessment will be required as to whether any cognitive deterioration is related to the epilepsy, and therefore potentially reversible, or results from underlying neurodegenerative disease. Targeted investigations are required if the latter is suspected.

References

1. ⊞ www.nice.org.uk/guidance/CG20, Appendix A.

2. ILAE website: ⟨⊕ www.ilae.org

Seizures in childhood (1–12 years)

- Epilepsies presenting in older childhood are wider in their range of presentation and prognosis.
- Idiopathic focal epilepsies are probably the most common.

Benign occipital epilepsy

- Benign occipital epilepsy probably has two forms:
- **Early onset** (also called *Panayiotopoulos syndrome*): often presents with a single episode (may be status epilepticus) where autonomic features predominate: vacant look, colour change, vomiting. EEG in 40% may show posterior spike-wave on eye closure (fixation off sensitivity). This epilepsy will respond promptly to treatment, but whether treatment is required may depend on frequency of episodes (if indeed recurrent). Many may go undiagnosed. The majority of patients grow out of the tendency to have seizures. Seizures are often relatively long, lasting for longer than 5 minutes.
- **Late onset** (of *Gastaut*) is less common and has more visual symptomatology during the seizures. The children may be able to give a vivid description of this or even draw the visual symptomatology. Seizures may secondarily generalize and post-ictal headache is common. Seizures are shorter, usually lasting <5min.

Benign epilepsy with centrotemporal spikes

- This is the most common syndrome in children.
- Children typically present between 5–10 years with unilateral perioral/focal motor seizures occurring from sleep, although 24–80% of seizures secondarily generalize.
- EEG will show the typical features of centrotemporal (Sylvian) spikes that may be enhanced by sleep.
- Whether treatment is required depends on several factors including frequency of episodes and how the child and family feel about their recurrence. Seizures usually respond promptly to carbamazepine or sultiame. Children will grow out of the tendency to suffer seizures by 14 years of age.

Idiopathic generalized epilepsies

- In younger children (5–10 years) the commonest manifestation is absence attacks associated with 3Hz spike wave activity on EEG as part of childhood absence epilepsy (CAE). Generalized tonic–clonic seizures may also occur, and when present the epilepsy is less likely to remit. The biggest differential diagnosis is with simple day dreaming: in CAE absence attacks are usually provoked by hyperventilation and are associated with 3Hz spike-wave activity on the EEG.
- In older children, IGE may present with absence attacks (with or without tonic–clonic seizures) associated with slightly faster spike wave activity on EEG (4–5Hz) as part of JAE, or this may be the first manifestation of JME (where myoclonus may not manifest until teenage years).
- Earlier onset CAE is most likely to respond to broad spectrum agents such as sodium valproate, ethosuximide, or lamotrigine. Children have

a 70% chance of spontaneous remission. Later onset IGE (e.g. JAE, JME) is likely to respond promptly to AEDs but unlikely to remit.

Symptomatic focal epilepsies

- Symptomatic focal epilepsies may present at any age.
- Children present with focal seizures, the semiology of which will depend on the origin of the seizures (📖 see Types of epileptic seizures, pp.61–73). Seizures arise from a structurally abnormal area of the brain.
- The most common causes in children include
  - Focal cortical dysplasia.
  - Benign tumours.
  - Ischaemic damage—e.g. stroke.
  - Mesial temporal sclerosis.
- The epilepsy may prove resistant to medication and should be referred early for consideration of surgery, particularly in children <5 years where their epilepsy may be part of an epileptic encephalopathy.

Myoclonic-astatic epilepsy

- This is a syndrome presenting in a similar age range to Lennox–Gastaut syndrome which previously may have been included within this group. However myoclonus is by far a more prominent feature and prognosis for cognitive outcome is better.
- These children present typically between 2–6 years.
- Generalized jerks with astatic (atonic) falls may happen several times daily. Falls may be the result of atonic seizures, myoclonic jerks or so called myoclonic-astatic seizures.
- EEG shows bursts of spike wave complexes or polyspike waves at 2–4Hz. EMG shows that muscle contraction responsible for jerks is often followed by a brief period of EMG silence.
- Long-term outcome is highly variable but cannot be predicted from age, antecedents, or clinical presentation at onset.
- Medication of choice include: sodium valproate, ethosuximide, levetiracetam, and the ketogenic diet.

Lennox–Gastaut syndrome

- Children present between 3–7 years with multiple seizure types including atypical absences, tonic seizures, myoclonic jerks.
- This is another epileptic encephalopathy where development may plateau at seizure presentation.
- Some (30%) have a history of infantile spasms in the first year of life.
- The diagnosis is based on a clinical triad of drop attacks, atypical absence, and tonic seizures with an EEG showing slow spike and wave and fast rhythms in sleep.
- Medications of choice include sodium valproate, lamotrigine, topiramate, levetiracetam, rufinamide. However seizures may well be resistant and wider issues need to be addressed such as the associated cognitive and behavioural compromise.

Landau–Kleffner syndrome and epilepsy with continuous spike-and-waves during slow-wave sleep

- These are further examples of epileptic encephalopathies where disturbances of cognition, behaviour and motor control occur with epilepsy and are attributed to epileptiform activity which is often subclinical.
- *Landau–Kleffner syndrome* is by definition 'acquired epileptic aphasia'. Children present with a regression in language skills, with or without a history of epilepsy, after a period of normal language development. The EEG abnormalities consist of slow waves, spikes and spike-wave complexes in the centro-temporo-parietal region which become generalized during sleep; in some it is associated with continuous electrical status epilepticus of slow sleep.
- *Epilepsy with continuous spike-and-waves during slow-wave sleep* is defined as the association of various seizure types, partial or generalized occurring during sleep and atypical absences when awake, with a characteristic EEG pattern consisting of continuous diffuse spike-and-wave complexes during slow wave sleep (during at least 85% of slow wave sleep), which is noted after the onset of seizures. Some children present with a regression of language, after onset of seizures and therefore classic Landau–Kleffner syndrome. Others may have changes in cognitive performance, varying from the severe to the subtle. In children where there is a history of regression of cognitive or language skills, sleep EEG recording must be performed. Treatment is targeted at seizures, although this may be one of the few indications where we attempt to treat the EEG abnormality. Specific response may be seen to steroids and/or benzodiazepines.

Rasmussen's syndrome

- First described by Theodore Rasmussen, a Canadian neurosurgeon, who observed that in certain children undergoing hemispherectomy for the treatment of epilepsy, pathology showed findings suggestive of chronic encephalitis.
- The syndrome is now well described involving progressive unilateral focal motor seizures, progressive hemiparesis, and cognitive decline. Progressive cerebral hemiatrophy of the hemisphere contralateral to motor seizures documented on MRI is highly suggestive of the diagnosis. Children usually present between 5–10 years with focal motor seizures that become increasingly drug resistant. Epilepsia partialis continua (🕮 see Seizures in special circumstances, pp.492–493) is seen in about 60%; less typical presentations have also been reported.
- Aetiology is unknown although viral encephalitis or an autoimmune process is suspected.
- Ultimate cure with cessation of seizures can only be achieved with hemispherectomy, with functional compromise (hemiparesis and hemivisual field defect). Timing of surgery requires careful consideration and therefore early referral to a specialist unit is imperative if the diagnosis is suspected.

NICE guidelines for children
- The NICE guidelines are written as guidance for the diagnosis and management of children with epilepsy in primary and secondary care.
- The key points are:
  - Children following a first event should be reviewed within 2 weeks.
  - A diagnosis of epilepsy should be made by a paediatrician with expertise in epilepsy.
  - A decision about treatment should be made jointly with the family, and be considered after two epileptic seizures.
  - If a scan is required this should be an MRI scan and performed within 4 weeks of request.
- Summary and full guidelines can be found at: 🖳 www.nice.org.uk/guidance/CG20

Seizures in adolescence and young adulthood

Two main diagnostic considerations are:
- Is the epilepsy generalized or partial?
- Is the epilepsy idiopathic or symptomatic?

Idiopathic generalized epilepsy (IGE)

- Although IGE usually presents in childhood and adolescence, it can present in adulthood.
- Some syndromes are listed in 🕮 Epilepsy syndromes—summary of characteristics, pp.104–121, in this chapter, along with the main clinical features.
- A syndromic diagnosis can be very helpful in relation to treatment and prognosis
- Not all patients fit neatly into a syndromic classification and there is overlap between syndromes.
- Imaging is normal and there is no pre-existing neurological disease or deficit, non significant cognitive impairment.
- Generalized epileptiform discharges (generalized spike(s) wave) on EEG is the hallmark of IGE. This may occur spontaneously in a routine awake EEG or with hyperventilation. Sleep EEG, particularly after sleep deprivation, increases the likelihood of observing generalized discharges during sleep or on awakening. A photoparoxysmal response may be observed. Focal discharges and fragments of generalized discharges also occur. The background rhythm is usually normal.

It is important to make the diagnosis of IGE in view of the implications to treatment (🕮 see Choosing an AED in IGE, p. 270). Electroencephalography is invaluable here, and it is recommended that this is requested early in this age group. If negative, the EEG should be repeated with sleep, preferably following sleep deprivation, although patients would need to be warned of the small likelihood of triggering clinical seizures. Treatment with some drugs such as valproate can normalize the EEG and reduce the likelihood of observing generalized discharges.

Main seizure types

GTCS

These occur from the waking state or from sleep. In a small proportion of IGE cases, the vast majority of convulsions occur within an hour of waking. GTCS in IGE are usually symmetrical in terms of motor features. Asymmetry does not exclude IGE but, where present, focal epilepsy needs to be considered. Specific auras are not usually present, but brief non-specific auras are not infrequent. These often consist of a brief head feeling or rush. Repeated myoclonic jerks may also precede GTCS and should not to be confused with a focal motor onset. There may also be a prodrome of feeling vague or muddled for a variable period. GTCS in IGE are usually brief and self-terminate.

Myoclonic

These are usually proximal affecting the upper limbs but can affect lower limbs or be generalized. They are often but not invariably worse on waking and occur, less commonly, in the afternoon. Their frequency is variable. In many they occur independently of GTCS, but in a minority they precede them. Some patients report them as arising from sleep. If purely nocturnal, it maybe difficult to differentiate between them and normal sleep-related myoclonus on history alone without EEG / surface EMG / video recording. The EEG recorded during myoclonic seizures in IGE usually shows a spike or polyspike and wave generalized discharge intermixed with a substantial amount of muscle artefact. Other myoclonic patterns in IGE include eyelid myoclonia with absences, head nods in myoclonic-astatic epilepsy, perioral myoclonia and myoclonic absences. These usually have a younger age at presentation and are discussed elsewhere. They often persist to adulthood. Jaw myoclonus also occurs in reading epilepsy, the classification of which as partial or generalized is debated.

Absences

There is a misconception that true absences do not occur beyond childhood. This is untrue. Childhood absences can persist to adulthood and discrete absences can and do present in adulthood but are more likely during teenage years. They are usually spanioleptic (rare) and not pyknoleptic (very frequent) as in CAE. These may occur in a daily pattern of a few absences only. Alternatively, they may occur intermittently, with many per day. Absences can also be subtle and may not be as obvious to the observer as childhood absences. The person affected may complain of 'foggy' periods or days with poor memory or concentration, or of days of feeling vulnerable, and more at risk of having seizures. In some women such days are more likely around their period.

Sometimes, it is difficult or impossible to count absences. A witness is helpful in establishing if there are discrete events. EEG video recording may demonstrate clinical change during epileptiform discharges. So-called phantom absences refer to clinical absences recorded on EEG without there being a prior history of absences, the patient having been referred, most commonly, following GTCS. Absences are usually brief. They can be exacerbated by inappropriate medication. Where prolonged they can be mistaken for CPS. Non-lateralizing automatisms can occur with more prolonged absences but onset and offset are usually clearer than with CPS. There is no substitute to an ictal video EEG for demonstrating absences, but a careful history is also very helpful. During typical absence seizures, the EEG shows generalized spike and wave activity at 3–4Hz.

Known triggers of seizures in IGE

- Alcohol, sleep deprivation, stress, excitement, menstruation, and photic stimulation are all well recognized triggers.
- Although pure photosensitive epilepsy is uncommon, photic-triggered seizures are well recognized in IGE in general with a photoparoxysmal response on EEG seen in up to one third of cases depending on the syndrome. 📖 see Epilepsy with GTCS, p.121.

- Some medications generally lower seizure threshold and may precipitate seizures in those susceptible. Examples include certain anti-malarial, anti-psychotic, and antidepressant drugs.

Previous history

There may be a history of febrile seizures, usually simple, in about 10% of IGE cases. There may also be a history of CAE with remission with a family history of febrile seizures or epilepsy. Sometimes a recent history of closed mild head injury is reported, the significance of which is uncertain.

Focal epilepsies

These are discussed in the following section.

Seizures in the adult

General guidelines

- Most idiopathic syndromes (focal or generalized) start by early adulthood. Some patients with autosomal dominant nocturnal frontal lobe epilepsy are an exception to this rule. Idiopathic syndromes starting in adolescence and early adulthood have been described in the previous section.
- Some idiopathic syndromes (e.g., JME, JAE) persist into adulthood.
- Symptomatic (and presumed symptomatic) generalized epilepsies tend to start before adulthood and seizures persist into adulthood.
- Most epilepsies starting in adulthood are focal symptomatic (or focal presumed symptomatic).
- Some focal symptomatic epilepsies with onset of seizures during adulthood can be due to an earlier cause occurring before adulthood (for instance, focal cortical dysplasia, mesial temporal epilepsy, benign tumours, arteriovenous malformations) or to acquired lesions.

Most common causes of seizures starting in young adulthood—excluding idiopathic epilepsies and acute symptomatic seizures

- Mesial temporal sclerosis (Box 3b.4).
- Head injury.
- Tumours and hamartomas.
- Focal cortical dysplasia.
- DNET.
- Vascular malformations: arteriovenous malformations and cavernous angiomas.

Temporal lobe epilepsy

- Approximately 60% of symptomatic focal epilepsies.
- Seizures last for 2–10min, sometimes more—excluding post-ictal symptoms.
- It can be associated with material-specific mild memory impairment: in verbal memory if arising from the dominant hemisphere for language and in visuospatial memory if arising from the non-dominant hemisphere.
- It is debated if temporal lobe epilepsy is associated with particular personality (humour, obsessiveness, hyperemotionality, hyposexuality, hypergraphia, hyper-religiosity).
- Epilepsy arising from *medial temporal structures* (hippocampal or mesiobasal epilepsy) is the most common type of temporal lobe epilepsy, where:
  - Mesial temporal sclerosis is the most common cause followed by tumours, arteriovenous malformations, and focal cortical dysplasia. Mesial temporal sclerosis tends to be unilateral but can be bilateral.
  - Seizure types include: simple partial, complex partial and/or secondarily generalized seizures.
  - *Simple partial seizures*: the most common sensation during simple partial seizures (aura) is a *rising epigastric (abdominal-chest) sensation*. Other common auras consist of olfactory and gustatory

sensations, autonomic symptoms (flushing, pallor, tachycardia, changes in BP, piloerection, pupillary dilatation), affective symptoms (intense fear being the most common, but depression, anger or irritability, euphoria, and erotic thoughts can also occur) or memory symptoms (particularly *déjà vu*, less commonly *déjà entendu*). Olfactory auras are intense and usually unpleasant (for instance, a putrid smell) and are typically seen in seizures arising from Sylvian and temporal areas. Cephalic symptoms (strange feelings in the head, headache, dizziness), dreamy states and feelings of depersonalization can also occur more rarely.

- *Complex partial seizures:* these may or may not be preceded by an aura consisting of the symptoms described for simple partial seizures lasting a few seconds. There is motor arrest and staring for several seconds and this can be followed by automatisms: oro-alimentary automatisms (lip smacking and licking, chewing), fiddling and fumbling with objects, fidgeting, restlessness, undressing, walking. If unilateral, automatisms tend to be ipsilateral to seizure onset. Automatisms can coexist with a mild contralateral dystonic posture. Vocalization (automatic uttering of words) can occur in seizures starting in the non-dominant hemisphere.
- *Secondarily generalized seizures:* tonic–clonic convulsions occurring from seizure onset, or after a period of simple or complex partial symptoms.
- *Post-ictal symptoms to both complex partial and secondarily generalized seizures:* often longer than in other seizure types, lasting for several minutes to hours. Confusion, headache, and sleepiness are the most common post-ictal symptoms. Post-ictal dysphasia is said to occur in seizures arising from the dominant hemisphere. Post-ictal psychosis can occur, typically with paranoid features, auditory and visual hallucinations. Depression and hypomania have been described in seizures arising from the right temporal lobe.
- The *inter-ictal EEG* can be normal, or it might show temporal slowing and/or unilateral or bilateral independent temporal epileptiform discharges, usually of maximal amplitude at the anterior or mid temporal electrodes.
- The *ictal scalp EEG* might show a focal temporal onset, or a diffuse onset.
- In epilepsy arising from *lateral temporal structures:*
  - A non-atrophic structural lesion is more commonly found than in epilepsy arising from medial temporal structures: glioma, angioma, post-traumatic scarring, focal cortical dysplasia, DNET, hamartoma.
  - Seizures from medial and lateral temporal origin often show similar characteristics, possibly because of rapid propagation. Nevertheless, seizures arising from lateral temporal structures commonly show the following features:
    —consciousness is preserved for longer than in epilepsy arising from medial temporal structures.
    —auras also include: structured visual and auditory hallucinations (including hearing melodies, sentences, micropsia, or macropsia).
    —affective and psychic auras are less common.

—sometimes vertigo occurs as an aura in seizures arising from the posterior portion of the superior temporal gyrus.
  • The inter-ictal EEG often can show epileptiform discharges with maximal amplitude at the Sylvian, mid temporal, and posterior temporal electrodes.
• The term *dual temporal pathology* refers to the presence of hippocampal sclerosis and an extra-hippocampal lesion in the same patient. Dual pathology can be observed in as much as 20–30% of temporal lobes resected for surgical treatment. Extrahippocampal lesions tend to be tumours, developmental cysts, or trauma.

Box 3b.4 The syndrome of mesial temporal epilepsy

• The most common cause of temporal lobe epilepsy in adults.
• >30% of patients have a history of complex febrile seizures. It is unclear whether the febrile seizures may be the cause of epilepsy or a co-effect from a common cause.
• Mesiobasal seizures.
• Onset of seizures in the second or third decade.
• Mesial temporal sclerosis on MRI:
  • Decreased hippocampal volume (atrophy) and destruction of the anatomical structure of the hippocampus.
  • Increased hippocampal signal on t2 weighted imaging.
  • Increased volume of the temporal horn of the lateral ventricle.
  • There might be *mild* atrophy of all the affected temporal lobe or in extreme cases of the whole hemisphere.
• The inter-ictal EEG can be normal, or it might show temporal slowing, and/or unilateral or bilateral independent temporal epileptiform discharges, usually of maximal amplitude at the anterior or mid temporal electrodes.
• The ictal scalp EEG might show a focal temporal onset, or a diffuse onset.
• Examination might be normal or show a slight facial asymmetry.
• Pathology shows loss of hippocampal neurons, disruption of the hipocampal structure and hippocampal gliosis.
• Seizures may or may not be controlled by AEDs.
• Good response to surgical removal of the temporal lobe: 90% of operated patients improve significantly and 60–70% become seizure free.
• Mesial temporal sclerosis tends to be unilateral but can be bilateral.
• Dual pathology can be present.

Frontal lobe epilepsy

Suggestive features

• Simple partial motor seizures.
• Brief seizures (<1min).
• Frequent seizures, often in clusturs.
• Nocturnal predominance.
• Bizarre automatisms, thrashing, kicking, clapping, bicycling.

- Dystonic posture from onset.
- Forced eye deviation from onset—contralateral to the side of seizure onset.
- Consciousness may be preserved during convulsions, but usually isn't.
- 'Frontal absences' or blank spells.
- EEG can be normal, even ictal.
- When EEG abnormalities are present, they may be:
  - Superior frontal.
  - Prefrontal.
  - Bifrontal.
  - Midfrontal—SMA (Supplementary Motor Aura).
  - Generalized discharges—55%.
- Propensity to status epilepticus.

Frontal complex-partial seizures
- Nocturnal preponderance.
- Brief, little post-ictal confusion, with sudden, frenetic, frantic, agitated and dramatic automatism, bimanual-bipedal.
- Vocalization is common—humming or shouting obscenities.
- Non-specific auras if any.
- Can arise from any region of the frontal lobe.
- Inter-ictal and ictal EEGs are often unrevealing.

Anatomical classification
- Primary motor area—precentral.
- Supplementary motor area.
- Dorsolateral.
- Frontopolar.
- Orbital.

Pre-central seizures
- Focal motor seizures: clonic, tonic–clonic, myoclonic convulsions involving mainly the hand and face, particularly the corner of the mouth.
- Often simple partial.
- Rarely Jacksonian march.
- Rolandic spikes.
- Frequency—18–25% of frontal lobe epilepsy.

Seizures from supplementary motor area
- Clusters of brief, unilateral or bilateral, symmetrical or asymmetrical tonic convulsions.
- Extension and abduction of one arm with rotation of head to the same side and flexion of the other arm—fencing posture.
- Often preserved consciousness.
- Somatosensory auras in 45%
- Frontal automatisms.
- EEG abnormalities:
  - Brief, frequent, frequent bursts of fast activity.
  - Midline fast activity or spikes.
  - Generalized discharges.

Dorsolateral frontal seizures
- Forced thinking.
- Complex visual illusions—abstract, intellectual.
- Cephalic aura in 38%.
- Loss of consciousness.
- Tonic eye and head deviation—contralateral to the side of seizure onset.
- Tonic posture—often bilateral and asymmetrical.
- Bipedal automatisms, clapping, vocalization, laughter.
- Superior frontal or bifrontal EEG abnormalities.

Frontpolar seizures
- Most often due to trauma.
- Loss of contact.
- Fixed gaze.
- Loss of tone and fall followed by tonic–clonic convulsions.

Orbital/medial frontal seizures
- Olfactory hallucinations.
- Loss of consciousness and automatisms.
- May resemble temporal lobe seizures.
- No early oroalimentary automatisms.
- Automatisms involve limbs, often violent, kicking, thrashing, sexual, vocalization.
- Brief, repetitive, often in clusters.
- Sometimes aura of fear.

Pathological abnormalities in symptomatic frontal lobe epilepsy
- Trauma—frontopolar.
- Neoplasms:
  - Low grade astrocytomas.
  - Oligodendrogliomas.
- Vascular malformations:
  - Arteriovenous malformations.
  - Cavernous angiomas.
- Developmental lesions:
  - Focal cortical dysplasia—pericentral.
  - Hamartomas.

Inter-ictal EEG
- Focal epileptiform discharges or slowing depending on the site of origin:
  - At Fz in medial frontal epilepsy.
  - At F3/F4 in lateral frontal epilepsy.
  - At F8/F7 and prefrontal electrodes in orbital frontal epilepsy.
- Sometimes secondarily generalized discharges, particularly in epilepsies arising from medial frontal cortex.

Ictal EEG
- Often normal—as often as 58%.
- Unilateral or bifrontal slowing—need to be differentiated from eye movement artefacts.
- Abnormalities according to location.

Autosomal dominant (ADFLE)frontal lobe epilepsy

- Initially 5 families, 45 affected, linked to chromosome 20q.[1] Now known to be caused by mutations in CHRNA4, CHRNB2 and CHRN2.
- Clusters of nocturnal brief motor seizures: tonic stiffening, clonic jerking, vocalization, thrashing, consciousness often retained.
- Somatosensory auras, fear, déjà vu, autonomic sensations in 70%.
- Start at any age, mostly in childhood.
- Normal examination and imaging.
- Inter-ictal EEG: discharges only in 16%—bilateral discharges.
- Ictal EEG: normal or bifrontal discharges.
- Previous name: nocturnal paroxysmal dystonia.
- Treatment of choice: carbamazepine.

Epilepsia partialis continua

- Partial clonic motor status epilepticus: mainly face and hand.
- Kojevnikov syndrome (1895): epidemic, spring-summer, tic-borne, epilepsy several months after a febrile illness.
- Other causes: encephalitis (particularly Rasmussen's), neoplasms, cortical dysplasia (particularly hemimegalencephaly), infections, vascular lesions (stroke, haemorrhage, malformations), trauma, HHE, metabolic and mitochondrial disorders, iatrogenic (penicillin).
- EEG: focal central or fronto-central spikes, not always clearly correlated with jerks (?need to back average).
- Treatment: pharmacoresistant.

Parietal lobe epilepsy

General characteristics

- Uncommon: <5% surgical series.
- Auras in 94%: mainly somatosensory (numbness, tingling), also pain (burning, abdominal, and headache), disturbance of body image, sexual sensations, visual illusions, vertigo (temporo-parietal junction), aphasia, gustatory hallucinations (operculum), retching (insula).
- Less common auras: elementary visual illusions, auditory hallucinations, cephalic sensations, conscious confusion.
- Motor phenomena: focal motor clonus (57%), head and eye deviation (41%), tonic posturing (28%).
- Less common symptoms: oral and gestural automatisms (17%), complex automatisms (4%), postictal dysphasia (7%), Todd´s paralysis (22).
- Symptoms often reflect spread to other lobes.

Pathological abnormalities in symptomatic parietal lobe epilepsy

- Neoplasms: the most common.
- Vascular malformations.
- Hamartomas.
- Cortical dysplasia (postcentral)
- Granulomas.
- Porencephalic cysts.
- Old cerebral infarcts.

Occipital lobe epilepsy

Clinical manifestations
- Considered rare: 8% of some surgical series.
- Visual positive signs: 47–73%:
  - Simple: contralateral spots, geometrical forms, black or coloured.
  - Complex hallucinations (14–20%): ?limbic involvement.
- Unilateral (contralateral) or bilateral ictal blindness (amaurosis): up to 40%. Can produce permanent blindness.
- Status epilepticus amauroticus.
- Forced blinking or eyelid flutter.
- Contralateral tonic–clonic eye deviation and nystagmus: medial occipital involvement. Sometimes ipsilateral.
- Spread: temporal lobe automatisms (29–88%) and focal motor symptoms (38–47%).
- Blinking (17%).

Pathological abnormalities in symptomatic occipital lobe epilepsy
- Unknown (25%).
- Tumours.
- Head injury
- Vascular lesions.
- Birth injury with anoxia.
- Focal cortical dysplasia.
- Sturge–Weber, coeliac disease with occipital calcifications.
- Meningitis, encephalitis.
- Porencephalic lesions.
- MELAS.

References

1. Scheffer IE, Bhatia KP, Lopes-Cendes I, *et al.* (1995). Autosomal dominant nocturnal frontal lobe epilepsy. A distinctive clinical disorder. *Brain*, **118**, 1–73.

Seizures in the elderly[1,2]

- In the UK, 25% of people with epilepsy are >60 years.
- Epilepsy increases above the age of 50 associated with imaging evidence of *cerebrovascular disease*—which is considered by some authors as the most common cause of epilepsy in all age groups.
- *The incidence of epilepsy increases with age*:
  - Incidence in the general population: 69/100,000.
  - Incidence among people age 65–69: 87/100,000.
  - Incidence among people age 70–80: 147/10,000.
- *Epilepsy in the elderly will become a more important problem* as population ages.
- The *general principles* for diagnosis and management are similar to those for younger population.
- *Special attention* should be paid to:
  - Interaction with other medication.
  - Low protein levels: nutrition, liver or kidney impairment, free drug levels more informative.
  - Impairment of memory; simplify medication, use dosette boxes.
  - Effects of AEDs on bone metabolism.
  - Decreased creatinine clearance.
- *The elderly are often taking multiple medication*:
  - Pharmacological interactions between AEDs and other medication can occur.
  - Some common medication, such as antidepressants, might be proconvulsants.
- *Lower metabolic rate:* more susceptible to dose-related effects. For instance, sodium valproate can induce more pronounced tremor resembling parkinsonian symptoms.
- *Low protein levels* when concomitant liver and kidney conditions. Importance of determination of AED free levels!
- *Memory impairment:* simplify medication.

Impact of seizures in old age

- Longer seizures.
- Increased probability of status, particularly non-convulsive.
- Increased probability of fractures due to osteoporosis and/or falls. Often followed by decline in independence.
- Fear of further falls and fear of further fits.

Diagnosis of seizures in old age

- Difficult to differentiate from syncope, cerebrovascular disease, cardiac disease, dementia, confusion, hypoglycemia, vertigo, and dizziness.
- Problems in history taking as many old people live alone and sometimes have many iimpairment.
- To distinguish from syncope the speed of recovery is useful but it is often difficult as recovery can be slower in this age group.
- Syncope may be associated with incontinence, particularly in old age.
- Non-specific abnormalities are common in the EEG in old age.

Causes of seizures in old age
- Symptomatic cerebrovascular disease, particularly haemorrhage (more than infarct). Seizures may be the first manifestation of cerebrovascular disease: screening and prevention with aspirin.
- Associated with asymptomatic imaging evidence of cerebrovascular disease.
- Head injury (21%).
- Incidence of tumours is low (5–15%).
- Metabolic causes (10%): alcoholism, fever, pneumonia.
- Degenerative disorders: Alzheimer's and other dementias.

Investigation of epilepsy in the elderly
- FBC, erythrocyte sedimentation rate, urea and electrolytes, blood glucose.
- Chest X-ray.
- ECG.
- Gamma-glutamyl-transferase: marker for recent alcohol consumption.
- Thyroid function.
- EEG if performed (not indicated if diagnosis and cause of epilepsy is known):
  • Frequent non-specific abnormalities and slowing.
  • Supports diagnosis if clear epileptiform discharges are seen.
  • Inconclusive in the absence of epileptiform discharges.
  • Crucial for the diagnosis of non-convulsive status epilepticus(NCSE).
- MRI—as epilepsy is usually symptomatic.

Frequently asked questions
In most patients, epilepsy in itself.
- Does not imply serious brain damage.
- Does not imply dementia.
- Can usually be controlled by medication if no progressive disease present.
- Medication does not cause brain damage.

Starting treatment in the elderly
- Lack of studies compared to younger patients.
- Treatment of a single seizure has been recommended if an organic cause is identified.
- Driving considerations.

Choice of drugs in the elderly
This can be difficult as many drugs have problems in the elderly and drug trials are limited, so there is limited evidence base to guide recommendations. Choice of AEDs should be tailored to each individual case. In general, tolerance to AEDs is less and doses needed lower.
There are limited trial data regarding specific use of AEDs in this setting,[3] although some advocate the use of newer AEDs on the grounds of better tolerability. AEDs with no interactions have an advantage. Below are comments regarding a few individual AEDs. Other AEDs may also be used.
Carbamazepine: while this is very useful in younger patients, it is generally not well tolerated in older people. It is subject to drug interactions and has the propensity to precipitate heart block in those susceptible.

It is therefore not first line in this setting. If prescribed, make sure ECG is recorded, start on very low doses (50mg–100mg) and proceed cautiously. Check interactions with concomitant medication.

Phenytoin: we do not favour this as first line as it has difficult pharmacokinetics which complicate use and is subject to interactions. Furthermore, the elderly seem to tolerate less well phenytoin levels within the quoted 'therapeutic range'; if used lower levels can be aimed for in the first instance, which may well be effective. Check interactions with concomitant medication.

Valproate: This is relatively easy to use, but again moderate to high doses may result in drowsiness. It may exacerbate Parkinsonian features or tremor, and where these are present, it is best avoided. Use low starting doses, increasing only if tolerated. Check interactions with concomitant medication.

Lamotrigine: A study comparing carbamazepine with lamotrigine found a higher incidence of adverse events in the former, particularly rash. The study has been criticized for the choice of carbamazepine formulation and titration. Nevertheless the authors' conclusion that lamotrigine 'can be regarded as an acceptable choice as initial treatment for elderly patients with newly diagnosed epilepsy' is reasonable.[4] Another comparative Scandinavian study is reportedly in progress.[3] The Veteran's Administration study discussed below also included lamotrigine.[5] Check interactions with concomitant medication.

Levetiracetam: This has the advantage of low interactions. It can cause irritability and depression. Excretion is renal and doses used lower. Half-life is likely to be increased in the elderly in view of decreased creatinine clearance. We suggest starting doses of 62.5–125mg/day increasing slowly depending on tolerance and response.

Gabapentin: This too has the advantage of low interactions. It was included in the Veteran's Association Cooperative Study 5 comparing 3 treatment groups: gabapentin (GBP) 1,500 mg/day, lamotrigine (LMT) 150 mg/day and carbamazepine (CBZ) 600 mg/day. The results showed high early terminations (LTG 44.2%, GBP 51%, CBZ 64.5% ($p = 0.0002$)) of which, the following were due to adverse events: LTG 12.1%, GBP 21.6%, CBZ 31% ($p = 0.001$) with no significant differences in seizure free rates. The authors concluded that lamotrigine or gabapentin should be considered as initial therapy for older patients with newly diagnosed seizures. Once again, one may question whether doses used in the study were optimal. Many other new AEDs were not tested.

Dosage in the elderly

- Check interactions with concomitant drugs.
- Start with low doses and aim for low target doses in first instance.
- In view of lower protein levels and concomitant disorders, free drug fraction of blood levels is more appropriate, but may not easily be available.

Complications of epilepsy in old age

- Spontaneous and seizure-induced fractures.
- Status epilepticus after withdrawing sleeping pills (benzodiazepines): often non convulsive and difficult to recognize.
- Medication toxicity: poor memory, somnolence, ataxia.
- Complications secondary to drug interactions.

References

1. Clyd, JC, Kelly KM, Leppik IE, Perucca E, Ramsay RE (eds). Epilepsy in the elderly. *New Directions.* **68**(1) pp S1–S83.

2. Sheorajpanday RV, De Deyn PP (2007). Epileptic fits and epilepsy in the elderly: general reflections, specific issues and therapeutic implications. *Clin Neurol Neurosurg* **109**(9):727–43. Department of Neurology, ZNA - Middelheim, Lindendreef 1, 2020 Antwerp, Belgium.

3. Leppik IE, Brodie MJ, Saetre ER, Rowan AJ, Ramsay RE, Macias F, Jacobs MP (2006). Outcomes research: clinical trials in the elderly. *Epilepsy Res.* **68** Suppl 1:S71–6. Epub 2006 Jan 18.

4. Brodie MJ, Overstall PW, Giorgi L (1999). Multicentre, double-blind, randomised comparison between lamotrigine and carbamazepine in elderly patients with newly diagnosed epilepsy. The UK Lamotrigine Elderly Study Group. *Epilepsy Res* **37**(1):81–7.

5. Rowan AJ, Ramsay RE, Collins JF et al. (2005). VA Cooperative Study 428 Group. New onset geriatric epilepsy: a randomized study of gabapentin, lamotrigine, and carbamazepine. *Neurol* **64**(11):1868–73.

Key reading

1. ILAE Task Force on Epilepsy Classification and Terminology. A Proposed Diagnostic Schema for People with Epileptic Seizures and with Epilepsy: Report of the ILAE Task Force on Classification and Terminology. Available at ▣ www.ilae-epilepsy.org/Visitors/Centre/ctf/index.cfm

2. Roger J, Bureau M, Dravet CH, et al. (1992) *Epileptic syndromes in infancy, childhood and adolescence, 2nd* edn. John Libbey, London.

3. Panayiotopoulos CP (2007). A *Clinical Guide to Epileptic Syndromes and their Treatment, 2nd* edn. Springer, London.

4. Scheffer IE and Berkovic SF (1997). Generalized epilepsy with febrile seizures plus. A genetic disorder with heterogeneous clinical phenotypes. *Brain*,**120**, 479–90.

Chapter 3c

Is it epilepsy?

Epileptic seizures without epilepsy

There are a number of acute conditions (intoxication, encephalitis, metabolic problems, etc.) with seizures as part of their symptoms. In most cases, seizures disappear with remission of the underlying condition. This is not considered epilepsy, since the presence of such seizures do not necessarily imply a significantly increased tendency to suffer seizures once the underlying acute condition has resolved. Nevertheless, although this situation is not epilepsy, seizures are identical to those seen in epilepsy, and they are called 'epileptic' seizures.

Synonyms

- Acute symptomatic seizures.
- Reactive seizures.
- Provoked seizures.
- Situation related seizures.
- 'Gelegenheitsanfälle'.

Characteristics of acute symptomatic seizures

- They are epileptic seizures induced by an acute temporary situation.
- They look like epileptic seizures although they are not part of an epileptic syndrome.
- They are often wrongly considered as epilepsy in epidemiological studies.
- They may be treated as epilepsy in the short term, but do not usually require long term treatment because seizures tend to remit when the underlying acute situation ceases. Where the acute situation causes brain damage, epilepsy may later occur.
- Overall prognosis depends on the underlying condition. For instance:
  - Poor prognosis and raised mortality if associated with encephalitis.
  - Good prognosis if associated with drug withdrawal.
- Acute symptomatic seizures may not be seen by neurologists. EEG investigations may not be obtained.
- They are very common, representing perhaps 50–80% of newly occurring seizures

Causes of acute symptomatic seizures

The most common causes of acute symptomatic seizures are:
- Febrile seizures: age specific.
- Traumatic brain injury.
- Cerebrovascular disease.
- Drug withdrawal.
- CNS infections.

According to Annegers et al.[1] the causes and risk factors of acute symptomatic seizures (excluding febrile seizures) are:
- *Cerebrovascular disease* (16%): 5–10% of stroke patients have seizures. Higher risk with haemorrhage and age >55 years.
- *Head injury* (16%): more in men.
- *Infection* (meningitis, encephalitis) (15%): 5% of patients with CNS infections have seizures. Highest incidence in first year of life.
- *Drug withdrawal* (14%): ethanol, less frequently barbiturates, benzodiazepines. Peak at age 35–54 years.

- *Metabolic causes* (9%): highest incidence in first year of age (hypocalcemia, hypoglycemia), slight increase risk after 55 years of age.
- *Toxic* (6%): carbon monoxide poisoning, acetylsalicilic acid overdose, recreational drugs.
- *Encephalopathy* (5%).
- *Eclampsia* (2%): at present, 0.1–0.7 per 1000 deliveries.
- *Others* (10%).

Incidence of acute symptomatic seizures

- 39/100,000 person/year—Rochester study.[1]
- 29/100,000 person/year—French study.[2]
- 21% of newly occurring seizures—British study.[3]
- Approximately 40% of afebrile seizures.
- Higher risk in men than in women.
- Highest risk during first year of life—metabolic, infectious and encephalopathic causes.
- Incidence increases progressively with age after 35 years.
- Cerebrovascular disease is the cause in 50% of patients >65 years.

Cumulative incidence of acute symptomatic seizures

- 3.6% risk of having acute symptomatic seizures during an 80-year lifespan.
- 5% in men and 2.5% in women.

Prognosis of acute symptomatic seizures

- Depends on the underlying condition. Relatively high mortality rate.
- Slightly increased risk of later developing epilepsy, compared with patients who do not suffer seizures under similar conditions.

References

1. Annegers JF, Hauser WA, Lee JR, *et al.* (1995). Acute symptomatic seizures in Rochester, Minnesota, 1935–1984. *Epilepsia,* **36**, 327– 33.

2. Loiseau J, Loiseau P, Guyot M, *et al.* (1990). Survey of seizure disorders in. the French southwest. 1. Incidence of epileptic syndromes. *Epilepsia,* **31**, 391–6.

3. Sander JWAS, Hart YM, Johnson AL, *et al.* (1990). National General Practice Study of Epilepsy: Newly Diagnosed Epileptic Seizures in a General Population, *The Lancet,* **336**, 1267–71.

The role of the clinical history

Generalities

- Many symptoms and signs in epilepsy are paroxysmal, occurring during brief periods of time, and consequently difficult to observe.
- In most cases, the initial diagnosis of epilepsy rests entirely on the clinical history.
- Diagnosis requires detailed knowledge of the features to look for.
- History taking cannot follow strict rules—take advantage of opportunities during conversation.
- Casual details can be of great importance—for instance, clumsiness in the morning may point to morning myoclonus.

Background

- *Avoid disturbing factors:* telephone calls, repeated entrance of secretaries or colleagues.
- *Make patient feel that their history is being listened to.*
- *Allow sufficient time, even for relatively simple cases.* It may take time to dismantle the history.
- *Always ask patients in advance to come with at least one attack witness.* Patients are often unconscious during the events or are unaware of them. They may be unable to provide a reliable description of the attacks other than the warning sensations (aura) and symptoms on recovery.
- *Take into consideration the pitfalls of history taken from witnesses:*
  - Over-rehearsed accounts, descriptions sometimes conforming to pre-conceived ideas.
  - Contradictory history from different people.
  - Doctors and nurses are of great value but sometimes misleading— descriptions of what they think it should be, rather than of what actually happened.
  - Distinguish first-hand from second-hand witnesses.
  - Determine if the complete episode was witnessed.
- *Small children usually cannot provide an account of subjective sensations or feelings.* An aura of fear or strangeness might manifest as the child running scared to his/her parents, or withdrawing into a corner.
- *The style of history taking depends on the patient.* With some it is better to listen, whereas others are discursive and is better to ask direct questions avoiding medical terms.
- *If the history is incomplete at first presentation, reschedule an early appointment to speak to other witnesses if available.*

History of the complaint

- Obtain descriptions of all *seizure types*.
- Obtain descriptions of *specific attacks*:
  - *Last attack witnessed*: it is often better remembered.
  - *First seizure*: it may differ from the rest as in febrile seizures.
  - *Worst seizure*: to estimate the scale of the clinical problem, the risk to life, and sometimes the circumstances of occurrence.
- Inquire about the *settings* in which attacks occur: it may help in management (to avoid triggers) and in distinguishing from non-epileptic attacks.
  - Study the relation to sleep cycle: if occurring while asleep, is it at the onset, in the middle, before awakening or shortly after? Does a change in sleep pattern or abrupt awakening precipitate seizures?
  - If daytime attacks: establish if they occur in the morning/evening/ randomly, and the patient's activity at the time of the attacks—rest, in bed, exercise, playing, at school, in bath, fasting, eating, standing, reclining, at computer, television or video game, bored, emotional or pleasantly engaged in pleasant occupation.
- Obtain a description of the *prodrome*, which could indicate a forthcoming attack, such as:
  - Changes in behaviour (irritability, sleepiness) which may precede epileptic seizures or migraine by hours.
  - Hunger, sweating can suggest hypoglycemia.
- Obtain a description of the immediate *stimulus*, if any, which has a short-term regular association with attacks, and has major diagnostic value:
  - In syncope: blood letting, sight of blood, injections, prolonged standing in hot or confined places, standing after prolonged sitting or lying down, breath, holding pain from minor trauma. In some QT syndromes exercise and auditory triggers.
  - Epilepsy: flashing lights, startle (also for hypereplexia which is rare), striped visual patterns, reading.
- Obtain a description of the *aura if present*: visceral, motor, sensory, psycho-sensorial:
  - It can be present in migraine and syncope.
  - Not available in small children: sometimes manifest as screaming, looking terrified, stopping ongoing activity, running to their mother, looking preoccupied or as if concentrating.
  - Aura suggests partial seizures and has localizing and lateralizing value if specific. Non-specific auras (odd sensation in head or in all body, etc.) can occur in generalized seizures.
- *Reconstruction of ictal signs* may be difficult because many things occur in brief period of time.
  - Video monitoring in hospital or at home.
  - Incontinence and tongue biting: traditional but are not necessary or specific. Lateral tongue biting is unusual in disorders other than epilepsy (occasionally in syncope).
  - Ask witnesses to mime the attack as this often shows interesting details such as posture asymmetries or distinguishes jerks from tremor or shivering.

- *Duration* of attacks:
  - It is often exaggerated—obtain objective time-clues.
  - It is different from the duration of post-ictal confusion, sleepiness, or headache.
  - Ask whether all attacks are self-terminating.
  - Post-ictal phase is of interest as it can be lateralizing: Todd's paralysis, aphasia.
- *Frequency/pattern of attacks*: a common response is 'it depends' or 'not fixed'. Try to obtain:
  - Frequency for each seizure type.
  - Average frequency per week.
  - Highest frequency per week.
  - Longest attack-free period.
  - Whether attacks occur in clusters.
  - Whether attacks occur from sleep.
  - Relationship to menstrual cycle.

History of the patient

Developmental history
- Emphasis in peri-natal history: length of delivery, normal delivery, milestones—age of independent walking, first words, school performance.
- Any recent change in performance or loss of skills.
- Previous diseases: meningitis, encephalitis, febrile seizures (length, lateralization, localized post-ictal deficits). Ask about old notes if possible to obtain.
- *Previous history of seizures does not mean that present attacks are epileptic.*

History of the epilepsy
- Age of onset of seizures.
- Initial manifestations.
- Changes in frequency.
- Types of seizures.
- Deterioration or arrest of development, cognitive or behavioural.
- Developmental delay.
- Detailed drug history: difficult but essential, often requiring detailed copies of notes. Compile information about all AEDs taken—alone or in combination—preferably in chronological order with starting doses and rates of escalation, maximum doses, duration of treatment, benefits or side effects, and reason for discontinuing. Document previous drug levels and correlation with attacks.
- Family history of neurological disease and seizures. Often difficult, try to obtain copies of previous EEG reports, etc.

Knowledge of the patient as a person
- Assess the degree of disturbance caused by the epilepsy on the patient and family.
- Epilepsy may be more of a handicap for those with active life styles.
- Assess the extent of family help and family attitudes.
- Impact on emotional, professional, and social status is variable.
- Management decisions are often guided by on such assessments.
- *With children, assess how epilepsy affects the patient and the family, its impact on learning at school, and the parents' expectations. This will affect how the patient and the family cope with disease.*

Key reading

1. Aicardi J. and Taylon DC (1997). History and physical examination. In *Epilepsy: A Comprehensive Textbook*. Engel J Jr and Pedley T A (Eds), Lippincott, Raven Publishers, Philadelphia, pp.805–810.

The role of the physical examination

Although physical examination is often normal in individuals with epilepsy, it should nevertheless be carried out as it can be useful in several circumstances, as outlined below.

'Inter-ictal' examination in patients with a new presentation

The examination is directed at:

- *Systemic and neurological examination looking for any abnormality suggesting other causes of collapse.* Examples include: postural hypotension, abnormal cardiac examination (cardiac syncope), obstructive airway disease (cough syncope), obtunded patient with focal signs (coning), evidence to suggest hydrocephalus (obstruction of ventricular flow resulting in loss of consciousness), evidence of organ damage/failure to suggest metabolic encephalopathy.

- *Abnormalities that may suggest a condition known to be associated with epilepsy.* Examples include adenoma sebaceum and retinal tumours in tuberous sclerosis, café au lait spots in neurofibromatosis (📖 see Neurocutaneous syndromes, pp.470–477) and short stature or ataxia in mitochondrial disease, facial angioma in Sturge–Weber syndrome, linear naevus in the face or abnormal pigmentation in incontinentia pigmenti or Ito's disease, dysmorphic features in Angelman and other paediatric syndromes, cataracts and fundal cherryed spots in the sialidoses, and unusual head shapes in craniosynostosis, hydrocephalus, or meningioma. Other examples include: features associated with systemic infective, vasculitic or inflammatory diseases such as connective tissue disorders, sarcoidosis, or HIV.

- *Neurological or systemic findings that might indicate early onset focal CNS pathology.* Examples include: asymmetry in limb size or reflexes, slight facial asymmetry (UMN facial weakness is more likely to be observed when people are asked to show their teeth than smile), shift in dominance, unilateral apraxia, increased tone or weakness.

- *Indication of any new focal neurological findings that may suggest recent onset cortical pathology,* for example, a space-occupying lesion: Reflex asymmetry, pyramidal drift or weakness, facial asymmetry, visual field defect or inattention, cortical sensory loss, upgoing plantar responses and papilloedema should all be looked for.

'Inter-ictal' examination in patients with chronic treated epilepsy

The examination also includes screening for specific side effects of current and previous AED treatment as well as for damage consequent to the epilepsy. The latter includes evidence of previous seizure-associated injury and cognitive deficits.

Examples of drug side effects include:

- Nystagmus, peripheral neuropathy, ataxia, gum disease (Fig.3c.1), hirsutism and coarsening of features with phenytoin.
- Connective tissue change such as Dupuytren's contracture, particularly with phenobarbital.
- Weight gain, tremor, hair loss, and motor slowing with high-dose valproate.
- Reduced verbal fluency and weight loss with topiramate.
- Weight gain with gabapentin.
- Visual field defect with vigabatrin.

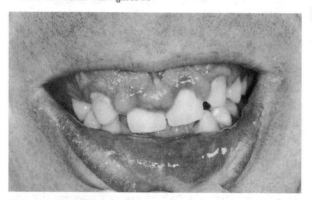

Fig. 3c.1 Gingival hypertrophy due to chronic treatment with phenytoin. (Reproduced with permission from Smith DF, Appleton RE, MacKenzie JM, et al. (eds.) (1998). *An Atlas of Epilepsy*. The Parthenon Publishing Group, New York and London.)

Ictal examination (examination during a seizure)

If the opportunity arises to attend to a seizure, it should be used:

- To ensure the person's safety (📖 see What to do during a seizure, pp.228–229) and provide rescue treatment if appropriate.
- To allow for the examination of the patient during the attack, e.g for responsiveness.
- To provide a reliable witnessed account of the episode.

The attack should be documented as carefully as possible with special attention to its evolution (📖 see example in Box 3c.1). If more than one episode is witnessed, document all in detail. Epileptic attacks, even if bizarre, are often stereotyped. If practical, video the attacks as early as possible after onset and continue recording into the post-ictal phase. Video recording would allow later careful review and the opportunity to consult a more experienced colleague.

Always take note of:

- Autonomic changes—BP, pulse, colour change, respiration.
- Responsiveness/orientation.
- Speech disturbance.
- Abnormal posturing.
- Loss of tone or fall.
- Tonic or clonic convulsions.
- Abnormal movement of eyes, lids, throat (swallowing), mouth (e.g. lip smacking), limb movement.
- Waxing and waning of any convulsive movements.
- Plantar responses and pupillary reflexes.
- How the episode subsides.
- Any confusion, weakness or dysphasia after the event.
- Any evidence of injury, tongue bite, or incontinence.

Box 3c.1 Example of seizure description

The patient seems to have a warning. He is vacant and unresponsive. His pulse is regular at around 100 beats per minute. He looks pale but not white. He shows lip smacking and swallowing movements. His right arm is flexed and stiff for 20sec while he picks at his clothes with the left hand. He then gets up and wanders around the room for 30sec, apparently confused. He gradually comes round and attempts to respond but his speech is unintelligible for a further 60sec. He is then clearly dysphasic and, although alert and cooperative, is unable to name objects. He recovers fully within 4min of onset. He confirms that he had his usual warning of a butterfly feeling in the stomach followed by a déjà vu feeling shortly before losing awareness.

A clear description such as this suggests a complex partial seizure of left mesial temporal onset in someone who is left dominant for language.

It is recommended that ECG is routinely performeed in patients with epilepsy.

Key reading

1. Smith DF, Appleton RE, MacKenzie JM, *et al.* (eds.) (1998). *An Atlas of Epilepsy*. The Parthenon Publishing Group, New York and London.

The role of the electroencephalogram (EEG)

What is the EEG?

The EEG is a record of variations in electrical activity recorded from different regions on the head. It is generated by neuronal function in the patient's brain. The EEG is thought to represent the compound electrical field mainly originating from postsynaptic potentials in the cerebral cortex. Because electrical fields attenuate with distance, electrical activity from deep brain structures (basal ganglia, hippocampus, amygdala) is hardly detectable on the scalp.

How is an EEG recorded?

- EEGs are most commonly recorded with electrodes on the scalp—scalp EEG.
- The EEG is displayed as simultaneous graphs of electrical activity versus time— 📖 see Fig. 3c.2.
- Most EEG recordings are currently digital, which allow reformatting, unlike previous paper recordings.
- Each graph (also called channel) represents changes over time in electrical activity in a region of the scalp.
- The standard EEGs used to study epilepsy show 10sec of recording at a time—i.e. 10sec per page or screen.
- Electrical activity is measured as voltage difference between two electrodes, showing negative polarity upwards—the opposite to the standard convention in physics.
- A typical EEG will record the electrical activity generated by the patient's brain for around 30min if not intended to include a sleep period (the so called awake or routine EEG), or for 60–90min if intended to include a period of sleep (a sleep EEG). The latter can be obtained during the day after sleep deprivation or with drug-induced sleep, using an agent that does not significantly affect the EEG (for instance, quinalbarbital)
- Most EEGs include a period of overbreathing (hyperventilation) and some stimulation with flashing lights (photic stimulation).
- Hyperventilation is achieved by asking the patient to breathe as quickly and deeply as possible for 3min. A toy windmill can be helpful to encourage children to hyperventilate.
- Photic stimulation is carried out by asking patients to look into a light that repeatedly flashes, located around 30cm away from the face.
- The frequency of the flashing light is measured in Hz (number of flashes delivered during 1sec). For each frequency tested, the patient is exposed to the flashing light for around 10sec. Several frequencies between 2–60Hz are used on each patient.
- There are reservations about performing photic stimulation on adult patients holding a driving licence, since there is a small risk of inducing a seizure in susceptible individuals, and consequently having the driving licence withdrawn. There is no need to carry out photic stimulation when epilepsy is not under consideration (e.g. hepatic encephalopathy) or is very unlikely (e.g. atypical psychosis). Some individuals find photic stimulation uncomfortable even if no photoparoxysmal discharges are recorded.

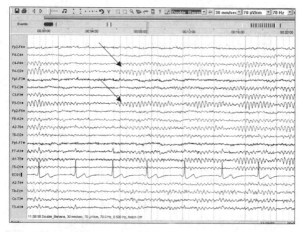

Fig. 3c.2 A normal EEG recorded with eyes closed, with clear α activity (arrows).

How to interpret an EEG

As cortical electrical activity changes with time, so does the EEG. EEG traces are always changing and these time variations appear as waves of different frequencies on the EEG record. EEG waves have traditionally been classified into frequency bands according to the Greek alphabet:

- α (read as alpha): waves of frequency between 8 –14Hz.
- β (read as beta): waves of frequency above 14Hz, also called *fast activity* or *fast rhythms*.
- θ (read as theta): waves of frequency between 4–8Hz.
- δ (read as delta): waves of frequency below 4Hz.

The ongoing electrical activity on the EEG is called the background activity. The α rhythm is an important part of the background activity in awake subjects. It is a sinusoidal rhythm that waxes and wanes, is blocked by eye opening, shows maximal amplitude over posterior regions of the head, and is fairly symmetrical, although often slightly larger on the non-dominant hemisphere (usually the right). The frequency composition of the background activity changes with age, level of consciousness, and disease. Background activity that contains mainly activity in δ and θ ranges is called slow activity. Normal children and teenagers tend to show more slow activity than normal adults, particularly posteriorly. Slow activity increases during normal sleep, confusional states or coma and in the presence of brain damage or abnormalities.

In addition to the ongoing background activity, the EEG can show brief waveforms that occur occasionally. These are called paroxysmal events, and are thought to result from sudden synchronization of neuronal activity. Some paroxysmal events are normal (e.g. vertex sharp waves and K-complexes often seen in sleep). Other paroxysmal events are abnormal (e.g. epileptiform discharges, as described in the next section).

Other useful EEG terminology
- Abnormalities that are unilateral and restricted to a localized area of the scalp are called *focal*.
- Abnormalities which can be recorded all over the scalp are called *diffuse* or *generalized*.
- Focal abnormalities seen over different regions at different times are called *multifocal*.
- Multifocal abnormalities restricted to one side or seen mainly on one side are said to be *lateralized*.
- The terms *regular* or *rhythmic* are often used to describe waveforms of similar shape occurring repeatedly, usually for several seconds.
- EEG artefacts: in the context of epileptology, artefact is an electrical signal that did not originate in the brain. EEG artefacts can have a variety of shapes and mechanisms. The most common are artefacts due to muscle activity (electromyogram), artefacts generated by movement of cables, eye movement, chewing and the electrocardiogram.
- In patients with epilepsy, the EEG can be recorded during periods free of seizures (inter-ictal) or during seizures (ictal).

How to interpret the inter-ictal EEG in epilepsy
Since seizures are relatively infrequent events, most outpatient EEG recordings obtained for the evaluation of epilepsy are inter-ictal.

Abnormalities of background activity:
- Persistent slowing of the background activity suggests a structural abnormality.
- In patients with idiopathic epilepsy, the background activity is normal—apart from medication-induced changes—as no underlying structural abnormality is present.
- Patients with symptomatic/cryptogenic epilepsy can show slowing of the background activity due to an underlying organic pathology.
- Slowing of the background activity would tend to be focal in partial (focal) epilepsy and diffuse in symptomatic/cryptogenic generalized epilepsy.

AED medication can induce diffuse slowing of the background activity. The degree of slowing is generally dose related, and is usually mild if no clinical signs of toxicity are present. This should be taken into consideration when interpreting the EEG, as patients suffering from any epilepsy type and treated with high doses of AEDs might show diffuse slowing of the EEG background, wrongly suggesting symptomatic generalized epilepsy. Drugs, particularly barbiturates and benzodiazepines, may also cause diffuse increase in fast rhythms (β activity).

Metabolic abnormalities can also cause slowing of background activity.

Paroxysmal abnormalities in epilepsy
Paroxysmal abnormalities in epilepsy are due to a sudden increase in synchronicity of neuronal discharges that can occur for brief periods (50–500msec) during the inter-ictal record. In patients with epilepsy, paroxysmal abnormalities are classified into sharp waves, spikes, polyspikes, and spike-and-wave discharges.
- *Sharp* waves are triangular waves lasting for >70msec.
- *Spikes* are sharper triangular waves lasting for <70msec.

- *Polyspikes* are runs of spikes, lasting for several hundreds of milliseconds, sometimes followed by a slow wave.
- *Spike-and-wave* discharges are spikes or sharp waves followed by a slow wave of opposite polarity, lasting for 300msec or longer.
- Polyspikes and spike-and-wave discharges are generically called *epileptiform* discharges because they tend to occur (although not exclusively) in patients with epilepsy.
- Examples of focal and generalized epileptiform discharges can be seen in Figs. 3c3–6.

The value of the inter-ictal EEG in epilepsy

Sharp waves and slow activity are rather non-specific abnormalities that can often be seen in conditions other than epilepsy (haemorrhage, infarcts, tumours, encephalitis, etc.).

Spikes and epileptiform discharges are the most reliable EEG abnormality to aid in the diagnoses of epilepsy. In general,
- 55% of patients with epilepsy will show epileptiform discharges in an awake inter-ictal EEG.
- 80% will show epileptiform discharges in a single sleep EEG.
- 92% of patients will show epileptiform discharges with a second sleep EEG

Thus, when first requesting an EEG with the diagnosis of epilepsy in mind, a sleep EEG, especially if performed relatively soon after an attack, is more likely to show abnormalities if the patient suffers from epilepsy.

Epileptiform discharges are very uncommon in normal subjects (0.2–0.3%). However, they are relatively common (5–20%) in patients with history of intracranial neurological disease or intracranial neurosurgery in the absence of epilepsy. Thus, epileptiform discharges should be interpreted with caution in these patients.

Epileptiform discharges associated with idiopathic epilepsy are age related and may remit beyond childhood/adolescence.

Photoparoxysmal responses (PPR)

(☐ also see Fig. 3b.12, p.108.)
- Some patients with epilepsy, and sometimes their relatives too, show spike-and-wave discharges when exposed to flashing lights.
- This is more likely to occur when the frequency of the flashing light is 18–20Hz.
- Spike-and-waves induced by flashing lights are called photoparoxysmal (or photoconvulsive) responses.
- They can be more or less restricted to the posterior regions of the head (grades I–III), or can be generalized (grade IV).
- If they are generalized, they have a strong association with epilepsy and are useful in the diagnosis of epilepsy.
- Patients showing generalized PPR are said to suffer from photosensitivity or to be photosensitive. In some epilepsy syndromes (for instance, JME), up to 40% of patients are photosensitive. In these syndromes, the presence of photosensitivity is a powerful diagnostic tool. PPR are more likely to occur, but not exclusively so, in generalized epilepsy syndromes.

Effects of hyperventilation

Hyperventilation can be associated with bilateral slowing of the EEG background activity, particulary over frontal regions. This is a normal phenomenon. It is more marked in children and young adults than in older people. It is probably due to a decrease in carbon dioxide blood levels, which induce cerebral vasoconstriction.

- Hyperventilation nearly invariably induces absence seizures in patients who suffer from the syndrome of Childhood Absence Epilepsy. This can be almost ruled out if no absence attacks are recorded during or shortly after well performed hyperventilation.
- Other forms of epileptiform discharges can also be activated by hyperventilation, but less consistently.
- Only clear epileptiform discharges should be considered to confirm the diagnosis of epilepsy, as different forms of δ waves and sharpened slow activity can be a normal response to hyperventilation.

Summary on interpretation of the inter-ictal EEG in epilepsy

The following general rules can be concluded with regard to the intepretation of the inter-ictal EEG in epilepsy,taking into consideration that not all patients with epilepsy will show abnormalities:

- Focal epileptiform discharges observed in the right age group without slowing of the background activity suggests *idiopathic partial epilepsy* arising from the area that shows discharges.
- Generalized epileptiform discharges without slowing of the background activity suggests *idiopathic generalized epilepsy*. Photosensitivity reinforces this diagnosis.
- Focal epileptiform discharges with focal slowing of the background activity suggests *symptomatic/cryptogenic partial (focal) epilepsy* arising from the area that shows discharges or slowing. Good quality imaging is advised.
- Focal, multifocal, or generalized epileptiform discharges with diffuse slowing of the background activity suggests *symptomatic/cryptogenic generalized epilepsy*.
- Mild slowing of the background activity, particularly in the theta range, can be due to antiepileptic medication.
- Abnormalities should be interpreted with caution in patients with history of intracranial neurological disease or neurosurgery.
- CAE can be almost ruled out if no absence attacks are recorded after vigorous hyperventilation.

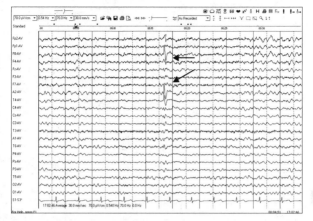

Fig. 3c.3 Example of right temporal focal epileptiform discharge (see arrows) recorded with maximal amplitude at F8, A2 and T4.

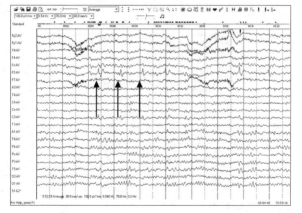

Fig. 3c.4 Example of focal epileptiform discharges over left frontal regions, with maximal amplitude at F3 (see arrows).

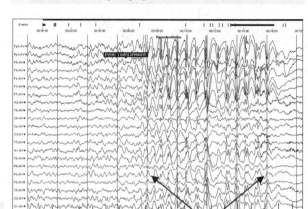

Fig. 3c.5 Example of generalized spike-and-wave during absence seizure induced by hyperventilation (see arrows for start and end of discharge).

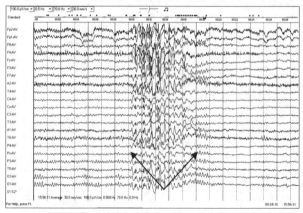

Fig. 3c.6 Example of generalized discharge in a patient with juvenile myoclonic epilepsy (see arrows for start and end of discharge).

Ictal EEG recordings

Ictal EEG recordings (EEG recorded during seizures) are more reliable than inter-ictal recordings to confirm the diagnosis of epilepsy, but are more difficult to obtain and are not usually possible for patients with infrequent seizures.

Ictal recordings can be obtained by chance if a seizure occurs during recording of a standard awake or sleep EEG. This is often the case in syndromes with frequent seizures, such as absence epilepsy or symtomatic generalized epilepsies.

If seizures occur less frequently but are still relatively frequent, prolonged EEG recordings might be necessary, usually in conjunction with simultaneous video recording (telemetry or EEG-video monitoring, 📖 see Role of video monitoring—video-telemetry, intensive monitoring, pp.190–195).

Indications of ictal recordings

Ictal recordings might be necessary in the following situations:
- Patients with frequent seizures and normal sleep EEGs where the diagnosis of epilepsy needs to be confirmed.
- Patients where the diagnosis of epilepsy is in doubt despite the presence of abnormal inter-ictal EEG findings, for instance, in patients with concomitant cerebral pathology.
- Differential diagnosis between epileptic and non-epileptic seizures.
- Classification of seizure types.
- To establish the frequency of seizures. For instance, to monitor the effects of therapy or in patients who have epileptic seizures in addition to non-epileptic events where it might be necessary to establish how many events are epileptic.
- During pre-surgical assessment in patients assessed for the possibility of surgery for the treatment of their epilepsy. In order to:
  - Establish beyond doubt that the patient has epilepsy.
  - Determine seizure type, which is necessary for choosing the surgical procedure and deciding if surgery is appropriate.
  - Identify the location and lateralization of seizure onset.

EEG findings during ictal recordings

EEG findings seen during seizures depend on the seizure type. Abnormalities can consist of:
- Rhythmic sharp waves.
- Rhythmic spikes.
- Slowing of the EEG in the θ or δ ranges.
- Flattening of the EEG—electrodecremental event.
- Low amplitude fast activity with frequency above 15Hz—high frequency or multiunit activity (Fig. 3c.7).
- A combination of the above patterns.
- Changes observed during a focal seizure usually evolve depending on seizure spread.

Some EEG changes are characteristic of certain seizure types:
- *Typical absence seizures:* generalized spike-and-wave activity at 2.5–3.5Hz.
- *Atypical absence seizures:* generalized spike-and-wave at frequency below 2.5Hz.

- *Generalized myoclonic jerks:* a generalized (poly-)spike-and-wave, usually intermixed with muscle artefacts.
- *Focal myoclonic jerks:* no EEG changes, or focal contralateral (poly-) spike-and-wave, usually over frontocentral regions.
- *Focal motor (clonic) seizures:* often show focal contralateral spike-and-wave synchronized with the jerks, usually over frontocentral regions. Sometimes no EEG changes.
- *Tonic and atonic seizures:* flattening of the EEG, usually diffuse, and often associated with diffuse fast activity.
- *Simple partial seizures:* EEG changes may be absent or are focal.
- *Complex partial seizures:* slowing of the background activity usually intermixed with sharp waves or epileptiform discharges. Although these seizures are focal in origin, the scalp EEG will show a clear focal onset only in around 30% of complex partial seizures, because substantial amounts of cortex might have been recruited bilaterally by the time EEG changes are seen on the scalp. Therefore, a diffuse or bilateral EEG onset on the scalp does not exclude a focal seizure onset (i.e. a diffuse EEG onset on the scalp does not necessarily mean that the seizure is generalized). Some complex partial seizures of frontal origin may not show EEG changes, or these may be buried among muscle and movement artefacts.
- *Generalized and secondarily generalized convulsive (tonic–clonic) seizures:* generalized spike-and-wave activity at around 3Hz obscured by or superimposed with rhythmic muscle and movement artefacts.
- *Post-ictal changes:* complex partial, generalized and secondarily generalized convulsive seizures are often followed by a period of confusion called post-ictal confusion. During this period, the EEG often shows focal or diffuse slowing in the δ and θ ranges, with superimposed focal or multifocal sharp waves and epileptiform discharges, sometimes with intermittent periods of EEG flattening.

How to interpret ictal recordings

EEG changes occurring during seizures will confirm that the seizures are epileptic. The opposite (the absence of EEG changes during seizures) is more difficult to interpret. Most epileptic seizures will show EEG changes but there are a few exceptions:

- *Simple partial seizures* may or may not show EEG changes, as the area of cortex involved in these seizures can be rather small and deep (hippocampus). Therefore, a normal EEG during a simple partial seizure cannot rule out epilepsy.
- *Focal myoclonic seizures* may or may not show changes on the on-going EEG for the same reason. If jerks are frequent, EEG back-averaging might show small brief EEG deflections associated with the jerks, preceding the jerks by a few milliseconds.
- *Some frontal complex partial seizures* may not show EEG changes, or these may be impossible to identify among muscle and movement artefacts.

If the EEG is normal while the patient appears unresponsive or with generalized convulsions, it can be assumed that the event is not an epileptic seizure. The reason for this assumption is that in order to lose consciousness (unresponsiveness) or to suffer generalized convulsions, a substantial amount of cortex needs to be recruited bilaterally, which will invariably generate EEG changes.

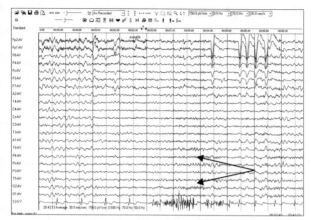

Fig. 3c.7 Onset of parietal seizure with diffuse EEG flattening associated with right parieto-occipital low-amplitude fast activity (at P4 and O2).

The role of neuroimaging

Modern neuroimaging is a rapidly evolving field, the fundamentals of which are beyond the scope of this book. We will focus on the principles relevant to the management of patients with epilepsy and summarize the neuroimaging findings occurring in some common conditions that can cause epilepsy.

Indications of neuroimaging in epilepsy

- Four major indications:
  - *Diagnosis* of the cause of epilepsy.
  - *Pre-surgical assessment:* localization of the epileptogenic lesion.
  - *Identification of complications:* e.g. brain injury, haemorrhage.
  - *Monitoring disease progression:* e.g. tumour.
- General guidelines:
  - Magnetic resonance imaging (MRI) is more sensitive than computerized tomography (CT) for the evaluation of most lesions affecting the brain.
  - CT is often useful in the assessment of bone detail and confirming acute haemorrhage.

Neuroimaging in the diagnosis of epilepsy and its causes

Generally, all patients with epilepsy or suspected epilepsy should have a brain MRI. An exception is children with a clear clinical and electroencephalographic diagnosis of idiopathic epilepsy, who do not require neuroimaging studies. Infants however should be imaged even if the working diagnosis is idiopathic epilepsy. Idiopathic epilepsies make up approximately 30% of patients with epilepsy, which means that neuroimaging is expected to be normal in a large proportion of patients with epilepsy.

Indications of skull X-rays and CT and contraindications to MRI

- Sick patients who need monitoring during scan (e.g. status epilepticus).
- Centres or countries where MRI is not available: mainly for financial reasons, as CT is cheaper than MRI.
- Calcified lesions: 📖 see below.
- Bleeding and head injury: CT is good in the acute phase of bleeding, which is not too relevant to epilepsy apart from bleeding after implantation of intracranial electrodes.
- Intracranial clips or implanted metals are a contraindication for MRI: metals can heat up in the brain during MRI acquisition and magnetic metals (basically, those containing iron, such as some steel) can move in the head.
- Heart pacemaker is a contraindication for MRI. VNS is a contraeindication to the latest generation of brain MRIs, (consult local neuroradiology department).
- Young children not requiring sedation for CT who may need sedation for longer MRI scan.

Disadvantages of CT

- Specific problems with CT in epilepsy:
  - Low sensitivity for soft tissue lesions. Small focal lesions causing epilepsy which are potentially curable by surgical resection can be readily detected by MRI but missed on CT.
- Exposure to X-rays: avoid in children and pregnant women.

Calcified lesions in head X-rays

- *Tumours:* calcification more often in seen benign tumours like meningioma (clouds on X-rays), glioma (curvilinear streaks on X-rays), oligodenroglioma, hamartoma.
- *Tuberous sclerosis:* brain lesions progressively calcify causing nodular and curvilinear densities, particularly around the ventricular system and basal ganglia.
- *Inflammatory disease:* old abscess, tuberculoma, congenital toxoplasmosis (curvilinear basal ganglia), cysticercosis.
- *Vascular lesions:* angioma, Sturge–Weber syndrome (often occipital calcifications), calcification is found in 15% of arteriovenous malformations.

King's MRI protocol for epilepsy

There are many MRI protocols that can now be used during image acquisition. As an example, the MRI protocol used routinely for patients with epilepsy at King's College Hospital, London, includes:

- Coronal fast spin-echo T2-weighted (TEeff 85 TR 4300) 3mm slice thickness, 0mm gap, perpendicular to temporal horn.
- Coronal FLAIR (fluid attenuated inversion recovery) (TE 115eff TR 8500 TI 1900) 3mm slice thickness, 0mm gap, perpendicular to temporal horn.
- Coronal IR-prepped SPGR T1-weighted (IR=inversion recovery, SPGR = spoiled gradient recalled) flip angle 30 TE 2.8 TR 14 1mm partition.
- Axial fast spin-echo T2-weighted (TE 75eff TR 3500) 5mm slice thickness 0mm gap, parallel to AC-PC line.
- Young children may require further alternatives to optimize grey–white matter contrast as myelination is not complete for at least the first 2 years of life, and lesions may 'appear' or 'disappear' as myelination is completed.

Other neuroimaging techniques

- *FDG-PET:* often shows inter-ictal hypometabolism, particularly in temporal lobe epilepsy. Useful in presurgical assessment but unclear other role in the diagnosis of epilepsy.

Other PET studies: largely experimental

- *SPECT, volumetric MRI, functional MRI, MRI spectrometry:* role unclear at present.
- *Magnetoencephalography:* largely as EEG in practice, although it has some advantages and disadvantages over the EEG.

Neuroimaging during pre-surgical assessment

MRI techniques used in epileptology have been constantly expanding. A summary of the use of the most relevant neuroimaging techniques present is the following:

- Skull X-ray:
  - To quickly identify skull fractures after head injury.
  - To identify calcifications which can aid in determining lesion type.
  - To check position of intracranial electrodes.
- Angiography: check cross filling during the amytal test.

- CT:
  - To check haemorrhage after implantation of intracranial electrodes.
  - To check position of non MRI-compatible intracranial electrodes and relation to cortical structures (particularly depth electrodes).
  - To identify calcifications which can aid in determining lesion type.
- Structural MRI:
  - For identification of lesions responsible for seizures.
  - To check position of MRI-compatible intracranial electrodes and relation to cortical structures (particularly depth electrodes).
  - Measurement of hippocampal volume: high sensitivity to confirm mesial temporal sclerosis in unclear cases.
- Inter-ictal PET (FDG, flumazenil): pre-surgical assessment of temporal lobe epilepsy.
- MRI spectroscopy: used to assess hippocampal sclerosis and is sometimes useful to characterize mass lesions.
- Inter-ictal SPECT: unclear indication.
- Ictal SPECT: role unclear, probably useful in pre-surgical assessment but not widely available.
- MEG: unclear.
- Functional MRI:
  - Localization of primary sensorimotor regions and primary visual cortex.
  - Lateralize (but does not localize) speech areas.
  - Unclear if able to lateralize (localize) memory function, although likely to do so in the near future.
- Diffusion tensor imaging with tractography can show location of important white matter tracts such as the optic radiation or corticospinal tract in relation to a lesion to aid surgical planning.

Imaging findings in the most common epileptogenic lesions

Here we summarize neuroimaging findings seen in lesions that can cause epilepsy. Neurodegenerative disorders can cause epilepsy and show neuroimaging changes and are described in the key references in the end of this chapter.

Stroke

The MRI characteristics of stroke are well recognized and will not be described in detail here.

- MRI can reliably show the location and extent of infarcts within 1 hour of onset.
- CT can detect acute focal haemorrhages of 1cm or larger in diameter, and MRI might not be necessary.
- Angiography can be useful if the cause or haemorrhage is not clear, particularly if the patient is not hypertensive.

Mesial temporal sclerosis (Fig. 3c.8)

- Hippocampal atrophy and sclerosis: suggested by:
  - Small hippocampus.
  - Loss of digitations hippocampi and definition of internal structure.
  - Increase in the size of the temporal horn of the lateral ventricle.
- Hippocampal signal hypointensity (darker) on T1-weighted inversion recovery images.

- Hippocampal signal hyperintensity (brighter) on T2-weighted inversion recovery images.
- Amygdalar sclerosis.
- Sometimes associated mild atrophy of the parahippocampal gyrus or of most of the temporal cortex.
- Changes are sometimes subtle and difficult to identify by eye. Quantified volumetric techniques might be necessary for diagnosis.
- Limboic atrophy(fornix, mamillary body and anterior thalamus in severe cases)
- Loss of grey–white boundary at temporal pole.

Dual temporal pathology

This term refers to the presence of hippocampal sclerosis and an extra-hippocampal lesion in the same patient. Dual pathology can be observed in as much as 20–30% of temporal lobes resected for surgical treatment. Extrahippocampal lesions tend to be tumours, developmental lesions, or trauma.

Astrocytic tumours

- Mass lesion with signal inhomogeneity.
- High signal on T2-weighted images.
- Solid and cystic components might be present.

Oligodendrogliomas

- In most cases are located within the frontal or temporal lobes.
- Predilection for medial structures in temporal lobes and superficial cortex in frontal lobes.
- Heterogeneous mass with cystic components and may have haemorrhages.
- Calcifications can be present and might be difficult to detect with standard spin-echo techniques. Gradient echo frequencies and CT are more sensitive to detect calcifications.
- Mild-to-moderate contrast enhancement, but oedema is rare.

Mixed glial lesions

- Frequent calcifications.
- Seizure onset at early age.
- Gangliogliomas are common in the temporal lobes.
- Solid mass lesion
- At times, partially cystic components.
- Inhomogeneous signals on T1 and high signals on T2
- High signals on T2.

Dysembryoplastic neuroepithelial tumours (DNET, Fig. 3c.11)

- High association with seizures.
- Usually located in the temporal lobes, often involving mesial structures or mesial structures plus neocortex.
- Cystic formations are uncommon.
- Usually involve grey and white matter.
- On CT they are hypodense lesions.
- Well localized.
- Hypointense on T1 images.
- Hyperintense on T2 images.
- Calcification is uncommon.
- Usually no enhancement with contrast.

Cerebral metastasis

- Relatively common, around 20% of brain tumours.
- Typical localization in grey–white matter junction.
- Often peripheral edema.
- Often multiple.
- Avidly enhance after contrast.

Arteriovenous malformations

- Presenting symptoms are intracranial haemorrhage or seizures.
- Dilated vascular structures with void signal on spin-echo sequences.
- High signal might be present with gradient-echo techniques.
- Adjacent gliosis and previous haemorrhage.

Cavernous angiomas (cavernomas)

- The most common vascular malformation.
- May be sporadic or genetic (autosomal dominant). In patients with multiple cavernomas (cerebral cavernomatosis) it is usually genetic.
- Calcification is common.
- Reticulated central core with T1 high signal ('popcorn' appearance).
- Haemosiderin deposits seen as a rim of hypointensity surrounding the central core.
- No mass effect or surrounding oedema, unless recent acute haemorrhage.

Focal cortical dysplasia (Figs. 3c.9 and 3c.10)

- The most common developmental abnormality.
- Frequently affecting peri-Rolandic cortex.
- Imaging can be normal.
- Usually solitary.
- Heterogenous T2 changes usually showing abnormal gyration and thickened cortex without mass effect, of variable size, ranging from small focal lesions to multilobar involvement.
- No enhancement with contrast.
- Often only subtle changes: abnormal grey–white matter patterns, thickened cortex, radial tracks in white matter, or fuzziness of grey–white matter junction. These features can be seen in T1 images but can be better identified with contrast inversion recovery sequences, which show better definition between grey and white matter.

Hamartomas

- Abnormal proliferation of neuronal, meningeal, glial cells, or a combination of them without evidence of neoplastic tissue.
- A common developmental lesion.
- More circumscribed lesion than focal cortical dysplasia, appearing as a mass lesion without mass effect.
- Isotense on T1 images.
- Hypertense signal on T2 images.
- Rim of hypointensity surrounding the hyperintense signal on T2 images.
- Often involve the cortical ribbon and the underlying white matter.
- In temporal lobe show predilection for medial structures.
- May flatten adjacent gyri.
- Calcifications are rare.
- In infants, may appear as hypointense lesions on T1 and hypertense on T2 images, in cotico-subcortical regions.
- None or mild enhancement with gadolinium contrast.
- Usually single lesions. If multiple, tuberous sclerosis should be considered.
- Hypothalamic hamartomas tend to be associated with gelastic (laughter) seizures.

Post-traumatic lesions

- Depending on the age of the lesion, haemorrhagic or gliotic (scarring) changes can be seen involving cortical and white matter.
- In temporal lobe tend to involve the pole and basal cortex, in contact with bone structures.
- In the frontal lobe, polar and orbital cortices are often affected.
- Bilateral lesions can be seen.
- Can be associated with subdural and epidural haematomas, or intraventricular haemorrhage.
- Intracerebral haematomas can be seen in the acute phase, often involving white matter and basal ganglia.
- Sometimes associated with skull fractures.

Porencephaly

- Generated by *in utero* necrosis before the hemisphere is formed, due to intracerebral haemorrhage or iscaemia secondary to occlusion of a major cerebral artery, usually the middle cerebral artery.
- Cysts that communicate with ventricles and subarachnoid space or both, with absence of much of the hemisphere affected.
- Often bilateral.
- Adjacent gyri can be abnormal.

Ulegyria (atrophic sclerosis)

- Often a consequence of birth injury due to emboli or thrombosis.
- Usually affecting the depths of sulci.
- High signal on T2 in the white-grey matter junction.

Hemiconvulsion–hemiplegia–epilepsy (HHE) syndrome
- Unilateral subcortical and cortical atrophy of most of one hemisphere, associated with ventricular dilatation.
- Porencephaly is not present.

Rasmussen's encephalitis
- Progressive unilateral hemispheric atrophy due to unilateral chronic encephalitis.
- Begins in the temporal insular region, causing enlargement of the temporal horn and sylvian fissure.
- Initially there are high-intensity signals from cortex with minimal cortical atrophy, due to gliosis and inflammation.
- Later, hemiatrophy and increased T2 signals from cortex.
- In late stages, massive unilateral ventricular dilatation and cortical destruction.

Sturge–Weber syndrome (encephalo-trigeminal angiomatosis)
- Changes are usually unilateral, with occipital or occipito-parieto-temporal preference.
- Cerebral atrophy.
- Sinus hypertrophy.
- Intracranial diffuse calcifications involving the cortex. Might be absent in small children.
- Abnormal choroid plexus vessels.
- Enhancement with contrast, which might be more accurate to show the extent of the abnormality.
- Gradient echo sequences useful in detecting calcification on MRI.
- Sometimes enlarged internal cerebral veins.
- Forme fruste: presence of cerebral angiomatosis with no skin lesions.

Hemimegalencephaly (Fig. 3c.12)
- Enlargement of at least one lobe of one cerebral hemisphere, but usually of the whole hemisphere.
- Thickened cortex.
- Broad gyri.
- Shallow sulci.
- Often increase T2 signal in abnormal white matter.
- Sometimes nodular heterotopias in white matter.

Subcortical heterotopia (singular: heterotopion)
- Islands of grey matter (?cortex) embedded in the white matter. Islands of grey matter are often round in shape (called nodules).
- Isotense lesions.
- Heterotopic nodules show irregular margins.
- Heterotopia can appear as:
  - Round nodules adjacent to, and often growing into, the lateral ventricles (subependymal heterotopia), or
  - Ovoid nodules in the middle of white matter (focal subcortical heterotopia), or
  - As large areas of grey matter replacing white matter (diffuse, band heterotopia or double cortex).
- Large heterotopic nodules may compress the ventricle.

- Absence of surrounding oedema (unlike some tumours).
- There might be thinning of the overlying cortex and diminished sulcus formation.
- Focal subcortical heterotopia can be differentiated from subependymal hamartomas of tuberous sclerosis because they tend to be isotense round or ovoid, rather than iso- to hypotense irregular or elongated lesions as seen in tuberous sclerosis.

Lissencephaly

- Gyri and sulci are fewer and less marked than normal.
- In the extreme form, there are no gyri or sulci (agyria).
- A milder form shows few, broad, flat gyri (pachygyria).
- Often associated with microcephaly and other severe syndromes (Walker–Warburg syndrome, Fukuyama's congenital muscular dystrophy, diffuse polymicrogyria).

Cortical dysplasia

- During development, neurones reach the cortex but distribute abnormally.
- The surface of the cortex can be smooth or have small bumps (microgyri), often multiple (polymicrogyri).
- Other abnormal cortical folding can be present.
- Isotense with respect to normal cortex.
- Prolonged T2 relaxation time might be present in underlying white matter.
- Calcification is rare (<5%)
- Anomalous venous drainage might be present as shown by the presence of large vessels in the region.
- Often perisylvian.
- In some patients, cortical dsyplasia is extensive involving most of one hemisphere (*extensive unilateral cortical dsyplasia*).
- Common manifestation of congenital cytomegalovirus infection.
- A bilateral opercular form (congenital bilateral perisylvian syndrome) sometimes is associated with pseudobulbar palsy (oropharyngeal dysfunction and dysarthria), cognitive dysfunction, and epilepsy.

Polymicrogyria

- A bilateral opercular form (congenital bilateral perisylvian syndrome) sometimes is associated with pseudobulbar palsy (oropharyngeal dysfunction and dysarthria), cognitive dysfunction and epilepsy.
- A bilateral occipital form is also seen, and unilateral localized regions.

Schizencephaly (agenetic porencephaly)

- Consist of grey matter-lined clefts that cross the entire cerebral hemisphere and connect the ependymal layer of the lateral ventricles with the pial lining of the cortex.
- The grey matter lining is dysplastic, often polymicrogyric.
- Unilateral or bilateral.
- The wall of the cleft might be in contact with one another (closed lip) or separated (open lips, porencephaly).

Tuberous sclerosis

Neurocutaneous syndrome that can have a variety of cerebral lesions:

- *Subependimal hamartomas*: usually along the ventricular surface of the caudate nucleous, calcify with age, and show variable contrast enhancement.
- *Giant cell tumours*: subependymal nodules near the foramen of Monro, tendency to enlarge non-invasively and induce hydrocephalus.
- *Cortical hamartomas or 'tubers'*: cortical or subcortical hamartomas with ill-defined inner margins.
- *White matter lesions*: islets of neurons and glial cells, of MRI characteristics of hamartomas. Occasionally, linear or curvilinear hyperintensity can be seen in T2-weighted images going from subependymal hamartomas to cortical tubers.
- *Cerebellar lesions*: less common than cerebral abnormalities.

CNS infections

- Signs of neuronal degeneration and inflammation: oedema, haemorrhages, and necrosis (particularly in herpes simplex), later gliosis.
- Temporal predominance in herpes virus encephalitis.
- Calcifications in congenital cytomegalovirus infection.
- Periventricular white matter lesions and cortical atrophy in subacute sclerosing panencephalitis.
- Bacterial infections show early hyperintensity on T2 images, later an abscess might appear (liquid cavity surrounded by gliotic tissue which enhances with contrast).
- Multiple septic emboli and infarcts in acute bacterial infections and endocarditis.
- Granulomas in tuberculosis.
- Multiple focal lesions in congenital toxoplasmosis or in immunosupressed patients.
- Round lesions, often multiple, in cysticercosis.

Key reading

1 Kuzniecky RI, Jackson GD (2005). *Magnetic resonance in epilepsy*, 2nd edn. Raven Press, New York.

2 Sartor K, Haehmel S, Kress B (2008). *Brain imaging*. Thieme Stuttgart, New York.

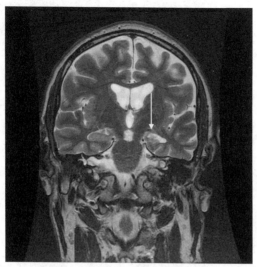

Fig. 3c.8 Left mesial temporal sclerosis. Note: shrinkage of the left hippocampus (arrow), destruction of its internal structure and increased volume of the temporal horn of the lateral ventricle, immediately lateral to the left hippocampus. T2 weighted full spin-echo sequence.

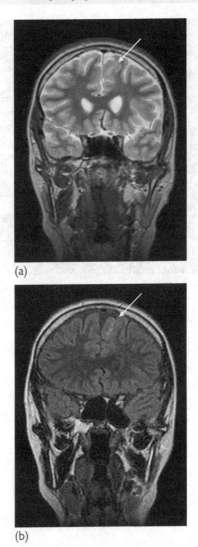

(a)

(b)

Fig. 3c.9 Focal cortical dysplasia over the medial and superior aspect of the left frontal lobe (arrow). (a) T2-weighted full spin-echo sequence. (b) FLAIR sequence. Note: cortical thickening, fussiness of the limit between grey and white matter, and increased brightness in the FLAIR sequence.

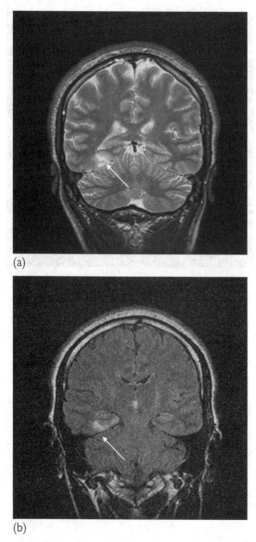

(a)

(b)

Fig. 3c.10 Right posterior subtemporal tumour or focal cortical dysplasia. (a) T2 weighted spin-echo sequence; (b) FLAIR sequence. Note: cortical thickening and increased brightness in FLAIR sequence.

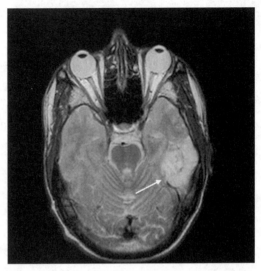

Fig. 3c.11 Left temporal focal lesion of uncertain aetiology.

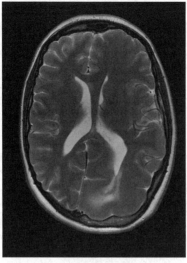

Fig. 3c.12 Left hemimegalencephaly. Note: enlargement of the left hemisphere with associated cortical thickening and some loss of gyral pattern.

The role of video monitoring—video-telemetry, intensive monitoring

Due to the intermittent nature of the clinical and electroencephalographic manifestations of epilepsy, establishing a definite diagnosis of epilepsy can be difficult unless an attack is witnessed and the EEG is recorded simultaneously.

The simultaneous recording of a video image of the patient and his/her EEG is a test of paramount importance in the diagnosis of epilepsy in many situations (📖 see Box 3c.2). It can be recorded continuously for hours to days until seizures occur in patients where seizures are sufficiently frequent. If the patient has an attack during the recording, the EEG and video image can be played back to allow correlations between clinical and electroencephalographic manifestations during attacks. Such correlations often allow a definite diagnosis of epilepsy and its type in patients where seizure history and inter-ictal or ictal standard EEGs are inconclusive.

This test is refered to as: video-EEG monitoring, video monitoring, intensive monitoring, intensive monitoring in epilepsy, epilepsy monitoring, video-telemetry and telemetry.

The term ambulatory EEG refers to the modality of EEG recording where the patient can walk freely, and carry out his/her normal every day activities at home or at work, while the EEG is being continuously recorded, usually without video image.

Box 3c.2 Main indications for video-telemetry

- Differential diagnosis of epilepsy: to establish whether the patient's attacks are due to epilepsy or to non-epileptic seizures, panic attacks, cardiogenic attacks, faints, movement disorders, sleep disorders, or other causes.
- Classification of seizures and epilepsy.
- Estimation of seizure frequency.
- Detection of seizure precipitants: reflex epilepsy, situational factors, self-induction.
- Presurgical assessment: localization of seizure focus.

Diagnosis of epilepsy

In the majority of patients, the diagnosis of epilepsy is obtained from an accurate seizure description (often obtained from witnesses) supported by an awake-sleep inter-ictal EEG and imaging. However, in some patients there remains doubt regarding the following:

- If they suffer from epileptic or non-epileptic attacks.
- The epileptic nature of the attacks is clearly established, but the type of epilepsy and seizures is unclear.

These issues can be established in most patients if attacks are observed during telemetry. Since in many cases treatment depends on diagnosis, video-EEG monitoring is sometimes crucial.

A suspicion of epilepsy may arise from events associated with impaired consciousness, temporary mental impairment, dizziness, fear, panic, aggressive outbursts, abnormal movements, behavioural disturbance, or fainting (📖 see Conditions that resemble epilepsy, pp.206–225). Sleep phenomena can also simulate epilepsy: somnambulism, apnoea, sudden arousals, night terrors, nightmares, eneuresis, crying, and vocalization. Non-epileptic attacks can be organic or psychogenic. Psychogenic attacks can be panic attacks, abreactive re-enactment of a traumatic event, or conscious or unconscious attempts to simulate epilepsy. In addition, it should be borne in mind that psychological factors can precipitate seizures in patients with epilepsy.

In many centres, a main reason for referral for video-EEG monitoring is the differential diagnosis between epileptic and non-epileptic seizures. In interpreting video telemetry it is useful to keep in mind the following:

- In most epileptic seizures, some form of EEG change occurs during the attack.
- Exceptions to this rule are some simple partial seizures and some frontal lobe seizures.
- EEG changes during epileptic seizures may not contain epileptiform discharges.

More specific details about EEG changes during epileptic seizures have been described in 📖 Role of the electroencephalogram, pp.166–175.

Diagnosis of psycogenic non-epileptic seizures

(📖 see also Conditions that resemble epilepsy, pp.206–225.)

Seizures that truly arise out of sleep cannot be psychogenic. In nocturnal non-epileptic seizures, there is usually an interval of some seconds between awakening and seizure onset.

Brief, frequent nocturnal attacks with bizarre frantic movements (automatisms) that may render the EEG unreadable, often occur in frontal lobe epilepsy. The strange, violent behaviour in the absence of identifiable EEG changes may be misdiagnosed as non-epileptic seizures.

For the diagnosis of psychogenic non-epileptic attacks, some authors recommend the use of intravenous injection of saline to precipitate their occurrence. This is an effective method but carries the risk of inducing non-epileptic attacks in patients who do not habitually suffer from them. 📖 see Activation methods, p.212.

Prolactin levels: prolactin blood levels can be obtained during or shortly after attacks in order to help establish if attacks are epileptic or psychogenic. They are not widely used. In interpreting prolactin levels it is important to keep in mind the following:

- An increase in serum prolactin levels above 500IU/mL occurs 15–20min after 80% of generalized convulsive attacks and in many complex partial seizures with automatisms but seldom in simple partial seizures.
- Studies of patients with intracerebral electrodes suggest that partial seizures with limbic discharges (either simple or complex) are associated with elevation of prolactin serum levels.
- Prolactin levels do not appear to increase in complex partial seizures of frontal lobe origin, although this is controversial.

- Elevations of prolactin levels after presumed seizures have been used to differentiate between epileptic and non-epileptic events.
- Reliable prolactin estimations can be made from capillary blood collected on filter paper that can be stored for up to a week, a technique suitable for outpatients.
- The specificity of this test has, however, been questioned, as marked elevations can occur with emotional stress.
- Prolactin levels can be useful in the diagnosis of epilepsy if they are obtained within 20min of the event and if they are clearly elevated.
- A non-elevated prolactin level is not useful, as it does not exclude the possibility of epilepsy.

Differential diagnosis of epileptic and non-epileptic seizures is particularly difficult in patients who suffer both. In this scenario, care must be taken not to make assumptions about other attacks from the few seizures recorded during video-monitoring, since observation of a non-epileptic attack does not exclude epilepsy, or vice versa. Careful questioning of patients and relatives should be carried out to disclose the presence of attacks different from those observed and to confirm that the attacks recorded are habitual.

The *clinical manifestations* of the attack are often conclusive in establishing whether a seizure is epileptic or not, but may also be misleading. Keep in mind the following:

- Automatisms, swallowing, sialorrhoea, dystonic postures or clonic movements are unlikely to be simulated by patients who have never witnessed true epileptic seizures.
- Clonic convulsions are virtually impossible to replicate in non-epileptic events, as simulated movements tend to have an irregular flapping quality unlike the regular alternating rapid contraction and slower relaxation seen in epileptic clonic movements.
- Epileptic clonus is rather regular with a frequency that often gradually slows down during the course of the seizure.
- Simulated clonus is less regular and does not gradually evolve, but may wax and wane or may stop for a few seconds and then continue, possibly at a different frequency or in different muscle groups—'reprise' phenomenon.
- Cyanosis is rare in non-epileptic seizures but common in tonic–clonic seizures.
- Convulsive movements in non-epileptic attacks might have a non-physiological flavour, such as jerking limited to one arm and the contralateral leg. Movements in either side might occur asynchronously whereas bilateral epileptic clonic convulsions occur simultaneously on both sides. Epileptic clonic movements are brisk, fast, repetitive, and regular at about 2–3Hz, consisting of a fast contraction followed by a more gradual movement in the opposite direction during the subsequent relaxation. Convulsive movements in non-epileptic attacks are more irregular, less repetitive, with similar speed in both directions, and less brisk, often consisting of flapping or flailing of limbs.

The inexperienced observer may not appreciate the wide range of ictal manifestations often seen in epileptic seizures. Particularly subject to misinterpretation are the bizarre behaviours often seen in frontal lobe seizures, such as clapping, bicycling movements, playing pat-a-cake, kicking, stamping, running, rocking, pelvic thrust, swearing.

By contrast, other behaviour is typical of non-epileptic attacks, such as prolonged asynchronous jerking of all limbs in full consciousness, sliding gently off a chair without injury with legs extended, arc de cercle posturing (opisthotonus), jerking of one arm and contralateral leg (which cannot be explained in terms of ictal physiology). It should be noted that there have been rare reports of reliably documented cases with bilateral tonic–clonic movements or of ictal automatisms without loss of consciousness in epileptic seizures.

Intervention by an observer during a seizure might establish that the event is non-epileptic:

- When a jerking limb is held and its movements restricted by the observer, another limb may begin to shake in non-epileptic attacks.
- A patient staring vacant may fixate his/her gaze when a mirror is held in front of his/her eyes if the attack is not epileptic.
- Patients in non-epileptic attacks can resist examination, screwing up their eyes if attempts are made to open them. If their own hand is held above their face and then released, the hand falls deviating to one side, missing the face. Care must be taken to avoid the patient's hand hitting his/her face during this manoeuvre. If a jerking limb is restrained by the examiner, the restricted limb might stop moving while the other limbs increase their jerking.

No EEG changes should be seen in non-epileptic psychogenic attacks, although sometimes it is difficult to establish the absence of EEG changes due to artefacts. In this case, the presence of alpha activity while the patient is apparently unconscious will establish that the attack is not epileptic.

Behavioural manifestations such as impulsive or aggressive behaviour, particularly in children and in the mentally handicapped often leads to referral to exclude complex partial seizures, which are rarely observed in this context (📕 see Diagnosis of status epilepticus, pp.198–205).

Attacks of daytime sleep and cataplexy accompanied by the characteristic sleep patterns in the EEG (multiple sleep latency test) allow the diagnosis of narcolepsy (📕 see Conditions that resemble epilepsy, p.216).

Episodic episodes of abnormal nocturnal behaviour with normal EEG should raise the question of night terrors, benign myoclonus of drowsiness, sleep apnoea, or restless legs syndrome (📕 see Conditions that resemble epilepsy, pp.214–216).

Cerebral anoxic episodes can induce EEG changes and, conversely, epileptic seizures can be associated with autonomic changes including tachycardia, bradycardia, and asystole. Thus, the temporal relationship between EEG and ECG changes is crucial in determining the aetiology.

Similarly, EEG changes may occur in hypoglycaemia and hypocalcaemia, and a blood sample may be necessary to establish if metabolic abnormalities are a possible cause of the attacks.

Telemetry with EEG, ECG and sometimes polysomnography can establish the nature of the attacks in around 80% of patients.

Classification of seizures in known epilepsy

The distinction between focal and generalized seizures has implications for medical and surgical treatments. In patients where epilepsy has been confidently diagnosed by history and/or previous inter-ictal EEGs, video monitoring might be necessary to distinguish between absence seizures (spike-and-wave activity) and brief complex partial seizures (focal discharges or diffuse EEG slowing), or between generalized and secondarily GTCS.

Focus localization

Patients suffering from drug-resistant epilepsy may be suitable for surgical resective treatment if a single source is identified as the origin of the seizures. Video monitoring might be necessary to establish if there is a single focus and where it is (see Surgical assessment, pp.414–433). Recording of seizures is crucial, but the study of inter-ictal abnormalities might also be helpful. In focal seizures, scalp EEG changes at seizure onset might be lateralized, but more frequently they are bilateral and start after the onset of clinical manifestations. In a relatively small proportion of patients, intracranial electrodes are necessary to identify the focus.

Evaluation of clinical syndromes

A number of syndromes can be first identified, or their clinical manifestation fully characterized, after patients have been observed on video-EEG monitoring.

Subtle seizures

Video monitoring can establish the occurrence of seizures not previously recognized or thought to be infrequent, particularly if ictal signs are subtle or consisting of normal behaviour (blinking, head movement, smiling, etc.). Subtle events are a particularly frequent problem in neonates and young children who cannot report subjective symptoms, and in older children who are thought to under-perform at school because of suspected frequent absence seizures. Seizures with negative symptoms (aphasia, motor slowing) will not be identified during video telemetry unless the patient is kept active, often by talking to visitors or other patients. The epileptic nature of subtle seizures will only be established by a consistent association with EEG changes.

Estimation of seizure frequency

Estimation of seizure frequency with video-EEG monitoring can be used to adjust medication dosage and the regimen of administration, particularly if seizures are occurring frequently as is in absence epilepsies. In a minority of patients, estimation of seizure frequency may be necessary to establish the effects of surgical treatment.

Detection of precipitating factors

Poor response to treatment may be due to external factors precipitating seizures. These can be highly specific, such as in reflex epilepsies (flashing lights, visual patterns, eating, reading, music, calculation), or more general such as sleep deprivation, alcohol consumption, stress, emotion, or menstruation. While some patients have learnt to recognize these factors, in others it might be important to assess such potential precipitating factors. Sometimes ambulatory EEG might be necessary, since the situational factors may be rather specific. For instance, physiological as well as emotional factors can be involved in eating epilepsy, so that the patient may have seizures when eating at home and not at the hospital.

Self-induced seizures in reflex epilepsies might be difficult to recognize in part due to patients' reluctance to discuss their habit. This is particularly common in photosensitive epilepsy, where the proportion of patients who self-induce seizures may be as high as 30%. Manoeuvres used to trigger seizures can be rather subtle, such as slow eye closure with upwards deviation of the eyes, waving the outstretched fingers in front of the eyes while looking at a bright light, or gazing at striped patterns. Where there is doubt as to whether such manoeuvres are the precipitating factor or an ictal phenomenon, the dilemma can be solved by darkening the room, since patients will initially continue to perform the manoeuvre but seizures and EEG discharges no longer occur.

The role of cognition and neuropsychometric testing

Neuropsychology is the discipline that studies the relationship between brain and behaviour. In humans, neuropsychology is particularly concerned with the effects of pathological conditions on the skills, behaviour, and adjustment of the patient.

In epilepsy, the brain or parts of the brain are known to be dysfunctional, at least during seizures. It has gradually become clear that patients with epilepsy may also show a degree of brain dysfunction between seizures (inter-ictal).

The causes of inter-ictal brain dysfunction in epilepsy are probably multiple:

• Brain damage caused by the underlying lesion(s).
• Intermittent inter-ictal epileptiform discharges.
• Carry-on post-ictal effects from previous seizures.
• Effects of antiepileptic medication.
• Brain damage due to severe seizures or status epilepticus.

In neuropsychology, brain function can be assessed by asking patients to carry out psychological tests that measure specific mental tasks relating to verbal and visuospatial skills, memory, attention, and executive function. Many tests have been designed over the years to measure particular skills but the following, for example, are widely used:

• Wechsler Adult Intelligence scale-III (WAIS-III) to measure intellectual level, including general intelligence (intellectual quotient or IQ).
• Wechsler Memory Scale-III (WMS-III) to measure memory.

In these tests, the higher the scores the better the intellectual function or memory ability.

Neuropsychology and epilepsy

In general with neuropsychological scores lower:

• Patients are more likely in symptomatic or presumed symptomatic epilepsy.
• Early onset epilepsy.
• Longer duration of epilepsy.
• Epilepsy with higher seizures frequency and multiple seizure types.
• These associations can in part be explained because many patients with younger age of onset, longer duration of epilepsy, higher seizure frequency, and multiple seizure types suffer from symptomatic (or presumed symptomatic) generalized epilepsy with widespread brain damage.

Neuropsychology and laterality of epilepsy

Many neuropsychological tests include subtests to specifically measure verbal and non-verbal function. For example:

- WAIS-III Verbal IQ: estimates verbal intelligence.
- WAIS-III Performance IQ: estimates non-verbal intelligence.
- WAIS-III Full Scale IQ: estimates global intelligence and is usually calculated from the above two scores.
- WMS-III Logical Memory and Verbal Paired associates: estimates verbal memory.
- WMS-III Visual Reproduction: estimates visual (non-verbal) memory.

Discrepancies between verbal and non-verbal abilities can be used to lateralize brain dysfunction with the assumption that the hemisphere with relatively low scores is likely to be the hemisphere that generates seizures.

In patients with epilepsy, 96% of right-handed patients have language dominance in the left hemisphere. Consequently:

- Deficits in performance IQ or in visual memory suggests epilepsy arising in the right hemisphere.
- Deficits in verbal IQ or in logical (verbal) memory suggests epilepsy arising in the left hemisphere.

However, only about 70% of left handed patients with epilepsy have language dominance in the left hemisphere. Consequently, the relation between laterality of epilepsy and verbal/non-verbal function is less reliable.

In patients with early brain damage, the proportion of right- or left-handed people with left language dominance is reduced (approximately 80% for left- and 30% for right-side dominance).

Neuropsychology and treatment

- Medical and surgical treatment of epilepsy can affect memory and language. Thus, neuropsychological tests can be used to monitor the effects of treatment on brain function.
- The effect of treatment on memory and language is not always negative. Many patients improve neuropsychological scores after surgical treatment, particularly if the number of seizures and epileptiform discharges decrease after surgery, or if antiepileptic medication is reduced or withdrawn.
- Patients with higher pre-surgical scores show higher risk of neuropsychological deterioration after surgery.
- Patients with lower pre-surgical scores are more likely to improve after surgery.

Diagnosis of status epilepticus

- Status epilepticus can be defined as a situation where seizures occur repeatedly or persist for an extended period of time.
- For practical purposes, status epilepticus can be defined as the occurrence of a seizure lasting for >30min, or of two or more seizures without full recovery of consciousness between seizures lasting for a period >30min.
- Seizures of any type, if persisting for long or occurring sufficiently frequently, constitute status epilepticus.
- Status epilepticus can induce brain damage (particularly if convulsive) and should be managed as a medical emergency.

Types of status epilepticus

Status epilepticus can be classified according to the type of seizure involved:
- Generalized convulsive status epilepticus:
  - Primarily generalized.
  - Secondarily generalized.
- Focal convulsive status epileticus (epilepsia partialis continua)
- Other simple partial status epilepticus
- Complex partial status epilepticus
- Absence status epilepticus
- Clonic status epilepticus
- Tonic status epilepticus
- Myoclonic status epilepticus

Status epilepticus can also be classified according to whether the onset is focal or generalized:
- Partial (focal) status epilepticus: complex partial status, simple partial status, secondarily generalized convulsive status.
- Generalized status epilepticus: absence status, clonic status, tonic status, primarily generalized convulsive status.

Status epilepticus can also be classified according to the presence or absence of convulsions:
- Convulsive status epilepticus: generalized convulsive, clonic or tonic status epilepticus.
- Non-convulsive status epilepticus: complex partial, simple partial or absence status epilepticus.

Sometimes, in the absence of clinical symptoms or signs of seizures, EEG recordings show a persistent pattern identical to those patterns seen during seizures. This is called *electrical status epilepticus* or *subclinical status epilepticus*.

Convulsive status epilepticus

The diagnosis of convulsive status epilepticus is reasonably straight forward on the basis of clinical and EEG findings:
- The patient shows tonic, clonic or tonic–clonic convulsions, similar in nature to those that can be seen during individual seizures, but lasting for >30min. Convulsive movements might wax and wane without full patient recovery between bursts of convulsions.

- During clonic movements, the EEG shows regular generalized spike-and-wave activity, muscle activity and movement artefacts associated with each clonic jerk.
- Tonic convulsions are often associated with EEG flattening, diffuse fast activity, and muscle activity.
- It might be difficult to establish if convulsive status is primarily or secondarily generalized, as the onset may be witnessed or even if focal may not be evidently so. Classification usually relies on the epilepsy type that the patient suffer from, or on the presence of asymmetries in the clinical and electroencephalographic manifestations of the convulsions. The presence of persistent ictal or postictal asymmetries suggests a focal onset (secondarily generalized).
- In practice, the distinction between primarily or secondarily generalized convulsive status epilepticus is not essential, since medical management is similar.
- Commonly, status epilepticus occurs in patients with a history of epilepsy, but can also occur de novo in patients with no history of epilepsy, often after drug withdrawal or in the context of an acute neurological insult such as stroke.
- Caution: 'pseudostatus' may be misdiagnosed as convulsive status with secondary iatrogenic complications.

Non-convulsive status epilepticus

Non-convulsive status epilepticus can be classified into simple partial, complex partial, and absence status epilepticus.

The clinical manifestations of non-convulsive status epilepticus can resemble psychiatric illness. Once considered in the diagnosis an EEG recorded during the episode will usually establish the diagnosis of status.

Simple partial status epilepticus

Simple partial status epilepticus refers to continuous or repetitive focal seizures lasting for >30min without impairment of consciousness.

Clinical manifestations depend on the location of the focus. There may be:

- *Focal motor convulsions* (epilepsia partialis continua), if the focus is largely restricted to the primary motor cortex: most commonly affecting the hand and face since these are the body parts with the largest cortical representation.
- *Somatosensory sensations*, if the focus is restricted to the somatosensory cortex: unilateral tingling, numbness, burning sensations, most commonly the hand and face are involved, since these are the body parts with the largest cortical representation.
- *Visual sensations* if the focus mainly involves posterior cortex: flashing lights, vision of coloured circles, blindness(status epilepticus amauroticus), misperception of size, shape and colour of objects, structured visual hallucinations (seeing unreal scenes, objects, animals, or persons).
- *Auditory sensations* if the focus involves the auditory cortex: tones or melodies.
- *Taste*: often a 'metallic' taste. Common in temporal lobe foci.
- *Smell*: often a 'putrid' smell. Common in temporal foci.

- *Aphasia* in full consciousness (epileptic aphasia), if the focus involves speech areas. Speech arrest may also occur with arrest of activity in general in seizures secondary to other foci.
- *Autonomic symptoms*: rising epigastric sensation (often described as 'butterflies' in the stomach). Common in temporal lobe foci.
- *Psychic symptoms*: the most common psychic symptoms are fear and déjà vu. Sometimes they may consist of thought disorders or complex hallucinations. They can be seen in temporal or frontal lobe foci.

Symptoms can be prolonged, lasting for up to weeks or months, sometimes leading to a more overt seizure or cluster of seizures.

Prominent psychic symptoms during simple partial status may present as an affective or anxiety disorder, or psychosis, or may resemble those reported in various psychiatric disorders. When lasting for several hours or days, patients may become irritable or depressed to the extent of experiencing suicidal thoughts.

When presenting de novo with dysphasia, mutism, language disorder or structured visual hallucinations, schizophrenia may be considered before the diagnosis of status epilepticus is reached.

Blindness lasting for up to several days is a relatively common symptom of occipital focal status (status epilepticus amauroticus) and the EEG will prove valuable in differentiating it from hysterical blindness.

The EEG during simple partial status epilepticus may be no different from the inter-ictal EEG if the cortical area involved is small or deep, or may show unilateral rhythmic sharp waves, spike-and-wave activity, or slowing.

Complex partial status epilepticus (Fig. 3c.13)

Complex partial status was initially thought to be a rare manifestation of epilepsy. However, it is often under-recognized, particularly in the elderly.

Two clinical forms can be recognized:
- Discontinuous form: frequent recurring complex partial seizures with partial or almost full recovery of consciousness in between.
- Continuous form: a long lasting episode of mental confusion and/or psychotic behaviour.

Confusion is a cardinal clinical characteristic of complex partial status. The level of consciousness may vary from profound stupor with little response to external stimuli, to minimal impairment where only careful cognitive testing may show subtle deficits. Patients are usually, but not always, fully amnesic for the episode.

Motor manifestations are also common in complex partial status. Convulsive movements and tonic spasms may occur intermittently. Adversion of the head and eyes are common, may persist for hours, and result in some patients walking in circles. Automatisms (lip smacking, swallowing, gesturing, fiddling and wandering) are less common and usually not as prominent and structured as in isolated complex partial seizures.

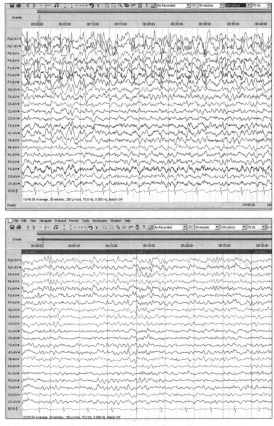

Fig. 3c.13 Non-convulsive (complex partial) status epilepticus. Patient with intractable focal seizures, age 46, who referred episodes of looking dazed and acting slow for several hours, occurring independently from his seizures. An EEG during one of these episodes showed continuous bilateral frontal slowing with superimposed frequent high-amplitude sharp, often rhythmic, epileptiform discharges, confirming that they are periods of status epilepticus (top). The EEG in the absence of these episodes shows much less slowing and no frequent discharges (bottom).

Occasionally, prolonged ambulatory episodes can resemble psychogenic fugues. Behavioural changes range from agitation, excitation, and occasional mania to severe psychomotor retardation and stupor. The patient may appear alert but rather sluggish or restless. This may manifest as delay in reactions and slowness of thought and/or speech. Speech may also be qualitatively abnormal, with marked perseveration, confabulation, echolalia, repetitive utterances or stereotyped responses. The patient may respond to simple commands, often in an automatic fashion, and can be guided to sit or walk.

Various psychotic symptoms can be present, including inaccessibility, complex visual or auditory hallucinations, delusions, ideas of reference, paranoia, thought disorders, and illogical responses. Severe catatonia is very rare, but mild degrees are common. Anxiety, depression, or dreamy states with altered perception of time or space can occur. Even in patients with chronic epilepsy, misdiagnosis of complex partial status as a psychiatric disorder may occur and some patients have long histories of repeated psychiatric hospital admissions and chronic treatment with antipsychotic drugs (which can decrease seizure threshold) before status is identified.

An ictal EEG obtained at least once during episodes of status is necessary to confirm the diagnosis. The range of abnormalities in complex partial status is wide. Experience, correlation with clinical state and comparison with inter-ictal EEG are required for assessment. Scalp EEG findings, although seldom normal, may be similar qualitatively to those seen in the inter-ictal record for the same patient, particularly if inter-ictal abnormalities are prominent. More often variable widespread changes can be seen, usually bilateral. Ictal patterns include continuous or frequent spikes, sharp waves, spike-and-wave, periodic electrodecremental events, or a significant excess of bilateral slow activity.

Absence status epilepticus

Occasionally absence seizures may be prolonged or may present in frequent clusters without clear cognitive recovery for several minutes to hours (absence status epilepticus).

Absence status epilepticus is more common in children.

Two main types of absence status epilepticus can be distinguished:

- *Typical absence status (petit mal status)*: consisting of runs of typical absence seizures (spike-wave activity at 2.5–3.5Hz), occurring in the syndrome of primary generalized epilepsy.
- *Atypical absence status*: consisting of runs of atypical absence seizures (spike-wave activity at <2.5Hz), occurring largely in symptomatic/cryptogenic generalized epilepsies, such as Lennox–Gastaut syndrome.

The two types are not always easily distinguishable on clinical grounds, and the EEG and clinical context are helpful in differentiating between them.

Between 2.6–9.4% of children with absence epilepsy or with 3/sec spike-and-wave activity on the EEG have a history of absence status.

The cardinal clinical manifestation of absence status is a variable degree of clouding of consciousness. Interestingly, in contrast to isolated absence seizures, consciousness may be only partially impaired during absence status, giving rise to symptoms resembling psychiatric conditions (as described for complex partial status).

In cases with a lesser degree of impairment in consciousness, the patient may only show slowed thinking and speech, poor concentration, and little if any amnesia. Surprisingly, such mild behavioural changes can take place in the context of continuous generalized spike-and-wave activity and formal psychometric testing may be necessary to disclose mild cognitive deficits.

In contrast to complex partial status, verbal abilities may be relatively preserved in absence status.

Patients with more severe symptoms may appear immobile, mute, sluggish, with delayed response to simple commands which may require repeated requests. They may appear expressionless or puzzled, their eyes partially closed, or as if in a trance. Automatisms may occur although less frequently than in complex partial status. Amnesia is common but may be fragmentary, with short patches of recall that may lead to a diagnosis of dementia. Other patients may show severe somnolence and lethargy (epileptic stupor), remaining immobile, their eyes closed and rolled upwards, with little spontaneous motor activity, reacting only to painful stimuli, unable to feed and incontinent. Such cases can be mistaken for a catatonic state.

About half of patients with absence status show motor manifestations such as myoclonus, atonia, eyelid fluttering, lip quivering, grimacing, or smiling. Facial myoclonus (especially involving the eyelid) occurs frequently in absence status but is rare in complex partial status. Termination of typical absence status with a tonic–clonic convulsive seizure may occur. Psychotic manifestations can occur but are neither as frequent nor as severe as in complex partial status.

The EEG is characteristic and frequently diagnostic in absence status. In typical absence status, continuous or almost continuous bilaterally synchronous and symmetrical spike-and-wave activity occur at 2.5–3.5Hz, with little or no response to sensory stimulation. In atypical absence status, continuous or almost continuous generalized spike-and-wave activity occur at <2.5Hz. Other electroencephalographic variants have been described such as irregular and slower spike-wave activity (<2.5Hz), prolonged intermittent bursts of spike-and-wave activity, generalized polyspike, and polyspike-wave activity at 2–6Hz. The degree of impairment in consciousness does not appear to correlate strongly with the type of EEG abnormality.

Status in patients with learning difficulties

Non-convulsive status epilepticus is particularly under-diagnosed in individuals with learning disabilities as it may manifest only as changes in affect, behaviour, or subtle cognitive deterioration. In addition, patients may suffer from on-going symptoms that resemble non-convulsive status, such as incontinence, cognitive deterioration due to AED toxicity, behavioural disturbances, automatic movements, and non-epileptic seizures. Episodic behaviour such as aggression, auto-mutilation, and masturbation or self gratification may present problems of differential diagnosis from epilepsy.

Atypical absence status, subclinical status and tonic status occur more frequently in patients with learning difficulty than in other populations. Generalized tonic–clonic, as well as simple and complex partial status epilepticus may also be more common in this population.

Ring chromosome 20 presents with epilepsy associated with variable learning difficulty and a tendency to non-convulsive status epilepticus, either complex partial or absence.

Epilepsy with status epilepticus during slow sleep (ESES)

ESES is defined as the presence of continuous generalized spike-and-wave activity during >85% of slow wave sleep. The term ESES is usually given to the electrical abnormality seen on the EEG. When combined with the clinical presentation, the syndrome may be known as continuous spike wave of slow sleep (CSWS). The clinical presentation may vary. Those with predominantly a regression in language often have a temporal emphasis on the EEG and a clinical presentation of Landau–Kleffner syndrome. Others with a more frontal emphasis may present with more global regression in cognitive ability. Overt seizures may be rare. It is one of the few situations where treatment is aimed at the EEG abnormality and requires careful monitoring.

Whatever the underlying disorder, long persistence of ESES tends to be associated with severe neuropsychological impairment.

The neuropsychological deficits may be secondary to the disruption of normal sleep, to the epileptogenic process and/or to the underlying aetiology.

Landau–Kleffner syndrome

Landau–Kleffner syndrome is a rare but fascinating childhood disorder that presents with acquired aphasia (starting after the child has already experienced a period of normal language development). The EEG may demonstrate one of several abnormalities, which range from ESES to multifocal epileptiform discharges in the awake EEG, more prominent over the temporal, parietal, and occipital regions.

Aphasia appears to be related to verbal auditory agnosia, which is followed by a reduction in spontaneous oral expression. During the early aphasic stage the child still communicates by gestures, but later all social interaction is lost, the child's behaviour often resembling those of autistic children. The behavioural difficulties demonstrated are often the most challenging part of management.

The nature of the relationship between discharges and the aphasia is much debated. The epileptiform discharges and aphasia may be epiphenomena related to the same underlying cause, or, alternatively, dysphasia may be a direct consequence of focal discharges involving speech areas. The aphasia may be reversed by treatment of the epilepsy; this may be medical with AED such as steroids, benzodiazepines, lamotrigine or levetiracetam. In resistant cases improvement may be seen with surgery (perisylvian multiple subpial transections deep into the Sylvian fissure), which supports an epileptic origin of the aphasia.

Angelman syndrome

Angelman syndrome is characterized by learning disabilities, profound speech delay, wide mouth, pointed chin, prominent jaw, ataxia, jerky movements (similar to those of puppets), affectionate nature and unprovoked episodes of laughter (thus the term 'happy puppet syndrome'). Neuroimaging usually shows no abnormality with the exception of occasional cerebral atrophy. The syndrome is associated with deletion of 15q11–13 on the maternally-inherited chromosome.

Severe EEG abnormalities are seen in Angelman syndrome: slow background activity, prolonged runs of high amplitude rhythmic delta of larger amplitude anteriorly with superimposed ill defined bursts of spike-and-wave activity and spikes superimposed on delta activity, mainly posteriorly, particularly with eyes closed. Such EEG abnormalities are often interpreted as epileptiform discharges and children are often treated with large doses of AEDs without benefit.

Patients often fail to establish eye contact and have short attention span. Usually the EEG during these episodes is not different from that seen at other times. Nevertheless, occasionally EEGs taken during periods when patients appear 'out of touch' may show features of non-convulsive status epilepticus which may respond, both clinically and electroencephalographically, to AEDs.

Seizures are common in this syndrome, affecting about 90% of individuals, about half of whom are refractory to AED treatment.

Status epilepticus in the elderly

Non-convulsive status epilepticus is common in the elderly and often manifests as confusion. This often occurs de novo in the elderly, secondary to electrolyte imbalance, treatment with psychotropic drugs, or withdrawal of benzodiazepines. Neuroimaging is mandatory, since de novo status epilepticus may be the first manifestation of tumours or undetected strokes. The diagnosis, once considered, is confirmed on EEG.

Diagnostic considerations

- EEG patterns seen in the different forms of status have been described above. Convulsive status epilepticus can often be diagnosed clinically by observing the patient's movements. An urgent EEG during status confirms the diagnosis.
- An urgent EEG is usually definitive in differentiating between non-convulsive status epilepticus and acute psychotic episodes or delirium in a patient who suddenly shows a state of mild-to-moderate cognitive impairment, partial responsiveness, confusion, or apathy.
- The scalp EEG can be normal or abnormal in simple partial status.
- A sleep EEG showing electrical status will support the diagnosis of certain epileptic syndromes such as Landau-Kleffner syndrome and ESES.

Conditions that resemble epilepsy

Because the cardinal symptoms of epilepsy ('the epileptic seizures') are relatively infrequent events in most patients, the health professional will seldom be able to diagnose epilepsy on the basis of direct observation of seizures. This means that when confronted with events that could be seizures, the most crucial part of the evaluation is the history taken from the patient and from witnesses to the events.

• *What to do:* you need a careful history. If the patient is unconscious, dysphasic, confused, or unaware of the details related to the event, ask a relative, friend, or any other potential witness. If none are present, use the telephone. If there are old hospital notes, look at them and summarize useful information.

• *What to avoid:* try not to rely on history from the patient alone. Often patients have limited memory of the events due to loss of consciousness. Some patients may not know they had an event at all.

Video recording of the events is usually invaluable, even if handheld or low in quality. Any event occurring suddenly (paroxysmal) and lasting for a few seconds to several hours can be mistaken for epileptic seizures. (Box 3c.3).

> **Box 3c.3 Transient episodes that can simulate epileptic seizures**
>
> *Loss of consciousness:* syncope, cardiac disorders, transient cerebral ischaemia, microsleeps, panic attacks, hypoglycaemia, non-epileptic seizures, head injury, drug and alcohol abuse, Arnold–Chiari malformation, tumours of the third ventricle.
>
> *Resembling generalized convulsions:* syncope with secondary jerking, movement disorders, hyperekplexia, non-epileptic seizures.
>
> *Resembling focal convulsions:* tics, transient cerebral ischaemia, tonic spasms of multiple sclerosis, movement disorders.
>
> *Drop attacks (sudden falls):* cardiovascular disorders (syncope, Stokes–Adams attacks, transient brainstem ischaemia or vertebro-basilar insufficiency, prolonged Q–T syndrome), movement disorders (hyperekplexia, Steele–Richardson–Olszewski syndrome, Parkinson's disease, multi-system atrophy, paroxysmal kinesogenic choreoathetosis, subcortical myoclonus), brainstem and spinal abnormalities (Arnold–Chiari malformation, cervical disc disease, spinal angioma), lower limb abnormalities (cauda equina disease), third ventricle tumours, vestibular disorders, cataplexy, metabolic disorders (hypokalemia, hyponatraemia), idiopathic drop attacks, non-epileptic seizures.
>
> *Focal sensory attacks:* transient ischaemic attacks (TIAs), transient vestibular symptoms.

Facial and eye movements: movement disorders, cranial nerve disorders, blindness, tics.

Psychic experiences: migraine, panic attacks, post-traumatic flashbacks, hallucinations and illusions due to sensory loss or psychosis, non-epileptic seizures.

Aggressive outbursts.

Prolonged confusional states and fugues: non-convulsive status epilepticus, acute encephalopathy, acute psychosis, transient global amnesia, hysterical fugue.

Sleep phenomena: normal movements, fragmentary myoclonus, non-REM parasomnias, REM parasomnias, sleep apnoea, other sleep movements.

Syncope (fainting)

Syncope is the most common cause of brief episodes of loss of consciousness.

Definition

Syncope consists of a sudden loss of consciousness and muscle tone due to brain hypoperfusion associated to a sudden drop in BP. The patient falls to the ground due to loss of muscle tone.

Mechanisms and precipitants

Simple faints (vasovagal syncope) are due to an excess of vagal autonomic tone resulting in a drop in BP. Vasovagal syncope is often related to clear precipitants: getting up quickly, standing for prolonged periods, particularly if associated with factors that induce vasodilation (hot and stuffy environments, crowded rooms or trains), drug or alcohol use. Syncopal attacks can also be induced by Valsalva procedures (coughing, straining), emotional stress, frightening or unpleasant scenes especially involving blood, painful stimuli, and 'sight of needles or blood'. Micturition syncope most often occurs in older patients suffering from prostatic hypertrophy. Syncope can also occur while sitting or lying.

Clinical manifestations of syncope

Syncope attacks often begin with clouding of consciousness, lightheadedness, imbalance, nausea, and waxy-pale skin. Immediately before the fall, some patients experience ringing in the ears and their vision 'going black' or 'grey'. Loss of consciousness is usually brief, lasting for about 10sec. The brief duration is due to quick recovery of BP and cerebral blood perfusion due to the patient falling to a horizontal position. If a horizontal position cannot be reached, such as when patients are sitting in an armchair or standing in a crowded place or telephone booth, re-assumption of cerebral circulation is slower and convulsive syncope can occur due to hypoxia. Convulsive syncope has similar onset but is followed by a tonic spasm (the back, head, and legs bend backwards while the fists are clenched). This is can be associated with nystagmus, midriasis, drooling, and incontinence. Tongue biting rarely occurs. Syncope can also be associated with brief myoclonic twitches that are often under-recognized, or with more prominent jerking, often leading to misdiagnosis as an epileptic seizure.

Differential diagnosis

The differential features between syncope and epileptic seizures are summarized in Table 3c.1.

- Epilepsy and syncope can occur in adults or children, and there may be family history in both.
- Loss of vision is uncommon in epileptic seizures. It can rarely be seen in occipital epilepsies—ictal and post-ictal amaurosis.
- Syncopal attacks tend to be much shorter than epileptic seizures with the exception of absence attacks, which can last for only a few seconds. However, this seizure type is rarely mistaken with syncope, since falls do not usually occur.
- Heart rate changes can occur in epileptic seizures due to autonomic changes associated with seizures. Asystole is exceedingly rare in epileptic seizures but can occur as part of ictal semiology.
- Myoclonic jerks are not infrequently seen in syncope and are often mistaken for epilepsy. In contrast to what is seen in tonic–clonic seizures, jerking in syncope is sporadic, irregular, lasting for a few seconds.
- Following a syncopal attack, pallor may be replaced by flushing and sweating.
- In syncope, consciousness is usually quickly recovered (within a minute or two). A long period of confusion after the episode would suggest an epileptic seizure (post-ictal confusion). A very useful question is to ask the patient what they remembered on first coming around. If circumstances are very different before loss of consciousness compared to when coming around (for instance, coming around in an ambulance), it can be assumed that the duration of loss of consciousness was relatively long, suggesting a seizure with a period of post-ictal confusion which can last for many minutes.
- Syncopal attacks occurring in the toilet tend not to be witnessed, and the patient may be prevented from lying down within the confined space of the toilet. If witnesses arrive after hearing the fall, there might be little to see or the patient may suffer jerks leading to the erroneous diagnosis of epilepsy.

Table 3c.1 Differential diagnosis between syncopal attacks and epileptic seizures

Feature	Seizures	Syncope
Immediate precipitant factors	Rare, present in reflex epilepsies, hyperventilation in absences	Frequent—heat, Valsalva, drug abuse, alcohol, pain, sight of blood
Warning	Specific motor, sensory or psychic auras, blackout of vision rarely seen (occasional in occipital seizures)	Lightheadedness, dizziness, nausea, ear ringing, blackout of vision
Muscle tone	Usually normal or increased, decreased in atonic seizures	Decreased if not convulsive, although increase tone and irregular jerking can occur
Duration	1–2min, only few seconds in absences, some tonic or atonic seizures.	10sec—longer if patient is prevented from lying
Occurrence during sleep	Common, particularly in frontal lobe seizures	Rare
Incontinence	Frequent	Rare
Tongue biting or injury	Common in convulsive seizures	Not likely
Skin colour	Flushed or pale	Pale, can be sheet white
Respiration	Apnoea and gasping if convulsive	Slow unless caused by hyperventilation
Perspiration	Hot, sweaty	Cold, clammy
EEG during event	Slowing often asymmetrical, spike-wave, sharp waves	Non-specific diffuse slow
EEG between events	Epileptiform discharges in 50–80%	Normal
ECG	Heart rate changes frequent, most commonly sinus tachycardia	Abnormal—arrhythmia, premature ventricular contraction, asystole
Post-confusion	Frequent	Rare

Cardiac disorders

Transient arrhythmias can cause episodes of abrupt loss of consciousness. They may show initial symptoms similar to those seen in syncope in addition to palpitations, chest pain, short of breath, and signs of cardiac insufficiency. These episodes may be associated with secondary epileptic seizures due to anoxia. The duration and severity of the attacks depend on the arrhythmia.

- Stokes–Adams attacks: due to transient complete heart block an abrupt and brief loss of consciousness with extreme pallor followed by flushing can occur, usually lasting for <1min, sometimes with associated confusion. The ECG often shows conduction block. Similar attacks can be due to ventricular tachycardia and ventricular fibrillation.
- Aortic stenosis and hypertrophic obstructive cardiomyopathy: can present with episodes of loss of consciousness, sometimes with focal neurological signs, due to brain hypoperfusion, particularly during exercise.
- Prolonged Q–T syndrome: can mimic idiopathic epilepsy. This is a serious condition associated with prolonged repolarization of the cardiac ventricles which can lead to ventricular fibrillation, syncope, and sudden death. Any child with unexplained episodes of loss of consciousness should have an ECG, particularly if there is family history, or if attacks are induced by exercise, fright or excitement.

Patients with unexplained blackouts should have detailed cardiovascular evaluation, including baseline ECG, 24-hour ECG, chest X-Ray and echocardiogram. Tilt-table tests and implantable loop recorders may also be considered.

Transient cerebral ischaemia

- The term transient ischaemic attacks (TIAs) refers to a situation where the blood supply to a region of the brain, is temporarily decreased for longer than a few seconds.
- Relevance: transient cerebral ischaemia can generate symptoms that simulate epileptic seizures and may be the cause of true epileptic seizures and epilepsy due to anoxia or to secondary cortical scaring.
- Mechanisms: transient cerebral ischaemia might be a consequence of impaired cardiac output, or may be due to focal cerebrovascular disease due to thrombosis, emboli, or haemorrhage. If due to impaired cardiac output, it usually causes loss of consciousness lasting for longer than a few seconds. If due to focal cerebrovascular disease, it can cause sensory, motor, speech, vestibular, or memory symptoms that can resemble simple partial seizures.
- Manifestations: in general, focal neurological symptoms in cerebrovascular disease tend to be negative (paralysis, loss of sensation, speech arrest) although paraesthesiae can also occur. Symptoms are not as stereotypical as in epileptic seizures. Involuntary movements can be seen if basal ganglia ischaemia is present. TIAs can last from a few minutes to 24 hours. If TIAs are suspected, a source for emboli should be sought (e.g. atrial fibrillation or carotid atheroma).

- Sudden drop attacks can occur in the elderly with vertebrovascular ischaemia. Attacks may be associated with head turning or neck extension. There may be signs of brainstem ischaemia (diplopia, vertigo, bilateral sensory or motor deficits in face and limbs).
- Differential diagnosis:
  - *Features that suggest seizures:* onset of attacks in childhood, loss of consciousness, automatisms, pos-tictal confusion or headache, hemianopia, scotoma, positive visual symptoms (flashing lights, coloured forms), duration <3min (although simple partial status can last for several hours), epileptiform discharges on the EEG.
  - *Features that suggest TIAs:* duration >3min, monocular blindness, signs or symptoms suggesting carotid artery distribution (hemiparesis, hemisensory loss, unilateral neglect, aphasia without loss of consciousness), signs or symptoms suggesting vertebral artery distribution (vertigo, dysarthria, deafness, diplopia, dysphagia, fall), cardiovascular risk factors (atrial fibrillation or carotid bruit or weak pulse, may also be present in the elderly with seizures), negative symptoms (paralysis, loss of sensation, speech arrest) normal inter-ictal EEG or absence of epileptiform discharges.

Non-epileptic seizures

Synonyms

Pseudoseizures, psychogenic seizures, (psychogenic) non-epileptic attack disorder, dissociative seizures. The terms 'pseudoseizure' and 'non-epileptic attack disorder' refer to psychogenic non-epileptic seizures. The term 'non-epileptic seizures' is sometimes used to refer to all attacks that can be mistaken with epilepsy, whether psychological or organic in origin. Nevertheless, the term 'non-epileptic seizure' is often used as a convenient shorthand for episodes with a psychological origin and this convention will be followed here.

Thus, in this chapter, non-epileptic seizures are defined as episodes of abnormal behaviour, due to a psychiatric disorder that may be mistaken for epilepsy but are not accompanied by any significant change in EEG brain activity. Broadly, they that can take two forms:
- Motor attacks: shaking and flailing of limbs, head and/or body.
- Motionless attacks: lying immobile, floppy, unresponsive or partially responsive.

Pathophysiology

Most often they are due to a psychiatric conversion disorder and are referred to as dissociative seizures. Less commonly they represent deliberate (conscious) attempts to feign illness. In this situation, a distinction is made between factitious disorder (Munchausen's syndrome) and malingering. In factitious disorder the motivation for simulating illness reflects an abnormal psychological desire to be ill and receive medical attention. This contrasts with malingering (not a medical diagnosis), a term used to refer to deliberate simulation of illness motivated by a desire to achieve some obvious practical gain (e.g. to obtain insurance compensation or benefits, or to avoid prison or military service).

Differential diagnosis

Table 3c.2 shows a summary of the features found useful in distinguishing between epileptic and (dissociative) non-epileptic attacks.

- In contrast to epileptic seizures, non-epileptic attacks are usually, but not always, prolonged, lasting for several minutes or hours.
- Non-epileptic attacks are more common in females but can occur in males. They usually start in adolescence or young adulthood (often later in males).
- There might be an obvious reason for secondary gains, but often it is hidden within a more complex psychological basis.
- Patients often have a history of unexplained medical presentations (such as abdominal pain, sometimes leading to surgery), childhood abuse, and poor response to AEDs.
- The diagnosis of non-epileptic seizures should be considered in patients with drug resistant attacks and repeatedly normal EEGs (or with mild non-specific abnormalities).
- Motor non-epileptic seizures can be particularly difficult to distinguish from complex partial seizures of frontal origin, where there are often bizarre frantic movements, occasionally with some retained awareness, few ictal EEG changes that can be unidentifiable among the profuse muscle and movement artefacts, and no post-ictal confusion.
- If seizures occur most weeks, video-telemetry is the best diagnostic test. More details on how to distinguish epileptic from non-epileptic psychogenic attacks can be found in 🕮 Role of video monitoring— video-telemetry, intensive monitoring, pp.191–193.
- Often home videos of the attacks filmed by the relatives can be most useful in assisting diagnosis.

Activation methods

It is commonly accepted that inpatient video-telemetry is the ultimate tool for seizure classification. In the context of identifying and classifying non-epileptic seizures, verbal suggestion and/or intravenous saline injections, both in an inpatient or outpatient setting, with prolonged video EEG monitoring is effective. In an outpatient setting, it could yield a success rate of 50% of capturing or provoking non-epileptic seizures, and thus ultimately establishing the diagnosis without requiring a hospital admission.[1,2] Using intravenous saline injection as a provocation method increases the yield of capturing non epileptic seizures by 30% in the inpatient setting.[3,4] To avoid misdiagnosis, careful history taking and reviewing the 'seizures' in question with the patient and relatives is of utmost importance.

References

1. McGonigal A, Oto M, Russell AJ, et al. (2002). Outpatient video EEG recording in the diagnosis of non-epileptic seizures: a randomised controlled trial of simple suggestion techniques. *Journal of Neurology, Neurosurgery and Psychiatry*, 72, 549–51.

2. Dericioğlu N, Saygi S, and Ciğer A (1999), The value of provocation methods in patients suspected of having non-epileptic seizures. *Seizure*, 8, 152–6.

3. Bazil CW, Kothari M, Luciano D et al. (1994) Provocation of nonepileptic seizures by suggestion in a general seizure population. *Epilepsia*, 35, 768–70.

4. Ribaï P, Tugendhaft P, and Legros B (2006). Usefulness of prolonged video-EEG monitoring and provocative procedure with saline injection for the diagnosis of non epileptic seizures of psychogenic origin. *Journal of Neurology*, 253(3), 328–32.

Table 3c.2 Differential diagnosis between epileptic and psychogenic non-epileptic attacks

Feature	Epileptic	Non-epileptic
Immediate triggers	Rare, except in reflex epilepsies, hyperventilation for absence seizures	Emotional experiences and stress (some-times apparent to carers, but often denied by patients), sometimes suggestion (photic stimulation, injection)
Other triggers	Sleep deprivation, stress, drugs	See above
Attacks when alone or asleep	Common	Less common—actually around 10%
Stereotypical attacks	Very stereotypical within the same seizure type	Sometimes, often affected by environment.
Onset	Sudden	Brief or gradual build-up over minutes
Aura if present	Various but stereotypical for each patient	Feeling of detachment (derealization), hyperventilation, palpitations, headache, dizziness, variable
Sounds and speech	Mumble, cry, grunt, stereotyped words or sentences in automatisms	Sometimes voluntary speech, but with low voice, sometimes unintelligible
Movements	Tonic, atonic, clonic (regular, repetitive, with sudden contraction followed by gradual relaxation, symmetrically synchronous if bilateral)	Irregular, wax and wane, asymmetrical, non-physiological, flailing, pelvic thrusting, opisthotonous, semi-purpose movements
Injury	Common from sudden falls, tongue biting (usually lateral)	Serious injury rare from falls or tongue biting (if present, usually tip of tongue)
Loss of consciousness and responsiveness	In absence, tonic, tonic-clonic or complex partial seizures. Partial responsiveness may be present in complex partial seizures	Variable, often partial response to motor commands
Incontinence	Common	Less common (10%)
Duration	Variable, often 1–2min, unless it goes into status epilepticus	Typically prolonged: minutes to hours
Ictal EEG	Abnormal except in some simple partial or frontal seizures or when excessive artefacts	Normal. Normal alpha activity while unresponsive

(Continued)

Table 3c.2 Differential diagnosis between epileptic and psychogenic non-epileptic attacks (*continued*)

Feature	Epileptic	Non-epileptic
Recovery	Sudden in absence seizures and frontal lobe complex partial seizures. Otherwise, often followed by confusion, splitting headache, tiredness and sleepiness in complex partial and tonic-clonic seizures. Loss of memory during the attack in other than simple partial seizures or myoclonic jerks.	Variable, often faster than expected from the duration of the attack, usually no postictal confusion or severe headache. Tearful. May have memory of events during period of unresponsiveness.
Serum prolactin	Elevated after 91% of tonic–clonic	Normal
Eyes	Usually open	Usually closed

Panic attacks

Panic attacks can resemble temporal lobe seizures in that they start with a feeling of fear or anxiety, autonomic changes, epigastric sensation, tachycardia, and hyperventilation. Hyperventilation can lead to lightheadedness, dizziness, oral and bilateral hand or facial paraesthesia, carpopedal spasms, blurred vision, and nausea. In contrast to epileptic seizures, loss of consciousness is rare and paraesthesias are usually bilateral, although they can be asymmetrical. There is usually a clear precipitant (recall of a distressing experience, being in a confined or crowded place) but not always. Cognitive symptoms of anxiety (e.g. fear of choking, suffocating, dying) are characteristic of panic attacks and are rarely a conspicuous feature in epileptic seizures. Panic attacks tend to be longer (several minutes) than seizures (<2min), with symptoms settling down more gradually.

Sleep phenomena

History taking of sleep phenomena is often difficult because patients can have little or no recollection of the events and there might not be witnesses. Overnight EEG recording, often with video monitoring, might be necessary to establish the diagnosis. The following phenomena may resemble epileptic seizures but the EEG is normal during the attacks:

- Normal sleep phenomena: hypnagogic jerks are prominent myoclonic jerks involving most limbs and body, commonly occur in normal subjects when falling asleep. More focal myoclonic jerks (fragmentary myoclonus), involving face, hands and legs, occur during stages 1, 2, and REM sleep. Periodic limb movements of sleep consist of a dorsiflexion of the ankle and great toe associated with flexion of the knee and hip, lasting for a few seconds, and occurring repeatedly every 5–90sec. They tend to occur in clusters over several minutes in light sleep. Their incidence increases with age, affecting perhaps half of the elderly.
- Restless leg syndrome: characterized by an urge to move the legs, particularly in the evenings when lying or sitting. It tends to start in middle to old age except for the familial form, with onset in adolescent

or early adulthood. Most patients with restless leg syndrome also have periodic limb movements of sleep.

- Non-REM parasomnias (night terrors and sleep walking): usually present in childhood or adolescent, often associated with family history. They tend to occur in sleep stages 1 or 2, usually between 30min and 4 hours after going to sleep. Attacks are relatively infrequent, often spaced out by months or years. They seldom occur more that once a week and rarely more than once in a night. They are more likely when sleeping in a strange bed. They may be associated with incontinence and self-injury but seldom with directed aggression. Most patients grow out of these episodes. There are two types:
  - Night terrors: patients look fearful or terrified, sometimes scream, and appear panic stricken and confused, for several minutes before falling back to sleep. Patients show profuse autonomic changes (tachypnoea, diaphoresis, dilated pupils, flushing, sweating, palpitations) and are difficult to arouse during the episodes. Vocalization (uttering words or sentences) occurs frequently. The patient may recall a frightening scene after the attack. Onset between age 4–12 years.
  - Sleep walking: the patient may sit up in bed, fidget or play with objects, resembling a complex partial seizure, but the EEG is normal during these attacks. In more severe episodes, patients may get out of bed, walk about in a trance and carry out complex tasks such as dressing, opening doors, go up or down stairs, eating, or sleep talking. Patients may respond to questions during the attack, usually in a slow monosyllabic fashion, and it may be possible to lead them back to sleep without awakening. There is no memory of the attacks.
- REM parasomnias: during these episodes, patients may flail their limbs, cry out words or names, or display violent behaviour, sometimes appearing to act a vivid dream, lasting for a few seconds to minutes. They may resemble frontal complex partial seizures. They usually present during middle age or in the elderly, particularly in males. They tend to occur in the second half of the night, where REM sleep is more common. They may occur in healthy subjects, associated with drug consumption (tricyclics, alcohol), or in disorders affecting REM sleep such as multisystemic atrophy. REM parasomnias may precede the diagnosis or presentation of such late onset degenerative disorders.
- Sleep apnoea: patients usually complain of daytime sleepiness. Nevertheless, episodes of nocturnal apnoea may be associated with grunting or restlessness, simulating nocturnal complex partial seizures. Occasionally, cerebral hypoxia associated with these episodes may lead to true seizures.
- Movement disorders: although typically movement disorders remit during sleep, occasionally the abnormal movements may be seen during sleep, apparently in association with brief arousals. Nocturnal body and head rocking can be sometimes seen in patients with learning disabilities.

Daytime sleepiness and microsleeps

- Sleep deprivation can lead to loss of consciousness in the form of daytime naps, sometimes lasting as little as a few seconds, occasionally resembling absence attacks.

- In some patients, a history of poor or little sleep would suggest the diagnosis, such as in shift workers.
- In patients with obstructive sleep apnoea a history of poor sleep is sometimes difficult to obtain. It should be suspected in obese patients with short broad necks and history of snoring.
- More rarely, with sudden short daytime naps may be due to narcolepsy.

Cataplexy

Cataplexic attacks consist of a sudden loss of muscle tone induced by emotion, particularly laughter. There is no loss of consciousness. They can be subtle, involving the neck muscles with forward drop of the head, or more severe, with buckling of the knees and collapse to the ground. They often occur in the context of narcolepsy. Narcolepsy is a neurological condition characterized by excessive daytime sleepiness manifesting as sudden and unavoidable episodes of sleep. During the day, the patient may fall asleep anywhere at any time, creating significant work and social difficulties. In addition, symptoms of narcolepsy, which may not occur in all patients, are cataplexy, sleep paralysis, hypnogogic hallucinations and going into REM sleep immediately after falling asleep.

Head injury

Head injury can cause loss of consciousness with associated amnesia. If there is not a known external cause for an accidental head injury, the patient should be fully evaluated, since the accident might be secondary to an initial loss of consciousness due to other causes including epilepsy.

Neurological causes of loss of consciousness and drop attacks

Episodes of loss of consciousness and falls can be due to subcortical abnormalities affecting the structures that regulate cortical excitability, such as in Arnold–Chiari malformation which can affect the brainstem, or tumours of the third ventricle. An MRI scan including views of the foramen magnum is required if such abnormalites are suspected. Vascular malformations of the spinal cord and cauda equina lesions can be associated with lower limb weakness and falls without loss of consciousness, often after exercise.

Movement disorders and stereotypies

Movement disorders tend to show fairly stable symptomatology and do not usually occur as brief paroxysmal attacks. In severe stages, movement disorders can induce falls that can resemble drop attacks. Symptoms are then so prominent that the diagnosis of the specific movement disorder is usually clear.

Genuine paroxysmal movement disorders are rare and often familial. The hallmark in the differential diagnosis is that movement disorders show no disturbance of consciousness, since they are essentially subcortical in origin. The following movement disorders can occasionally be misdiagnosed as epilepsy:

- Paroxysmal kinesogenic choreoathetosis: attacks start in childhood or adolescent, they last from a few seconds to <2min, can occur in clusters and are usually triggered by certain movements. As in seizures, the abnormal movements in paroxysmal kinesogenic choreoathetosis can be unilateral or bilateral and are stereotypical within each patient, but vary considerably from patient to patient. If unilateral, the attacks may resemble focal motor epileptic seizures. If lower limbs are involved, falls can occur, resembling epileptic drop attacks. Inter-ictal and ictal scalp EEG recordings are normal. There is often family history of the condition, since if is usually autosomal dominant. It is most unusual for epileptic seizures to be induced by movements.

- Paroxysmal dystonia: attacks are longer, lasting for minutes to hours and are often induced by alcohol, caffeine or exercise.
- Idiopathic torsion dystonia and Wilson's disease: patients may suffer acute exacerbations, which can simulate convulsive movements.
- Chorea: movements occur randomly and persistently, affecting multiple muscle groups. Movements are not as fast, repetitive and stereotypical as epileptic tonic or clonic movements, which tend to affect the same muscle groups. Seizures lack the continuous flow of movement that is so distinctive of chorea.
- Tetanus: it is now very rare. After an incubation period of around 1 week, the patient shows lethargy, spasms of face, neck and body, followed by persistent rigidity of all limbs, neck, and body.
- Stereotypies in patients with learning disability: these stereotyped movements include head banging, body rocking, and more subtle movements that can be difficult to distinguish from the automatisms seen in complex partial seizures. They tend to occur in daytime, but occasionally can be seen during sleep. EEG video telemetry is very helpful in co-operative patients.
- Bruxism can simulate oral automatisms as it can occur during the day, particularly in patients with learning difficulties. Episodes tend to be longer than complex partial seizures and there is no change in the level of consciousness.
- Hemifacial spasm seen in the elderly and middle aged initially involve the eye and then spread to the ipsilateral hemiface. They may be associated with hemifacial weakness.
- Tremor is usually too persistent and smooth to simulate clonic seizures, but occasionally it can resemble epilepsia partialis continua.
- Subcortical myoclonus should be suspected when the muscles involved correspond to the territory of specific spinal segments or if there is sequential activation of trapezius, sternocleidomaster, orbicularis orbis, and masseter, which is seen in reticular (brainstem) myoclonus. Subcortical myoclonus does not show EEG activity linked to the jerks, even after back-averaging.

Hyperekplexia

Attacks are characterized by an exacerbated startle reaction that may cause stiffening and jerk of all limbs and may result in a sudden fall. Incontinence may occur. Rarely, respiratory arrest may cause cyanosis and anoxic seizures. All attacks are induced by unexpected stimuli, usually auditory. Hyperekplexia can be acquired but is usually familial and there is often history of hypertonia in infancy. Defects in the fifth chromosome (5q33.2–33.3) are associated to hyperekplexia.

Hyperekplexia is easily distinguished from most epileptic syndromes in that attacks are triggered by sudden stimuli, usually loud noises. The main diagnostic problem arises from startle epilepsy, a rare form of epilepsy where seizures can be triggered by a startled response to any cause, including an unexpected noise. This most commonly arises in the context of frontal lobe epilepsy. The main clue in epilepsy is that startle seizures are often associated with frequent spontaneous seizures.

Tics

They are very stereotyped sudden movements (e.g. eyeblink, grimacing, nodding, shrugging) often starting in childhood and adolescent. They tend to affect the head, neck, and shoulders. They can resemble focal motor seizures or myoclonic jerks but the patient can suppress them voluntarily for a limited length of time. Suppressing the tics leads to psychological uneasiness that is released by allowing tics to occur again. They are common in patients with learning disabilities and in Gilles de la Tourette syndrome (tics consisting of vocalization, swearing, arm thrusting, kicking, shoulder shrugging and jumping, in addition to sleep disturbance and obsessive–compulsive behaviour).

Episodic dyscontrol (rage attacks)

The episodic dyscontrol syndrome is characterized by recurrent attacks of uncontrollable rage, and physical and/or verbal aggression. There is usually a precipitant, which is typically disproportionate to the intensity of the aggression. It tends to occur in adolescents and young adults who often are irritable between attacks. Attacks occur suddenly and are explosive, with severe person-directed aggression (obscene language, kicking, scratching, hitting, spitting, biting). During the attacks, patients might appear psychotic, and may suffer fatigue, amnesia or remorse after the attacks. Incontinence is rare. It may coexist with epilepsy, since both can be a consequence of brain damage, particularly head injury. Both can show an abnormal inter-ictal EEG. Aggressive behaviour during epileptic seizures is rare, has no precipitant (although there might be a warning), aggression is not person-directed and is associated with loss of consciousness or confusion. The ictal EEG is normal during episodic dyscontrol and always abnormal during complex partial seizures.

Idiopathic drop attacks

This is a rare condition of unclear pathophysiology. It is most common in middle age females who suffer sudden falls without loss of consciousness (the patient remembers falling and hitting the ground). It is thought to be due to abnormalities in spinal reflexes related to the lower limbs.

Metabolic disorders

Hypoglycaemia: apart from patients with diabetes mellitus, hypoglycaemia is a rare cause of loss of consciousness. Loss of consciousness can occur in patients with insulin-secreting tumours, usually after missing a meal. It may also be fictitious due to self-administration of insulin. Attacks are preceded by lightheadedness, autonomic changes (tachycardia, sweating) or mood changes. Other causes include metabolic hypoglucaemias such as hereditary fructose intolerance.

Blood ion levels: a rare cause of drop attacks is periodic paralysis due to sudden changes in serum potassium, sometimes associated with carbohydrate intake, emotion, or after exertion. The onset is gradual and attacks last for hours. Low magnesium levels can cause falls due to weakness, muscle cramps, or cardiac arrhythmia. In addition, there may be athetosis, jerking, confusion, disorientation, hallucinations, and tetany. True epileptic seizures can also occur. Hypomagnesemia can be inherited or be secondary to other conditions. Hypocalcaemia can induce perioral tingling and paraesthesia ('pins and needles') in hands and feet, tetany, and carpopedal spasm are seen. Carpal spasm can be elicited by inflating the BP cuff and maintaining the pressure above systolic (Trousseau sign of latent tetany). Tapping of the inferior portion of the zygoma induces facial spasms (Chvostek's sign).

Acute encephalopathy

Acute encephalopathy of any cause (metabolic, infectous, toxic) is associated with different degrees of loss of consciousness, which can be difficult to distinguish from non-convulsive status epilepticus. In addition, true epileptic seizures can occur as a result of acute brain injury during encephalopathy. EEG recordings can be fundamental in the diagnosis (📖 see Seizures in the intensive care unit, pp.458–459).

Tonic spasms in multiple sclerosis

They usually occur in known multiple sclerosis, in patients already diagnosed, so that the question of differential diagnosis with epilepsy seldom occurs. Spasms last for seconds to 1min and often respond to low doses of antiepileptic drugs.

Peripheral nerve entrapment

Chronic compression of peripheral nerves usually presents with unilateral weakness, pain, numbness or tingling but can occasionally present with jerks or twitches due to nerve irritation. Tingling is usually too persistent to resemble sensory simple partial seizures.

Migraine

Migraine attacks may cause focal paraesthesias that can evolve to numbness. Attacks can be preceded by heightening of awareness and elementary or complex visual illusions. In migraine attacks, such symptoms are associated with or followed by pounding headache, photophobia, and nausea without total loss of consciousness unless the patient sleeps. Both headache and visual illusions can occur in some occipital seizures. Attacks typically last for hours whereas seizures last for minutes. Loss of consciousness can occur in basilar migraine. There are often recognized precipitants and family history.

Common features between epilepsy and migraine: episodic occurrence, headache, sensory aura (visual, paraesthesias), motor aura (weakness), loss of consciousness (basilar migraine), focal slowing on the EEG, common diseases that can co-exist on the same patient.

Features suggesting epilepsy: absence of headache or less severe headache, bilateral and non-pulsatile headache, epileptiform discharges on inter-ictal or ictal EEG, persistence of slowing in the inter-ictal EEG, fast spread of aura.

Features suggesting migraine: severe, unilateral and pulsating headache, nausea, vomiting, photophobia, phonophobia, malaise, family history of migraine, EEG slowing only during or shortly after the attack, slow spread of aura.

Abdominal migraine and abdominal disease

Recurrent childhood episodes of abdominal pain, vomiting, and autonomic changes are common features of abdominal epilepsy, abdominal migraine, and intra-abdominal disease.

* *Features suggesting epilepsy:* other features of seizures (may be absent), abnormal EEG, response to anticonvulsants.
* *Features suggesting abdominal migraine:* other clinical features of migraine (may be absent), family history of migraine, response to anti-migraine drugs.
* *Features suggesting abdominal disease:* most children with recurrent abdominal pain do not have epilepsy or migraine. Other causes should be sought vigorously.

Transient vestibular symptoms

Peripheral vestibular disease is a common cause of paroxysmal vertigo attacks. Ménière's disease is the name applied to recurrent vertigo attacks associated with tinnitus and progressive deafness. These attacks can in principle resemble the attacks of vertigo that can occasionally be seen in insular and peri-insular epilepsies (parietal and temporal) but they can usually be distinguished on the basis of associated symptoms:

* Common features between epilepsy and Ménière's disease: episodic vertigo, tinnitus, temporal slowing can be seen in 25% of patients with Ménière's disease.
* Features suggesting epilepsy: non-vestibular auras, language disorder, loss of consciousness, epileptiform discharges.
* Features suggesting Ménière's disease: hearing loss, ear pain, tinnitus. Tinnitus and/or deafness may be absent during the initial attack(s) of vertigo, but will appear as the disease progresses

Defects in eye movement

Defects in eye movements can occur in a variety of neurological conditions including cerebellar, brainstem and cranial nerve lesions. Episodes of bizarre eye movements can occur in blindness. Careful history and neurological examination often identifies the associated features and exclude epilepsy.

Transient global amnesia

Transient global amnesia refers to a sudden episode of amnesia for recent events presenting during middle and old age, with abrupt onset, preservation of self identity and consciousness, inability to recall recent events and to memorize new information, and partial retrograde amnesia for days to years. Patients may perform complex activities that are not remembered afterwards. Patients are alert with fluent speech. Such episodes may last for up to 24 hours, usually less. They typically occur in patients above 50. The patient's behaviour can appear relatively normal, except for those who know the patient well. After the episode, patients report a complete amnesia for events that took place during the attack and a variable degree of retrograde amnesia. The pathophysiology is poorly understood, but transient episodes of ischaemia or epileptic phenomena can be responsible if affecting both hippocampi. It appears that some cases of non-convulsive status epilepticus can present with a syndrome resembling transient global amnesia.

Hysterical fugue

This refers to episodes where patients carry out complex actions while cognitive function and EEG recordings are normal. Yet patients will have no recollection of performing these actions. They might be brief or prolonged (for hours or days). There is no organic cause. They are usually explained as a psychiatric conversion disorder. The question of malingering often arises, particularly in a forensic context (is the patient responsible for a crime committed during the episode?).

Differential diagnosis in children

- Misdiagnosis in children is common. It is the most common cause of failure in response to treatment.
- Common causes are lack of awareness of other possibilities, and lack of understanding of what is important in history.
- There is some overlap with adults, but some disorders are exclusive or more common in children.
- A trial of antiepileptic medication is not an appropriate diagnostic test in view of the fact that many movement and behavioural disorders can respond, and does not necessarily imply they are epileptic in origin.

Syncope and related disorders

Vasovagal attacks can occur in children but are rare as a cause of syncope under the age of 10 years. A cardiac cause should be excluded in all such cases, especially where there are atypical features to the history, e.g. syncope on exertion or from sitting. In any case it is recommended that all children presenting with episodes of loss of consciousness should undergo an ECG.[1] The key features of different types of attacks are shown in Table 3c.3.

Cyanotic breath-holding attacks

These are a relatively common cause of loss of consciousness in children age 6 months to 6 years. They are triggered by frustration, fright, pain, or minor injuries. The child then begins to vigorously cry. There is prolonged expiration, the child becomes cyanosed, and they then lose consciousness, go rigid and can assume an opisthotonic posture. Shortly afterwards the child loses tone and goes limp until breathing is restored. The marked lethargy and confusion often seen after convulsive seizures is usually missing. The period of apnoea is usually short (<1min), but if it is prolonged, a tonic–clonic epileptic seizure may occur secondary to cerebral hypoxia. There may be a family history of such attacks.

Reflex anoxic seizures

Synonyms: vagal attacks, white breath-holding attacks pallid infantile syndrome.

They are less common than cyanotic breath-holding attacks. They are also precipitated by frustration, fright, pain, or minor injuries. The child falls limply and quickly regains consciousness, or, if prolonged, convulsions may ensue. Pallor and cold sweats may precede loss of consciousness. Minor cyanosis might also be present. They usually occur in children between 3 months and 14 years but are particularly common between 12–18 months, coinciding with the onset of walking and frequent falls. Ocular compression has been advocated for diagnosis but is not commonly used: pressure on one ocular globe was applied during ECG and EEG recordings. Asystole for 2sec or longer was present in 50% of patients with white breath holding attacks and in 25% of children with cyanotic breath-holding attacks. If asystole lasted for >10sec, a convulsive seizure ensued.

Neurological

- As outlined earlier, many of the movement disorders that can be misdiagnosed as epilepsy may present in childhood and in adults.
- Benign paroxysmal vertigo and benign paroxysmal torticollis present before the age of 5 years. They involve sudden onset of vertiginous episodes (where the child will be unwilling to move or be unsteady on their feet) or torticollis, which last minutes to hours. Such episodes resolve with age.
- Alternating hemiplegia is a condition presenting in the first year with abnormal eye movements, subsequently characterized by intermittent episodes of hemiplegia that may last minutes to hours. Epileptic seizures may coexist, and there is a higher prevalence of learning disability.
- Abnormal movements of the upper body found in association with oesophageal reflux is termed Sandifer's syndrome. The movements are thought to be an attempt to relieve the pain of oesophagitis by changing intrathoracic pressure. Such movements would be particularly related to mealtimes, and are more frequently seen in children with neurological problems or developmental delay.

Table 3c.3 Differentiating features between cyanotic breath-holding attacks, pallid infantile syncope, and convulsive seizures*

	Cyanotic breath-holding attacks	Pallid infantile syncope	Convulsive seizures
Age	6 months to 6 years	12–18 months, but variable	Any
Precipitant	Frequent	Frequent	Occasional
Sequence of events	Crying, apnoea, LOC	Upset, pallor, LOC	Sometimes aura, LOC
Heart rate during ocular compression	See text	See text	Not available
Post-ictal symptoms	None	None	Confusion, headache, sleepiness, tiredness. Often absent in tonic seizures
Inter-ictal EEG	Normal	Normal	Often abnormal
Ictal EEG	Slow	Slow	Epileptiform activity can be present

LOC = loss of conciousnss

*Modified with permission from Browne TR and Holmes GL (2004). *Handbook of Epilepsy*, 3rd edn. Lippincott Willims & Wilkers, Philadelphia.

Neurological

- As outlined earlier, many of the movement disorders that can be misdiagnosed as epilepsy may present in childhood and in adults.
- Benign paroxysmal vertigo and benign paroxysmal torticollis present before the age of 5 years. They involve sudden onset of vertiginous episodes (where the child will be unwilling to move or be unsteady on their feet) or torticollis, which last minutes to hours. Such episodes resolve with age.
- Alternating hemiplegia is a condition presenting in the first year with abnormal eye movements, subsequently characterized by intermittent episodes of hemiplegia that may last minutes to hours. Epileptic seizures may coexist, and there is a higher prevalence of learning disability.
- Abnormal movements of the upper body found in association with oesophageal reflux is termed Sandifer's syndrome. The movements are thought to be an attempt to relieve the pain of oesophagitis by changing intrathoracic pressure. Such movements would be particularly related to mealtimes, and are more frequently seen in children with neurological problems or developmental delay.

Behavioural/psychiatric

- The most common cause of misdiagnosis of absence epilepsy is day dreaming or non attention, although the latter is by far more common. These should be relatively easy to exclude by their situational nature and the ability to be distracted out of them although this may require physical touch.
- Self-gratification behaviour is very common, especially in the very young child. Children during episodes may appear distracted, unaware of their surroundings, and flushed. Such events, although at diagnosis may be distressing to parents, have a good prognosis for resolution.
- Stereotypic and ritualistic behaviours are seen particularly amongst children with learning difficulty and/or autistic spectrum disorder. Concern may be expressed about a possible epileptic nature, especially in those who have this as an additional diagnosis.
- Overflow movements or shuddering attacks are distal movements seen in toddlers at times of excitement.

Parasomnias

- A wide range of sleep phenomena exist in children. Parents only become aware of this when forced to sleep with them.
- Benign sleep myoclonus seen in the first 6 months of life continues to be misdiagnosed as epilepsy. Key features are jerks that only occur in sleep and the child is developmentally normal.
- Hypnic jerks continue to occur at any age.
- Night terrors (🕮 see Sleep phenomena, p.215) may be characterized by sudden awakening at a similar time each night; the child may appear terrified, inconsolable and out of touch. They will eventually settle back to sleep. These may be aborted by waking the child at a time each night shortly prior to the time of a likely attack.

Table 3c.4 shows a summary of the differential diagnosis of epilepsy in children.

Table 3c.4 Differential diagnosis of epilepsy in children

Syncope and related disorders	• Reflex syncope • Cyanotic breath-holding attacks • Reflex anoxic seizures • Cardiac arrythmias
Neurological	• Tics • Paroxysmal dystonia • Hyperekplexia • Sandifers syndrome • Paroxysmal dyskinesias • Cataplexy • Benign paroxysmal vertigo/torticollis • Alternating hemiplegia • Eye movement disorders • Overflow movements • Migraine
Behavioural/psychiatric	• Daydreams • Dissociative states • Self-gratification behaviour • Hyperventilation • Panic/anxiety • Non-epileptic attack disorder • Stereotypies/ritualistic behaviour
Parasomnias	• Night terrors • Sleep myoclonus • Head banging • Confusional arousal

References

1. Scottish Intercollegiate Guidelines Network (SIGN) (2005). Diagnosis and management of epilepsies in children and young people. A National Clinical Guideline. March 2005.
🖰 www.sign.ac.uk

What do I do now?

What to do during a seizure

Don'ts! What not to do!

- *Do not introduce objects into the patient's mouth to prevent tongue biting:* teeth can be broken, your own fingers can be bitten, and most likely you will not be able to prevent patients from biting their tongue or cheek.
- *Do not automatically call an ambulance straight away in patients with known epilepsy:* most seizures stop spontaneously in 2–3min. If a convulsive seizure occurs for the first time, patients need to be assessed for possible underlying neurological or other causes; an ambulance *should* be called. Call an ambulance in all cases if the seizure does not stop spontaneously within 5min.
- *Do not restrict movement in convulsive seizures:* it can induce joint dislocations and bone fractures.
- *Do not try to move them unless in danger.*
- *Do not give the person anything to eat or drink until fully recovered.*
- *Do not attempt to bring them around.*
- *Keep the person under observation until fully recovered.*

What to do during a simple partial seizure—patient is fully conscious

- *Just wait!* Simple partial seizures are not life threatening and many remit spontaneously. Prolonged simple partial seizures may require treatment depending on the individual case.
- *Reassure patient and keep patient under close observation* in case the seizure evolves into more severe seizure types (complex partial or convulsive seizures).

What to do during a complex partial seizure or prolonged epileptic absence—patient vacant or confused, unresponsive or partially responsive, and may have automatisms such as chewing mouth movements, but not convulsions

Prevent danger!

Patients may continue activity including walking around in an automatic fashion, especially in the post-ictal phase which can be long. Therefore it is very important to prevent patients from getting into dangerous situations such as walking onto the road, falling off platforms in train or underground stations, grabbing knives or other dangerous tools, pouring boiling water onto themselves or others, getting burned with hot irons, etc. Gently direct them to safety, as some patients may show resistive aggression if forcibly restricted in the ictal and post ictal phase.

Record the precise behaviour during the seizure and its evolution as it may later aid classification of seizure type and assess the patient's cognitive state

This is important. Cognitive assessment should be relatively simple, as time is limited. Ask patients where they live, where they are, ask them to name objects shown to them (for instance, a watch, a tie, a coin, a key), ask them to remember a number or the objects shown. Carry on with the assessment even if the patient is unresponsive (you might be surprised how much some patients can remember later!). Carry out this assessment periodically in order to evaluate the evolution of the seizure and whether the patient is recovering. Record evidence of word finding difficulty as the patient recovers as this may suggest dominant hemisphere lateralization of the seizure.

Treatment may be required if prolonged depending on the individual case.

What to do during a convulsive seizure—patient unresponsive, stiff or jerking

- *Prevent danger and injury!* Make sure that the patient cannot fall, put up cot sides if available, lower bed, remove patient from the road, or from the edge of cliffs or platforms. Make sure that his/her head and limbs do not hit furniture, walls, or other objects while jerking by placing pillows etc. strategically, including to try and prevent 'carpet burns'. Do not try to move the person unless in danger
- *Once the seizure has stopped, make sure airway is clear:* uncover face, remove objects from mouth, including dentures if possible. Do not introduce objects inside the patient's mouth!
- *Prevent aspiration of secretions:* during convulsive seizures the reflex involved in swallowing is abolished, and mouth secretions can be aspirated. This increases the risk of pneumonia, a potentially fatal complication. Put the patient in the recovery position (Fig. 4a.1a–c), so that mouth secretions come out one side of the mouth due to gravity. If a mechanical aspirator is available, aspirate secretions from the mouth. If the seizure occurs in hospital, depending on patients colour and duration of attack, it may be appropriate to give oxygen.
- *Do not restrict movements:* it can induce joint dislocations and bone fractures.

What to do during very brief seizures—absence seizures, myoclonic jerks, atonic, and some tonic seizures

Myoclonic jerks, atonic and tonic seizures are momentary or last for a few seconds, whereas absence seizures can last up to 30sec or longer. Very brief seizures do not allow for specific treatment by the observer. They require chronic treatment with the aim of reducing seizure frequency, but no specific action is usually necessary during the seizure except in preventing injury in seizures associated with falls. Patients suffering from drop attacks (tonic or atonic seizures) can benefit from wearing a protective helmet to prevent head and facial injuries.

What to do after a seizure

Simple partial seizures, absence seizures, myoclonic jerks, atonic and brief tonic seizures are usually followed by quick recovery and do not usually require specific action. Patients can fall during seizures, resulting in injuries, which may require specific treatment (stop nose bleeding, suture cuts, etc.). Complex partial and convulsive seizures usually last for 2–3min and are followed by a period of gradual recovery. The patient may be still unconscious immediately after a convulsive seizure and is vulnerable during this period. It is important to make sure that breathing pattern and colour recover and patients should be monitored until they become fully alert. Seizures are often followed by a relatively long period of confusion (post-ictal confusion), which can last from a few minutes to several hours. During this period patients gradually recover their cognitive skills. They may complain of headache, tiredness, or be sleepy for several hours. Analgesia may be required. During post-ictal confusion, patients must be under close observation, as they might wander about aimlessly, sometimes getting themselves into dangerous situations. If disturbed, they might push you away or become mildly aggressive, so leave them alone if they are safe, but keep an eye on them. If patients are sleepy or tired, find a place for them to rest.

What to do if seizures do not stop

If the seizure is prolonged, or the patient suffers a cluster of seizures without regaining consciousness in the period between seizures, patients should be taken to hospital. This situation, status epilepticus, is a medical emergency (📖 see Diagnosis of status epilepticus pp.198–205 and Management of status epilepticus, pp.394–410).

How long should one let a seizure or a cluster continue before calling an ambulance? This depends on the patient's habitual seizures. If they normally cease spontaneously within a relatively short period, an ambulance is only called if the seizure continues beyond the usual duration. If on the other hand, the seizures are always prolonged and require intervention, an ambulance should be called immediately. In those with chronic epilepsy, an individualized protocol is often agreed between the patient/carers and care-providers and reviewed on a regular basis, and should be followed. The same applies for the use in the community of rescue medication, such as buccal midazolam or rectal diazepam (📖 see Management of status epilepticus, pp.394–410). Unless the individual care protocol says otherwise, an ambulance should be called if someone is still convulsing at 5min; if rescue medication has been given (usually if convulsive movements continues for 5min), then generally an ambulance should be called, if still convulsing 5min after the rescue medication.

Some simple partial seizures can last for long periods. Their management depends on the patient's history. Those where prolonged simple partial seizures tend to evolve to convulsive or complex partial seizures should be treated more aggressively. Again rescue medication can be useful in this situation and, if unsuccessful, the patient should be taken to hospital.

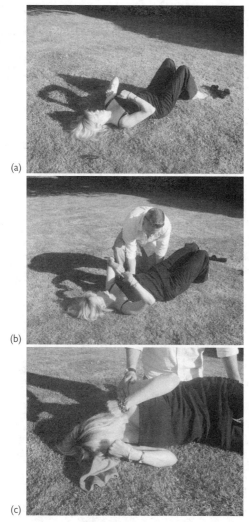

Fig. 4a.1 When a subject if found suffering tonic or clonic convulsions (a) try to roll him/her onto one side if possible (b) so that saliva dribbles down one corner of the mouth to prevent aspiration (c). Padding is placed under her face to avoid rubbing of the skin against the ground (c). Avoid introducing any objects into the mouth.

Early prevention of severe seizures and status epilepticus

Some patients or their relatives can predict from early seizure manifestations, that a severe or long-lasting seizure is coming. This is particularly true in patients with symptomatic generalized epilepsies and multiple seizure types. If severe seizures can be predicted at early stages, the patient or his/her relatives can administer an effective and fast-acting AED as soon as severe seizures are foreseen. Benzodiazepines appear to be ideal for this purpose as 🕮 discussed in Box 4b.14, p.398.

What to do if seizures are prolonged

Well-controlled GTCS

If a patient's epilepsy is well controlled on medication, seizures tend to be short lived (1–2min). It is unusual for such patients to have a prolonged seizure.

In all cases of prolonged seizure, admit to A&E for further investigation of the underlying cause (☐ see Boxes 4a.1 and 4a.2). If two or more seizures in <24 hours, admit until patient is assessed and is stable.

Box 4a.1

A generalized tonic–clonic seizure lasting >5min is a medical emergency—call 999 in the UK

Use rescue medication in the community if available. Patients with chronic epilepsy may have an individualized protocol (e.g. of buccal Midazolam or rectal diazepam).

Rescue medication can also be administered by ambulance crew who in the UK have rectal and IV benzodiazepines. Treat with 5–10mg diazepam intravenously/rectally or 1–3mg lorazepam intravenously.

Well controlled partial seizures

Certain circumstances may place a person at risk of increased seizure frequency (☐ see Box 4a.3).

Simple partial seizures

- Simple partial seizures are typically very brief (<30sec) and there is no loss of consciousness. Prolonged simple partial seizures are rare, but simple partial status epilepticus can occur (☐ see Simple partial status epilepticus, pp.199–200).
- Repeated simple partial seizures are more common and, although not dangerous, can be very frightening for patients. They can also lead to secondarily GTCS.
- Simple partial seizures can often be aborted using oral benzodiazepines (e.g. clobazam 10mg stat and a further 10mg after 30–60 min). If the seizures are not controlled (maximum 40–60mg in 24 hours) admission for IV benzodiazepines may be needed.

Complex partial seizures

Partial seizures with impaired consciousness. Confirm with family/carers the usual pattern and duration of seizures:

- It is unusual for a complex partial seizure to last > 3min but complex partial seizures are often followed by prolonged periods of confusion so identifying the end of the seizure can be difficult.
- Post-ictal (post seizure) confusion usually lasts 10–30min.
- Clusters of complex partial seizures are not uncommon. Treat with oral benzodiazepines (e.g. clobazam 10mg stat and a further 10mg after 30–60mins. if the seizure is not controlled - maximum 40-60mg in 24 hours). Admission for IV benzodiazepines may be needed.

- Prolonged complex partial seizures do occur but are usually not life-threatening except for the risk of leading to secondarily generalized tonic-clonic seizures. Admit to hospital for IV benzodiazepine to abort the seizure (📖 see Management of status epilepticus, pp.394–410)

Poorly controlled or drug-resistant epilepsy

- Some groups (e.g. patients with learning disability) may experience prolonged seizures sometimes lasting up to 10min. If this is habitual for the patient and the seizure is always self-terminating, then admission to hospital is not needed—admission can create more problems e.g. disruption of routine, risk of infection.
- *Consider prescribing rectal diazepam or buccal midazolam to patients with a history of uncontrolled prolonged tonic–clonic seizures for use when a seizure lasts >5min.* If either is prescribed, always ensure carers are adequately trained to administer it—the JEC[1] provides pre-prepared care plans and educational tools, and training can be obtained via the National Society for Epilepsy[2] and Epilepsy Action[3] in the UK. Training of use of buccal midazolam is also available in many units.

Box 4a.2 Factors which increase seizure frequency and/or make prolonged seizures more likely:

- Alcohol—e.g. an episode of binge drinking, particularly with sleep deprivation.
- Recreational drug use.
- Use of other medication that interacts with AEDs—e.g. antibiotics, contraceptive pills.
- Non-adherence to treatment or recent medication withdrawal reduction.
- Concurrent illness e.g. diarrhoea and/or vomiting, pyrexia/infection.
- Prolonged sleep deprivation.
- Stressful events/episodes—e.g. exams, bereavement, house move, divorce, unemployment.

Box 4a.3 Be aware of seizure types and usual patterns

It is not uncommon in certain patients—especially those with seizures arising from the temporal lobe or in patients with learning difficulties—to have multiple seizure types. If this is typical of their habitual pattern, do not admit to hospital.

Box 4a.4 When should I send a patient to hospital?

Often neurologists can provide an action plan for use in the event of poorly controlled seizures. When not available consider sending to hospital if:

- A patient has a prolonged tonic–clonic seizure lasting >5min if that is atypical for the patient.
- A patient has two or more complex partial seizures in <6 hours.
- A patient has two or more tonic–clonic seizures in <24 hours.
- The parents and/or carers cannot cope with the seizures.
- Any injury requiring medical attention is sustained during a seizure—there is a high risk of cerebral injury and limb fracture following falls.
- If there is no complete recovery after a seizure.
- If there are new neurological signs.

If in doubt, ask the specialist neurology or paediatric team on-call at your local hospital for advice.

References

1. Joint Epilepsy Council: 🖰 www.jointepilepsycouncil.org.uk
2. National Society for Epilepsy: 🖰 www.epilepsynse.org.uk
3. Epilepsy Action: 🖰 www.epilepsy.org.uk

When to refer patients to secondary or tertiary centres

Refer to a neurologist in the following circumstances:

First suspected seizure

NICE recommends referral of all patients with a first suspected seizure for urgent (within 2 weeks) assessment by a neurologist with training and expertise in epilepsy, to make an accurate diagnosis, classify epilepsy, exclude underlying causes (e.g. tumour), and receive clear guidance on medication, safety, work, and driving . Any decision to start treatment is usually postponed until two confirmed seizures have occurred and appropriate tests (i.e. EEG imaging and neurological assessment) have been performed.

It has been claimed that, in the UK, the misdiagnosis rate for epilepsy is as high as 20-30%—that equates to 105,000 people taking unnecessary antiepileptic medication. Although these figures might be an overestimate, differential diagnosis of epilepsy is a common and sometimes difficult issue.

Poor control

Failure of two or more first-line therapies and/or continuing seizures for more than 2 years despite medication

Refer for review. Diagnosis should be reconsidered and, if epilepsy is confirmed, those with partial epilepsy syndromes may be suitable for epilepsy surgery.

Re-emergence of seizures

Refer for neurological review all drug-resistant patients, in particular those who experience a re-emergence of GTCS or dramatic change in seizure frequency for neurology review.

If patients are well-controlled for several years and then experience a sudden re-emergence of their seizures, consider the following:

- **Non-adherence to treatment:** drug levels can be useful to confirm this. Explore the reasons for non-adherence e.g. forgetfulness, unacceptable side effects, patient beliefs (e.g. the patient feels the epilepsy has gone into remission so there is no need to take medication).
- **Alcohol:** patients are often anxious about taking AEDs and drinking so decide to omit their drugs in order to drink.
- **Recreational drug use:** most class A drugs increase seizure risk.
- **Other medication** that interacts with AEDs e.g. contraceptive pill, antibiotics, or lower seizure threshold e.g. antipsychotics.
- **Concurrent illness:** particularly diarrhoea and/or vomiting which interferes with absorption of antiepileptic medication and pyrexia/infection which can lower seizure threshold.
- **Prolonged sleep deprivation:** can lower seizure threshold e.g. if change in time zones or shift work.
- **Stressful event/episode** e.g. death in the family, exam stress.
- **Change from usual brand medication:** because bioavailability can be different for different brands. Changing medication brand, while fine for many patients, could result in reduced drug blood levels with loss of seizure control or increased levels and toxicity for some patients.

Generic prescribing may lead to changing of brand. With phenytoin, changing brand results in a 10% risk of worsening seizure control. The effect is less with other drugs.

- *Marked weight gain/loss:* can alter drug pharmacokinetics.
- *Pregnancy can alter seizure control:* refer all pregnant women with epilepsy for neurology review.
- *Progressive neurological disease*.

Suspected adverse side effects of AED

Arrange for neurology review if toxicity is evident even if unsupported by blood levels.

Proposed or actual pregnancy

Any woman with a diagnosis of epilepsy who is planning a pregnancy or who has become pregnant should be referred promptly for a neurological opinion and asked to take folic acid (5 mg/day).

Ensure all women of childbearing age with the diagnosis of epilepsy receive preconception advice and counselling. Antiepileptic medication increases the risk of fetal malformations. 📖 see Antiepileptic drugs in special situations, pp.364–374; Counselling in people with epilepsy, pp.524–527; Epilepsy, contraception, and pregnancy, pp.448–454.

Altered clinical circumstances

If pointers to a previously unsuspected cause for the fits appear, or concurrent illness (physical or psychiatric) complicates management, refer for specialist review—neurology or other depending on clinical circumstances.

Consideration and counselling for AED withdrawal

Consider if free of fits for 2–5 years. The longer the period of seizure freedom, the lower the risk of recurrence, but it remains significant. The decision to stop medication *must* be the patient's. Balance the problems and inconvenience of drug taking against the risks of fits returning with implications for safety, driving, employment, and family. Withdrawal of AEDs must be managed by, or be under the guidance of, a neurologist—refer.

Seizure recurrence is more likely if:
- History of GTCS.
- EEG with clear epileptiform discharges.
- Juvenile myoclonic epilepsy
- Infantile spasms.
- Taking more than one drug to control epilepsy.
- One or more seizures after starting treatment.
- Duration of treatment >10 years.

Seizure recurrence is less likely if: seizure free for 5 years or longer.

Who may benefit from being referred to sub-specialist care

- Patients where, after initial investigations there remains diagnostic doubt
- Patient with epilepsy with uncontrolled seizures.
- Patients with multiple medication or co-morbidity where prescribing requires extra caution—such as liver or renal failure, severe depression, metabolic disorders, severe learning difficulties.
- Women of childbearing age and pregnant patients, depending on the experience of current physician.
- Patients willing to try novel drugs or take part in drug trials.
- Patients who may be suitable for epilepsy surgery.
- Controlled or uncontrolled patients seeking specialist advise in personal issues such as:
  - Can I stop my tablets?
  - Can I drive?
  - Can I dive or practice other risky sports?
  - Can I have surgery?
  - Can I have children?
  - What is the risk of my children having epilepsy?
  - What is the risk of miscarriage?
  - Can the tablets affect my baby?

Referral to a tertiary centre

Some patients require referral to specialist units. Some physicians or general neurologists erroneously believe that they should only refer a patient with intractable epilepsy if MRI shows one potentially resectable lesion—such as hippocampal sclerosis, cavernoma, dysembryoplastic neuroepithelial tumour, focal dysplasia, or hemiatrophy. They may also believe that there is no added value to the referral because the same AEDs are available to all physicians. This is not so, as more expert selection use of the same available AEDs can lead to full control:

- All uncontrolled patients should be offered the opportunity of being referred. The patient may be referred to an epilepsy surgeon or more frequently to a neurologist with a special interest in epilepsy with access to tertiary assessment.
- Controlled patients may also be referred for specific advice, for instance, when contemplating the possibility of withdrawing AED medication.

In tertiary centres, multidisciplinary meetings which may include neurologists, neurophysiologists, neurosurgeons, neuroradiologists, neuropsychologists and neuropsychiatrists allow for a full assessment to be made. A disadvantage is that tertiary centres are often at a distance from the patient's local hospital.

Examples of possible benefits from a tertiary centre include:

- Review of the diagnosis, if appropriate with re-investigation, including EEG video telemetry—maybe it isn't epilepsy after all or maybe the classification is incorrect, with implications to choice of AED treatment.
- Not infrequently, control can be achieved by more expert use of previously tried AEDs. Patients may also want access to new medications or to take part in drug trials.

- Better quality MRIs or other imaging modalities, including an opinion from an experienced specialist neuroradiologist. This may identify focal lesions which are potentially respectable—e.g. identification of hippocampal sclerosis or cortical dysplasia may require dedicated sequences.
- Invasive intracranial video-EEG recordings in selected cases may identify candidates for possible surgical resection even where MRI is negative or shows more than one possible lesion.
- Some patients may benefit from functional (non-resective) surgery for epilepsy. Examples include callosotomy, deep brain stimulation, and vagus nerve stimulation—the latter an increasingly used technique.
- Patients may benefit from admission to medium-stay dedicated epilepsy units for a holistic assessment and medication adjustment under observation.
- Some may benefit from more sophisticated investigation of the aetiology of the epilepsy.
- Patients may seek to be more informed about their epilepsy and more expert advice with regard to lifestyle, driving, psychological or social problems.

Key reading

1. NICE (2004). The epilepsies: the diagnosis and management of the epilepsies in adults and children in primary and secondary care (2004). Available at: ⁂ http://www.nice.org.uk/Guidance/ CG20

Management of epilepsy

Optimal management requires:
- Accurate diagnosis and, whenever possible, syndromic classification.
- Treatment of underlying aetiology, where appropriate.
- Optimal treatment of the epilepsy.
- Proactive prevention and management of potential complications.
- Holistic care.
- Multidisciplinary care.

The following health care workers should be involved in epilepsy care:
- Neurologist or paediatrician with access to appropriate supporting services—clinical neurophysiology, neuroradiology, neuropsychiatry, neurosurgery, laboratory facilities, pharmacology.
- Epilepsy Specialist Nurse.
- Trained Epilepsy Counsellor.
- GP.
- Practice Nurse.

Treatment of the epilepsy involves:
- Patient/carer ongoing education on epilepsy, its treatment, and its implications to allow for active patient/carer involvement with management.
- Seizure prevention by avoiding seizure triggers.
- Seizure prevention with appropriate long-term AED.
- Prompt advice and review of medication as clinically indicated between routine appointments.
- Rescue treatment for acute attacks if prolonged or occurring in clusters.
- Identification of those suitable for non-medical treatment, such as resective surgery or vagus nerve stimulation (VNS).
- Diagnosis review and reassessment if there is a poor response to treatment.
- Advice and treatment review to special groups—e.g. preconception counselling.
- Management of associated disorders if present—e.g. depression or behavioural problems.

Follow-up of patients with epilepsy

It is only too easy to follow-up patients in clinic to no purpose and it is helpful to keep certain aims in mind. These include:

Aims of follow-up
- To diagnose and monitor the condition causing the epilepsy where appropriate.
- To prevent seizures.
- An important goal is that of seizure freedom since seizures carry a physical risk and since seizure freedom is associated with a better quality of life. There are exceptions, as in these examples:
  - If seizures are very mild without significant risk of injury i.e. without associated falls, significant impairment of function, or post-ictal symptoms, and if the patient does not care to drive, the patient may

prefer living with minor seizures, such as auras or myoclonic jerks, to further drug manipulation.

• If the patient has intractable epilepsy with multiple seizure types and previous many unsuccessful medical and surgical attempts at controlling seizures, then the chances of total seizure freedom with additional intervention are very small indeed. The goals may be then modified depending on the individual case. For example goals may be:

—to prevent convulsive seizures especially if prolonged.

—to abort prolonged seizures or clusters of seizures with rescue medication.

—to prevent injury, e.g. by preventing seizures associated with falls or by supervision when ambulant or the wearing of head protection.

—to prevent frequent emergency hospital attendance or admission.

—to prevent seizures on important days or outings.

—to achieve stability with a predictable pattern of seizures.

—to minimize medication side-effects.

• To prevent complications of treatment: there are potential side effects with all treatments as discussed in other sections. These can be short, medium, or long term. They can, amongst others, affect the individual's quality of life, educational attainment, cognition, employment and social prospects. There are also effects on the unborn child. Awareness of potential side effects and their proactive management helps in minimizing their impact.

• To maintain a record of the epilepsy and its treatment for current and future reference: we cannot over-emphasize how important this is. Documentation is essential in a long-term condition and is unfortunately largely deficient. Keeping accurate records of seizure frequency, responses to treatment, side effects, doses used and escalation rates, reasons for withdrawal, as well as the rationale behind therapeutic decisions can inform future treatment. Relying on the physicians or the patients' recall is insufficient.

• To provide support and continuity: this is best achieved by a multidisciplinary service as discussed earlier. Although occasionally a new 'fresh' assessment is helpful by another physician, in general continuity of care is advised and is favoured by both patients and physicians given the nature of management of a long-term condition.

• To identify and treat associated comorbidity.

What do we record at clinic visits during follow-up?

The following information is needed to aid treatment decisions and for future reference. We advise that this information is included in clinic letters and copied to patients and carers:

• Summary: epilepsy diagnosis, classification, date of onset, aetiology, summary of previous investigation results and treatments given.

• Seizures:
  • Seizure type, frequency and pattern: 1-year planners are best for easy reference. Some patients may wish to supplement with a more detailed diary
  • Seizure-triggers: this information is essential to guide management

- Medication/treatment:
  - Regular AED treatment, with information on preparation, dose schedule, last change in doses, adherence to treatment (on history and if appropriate blood levels), response to recent change, etc.
  - As required rescue treatment, with information on doses and how often this is used and in what circumstance.
  - Treatment for other conditions: This should include any recent change.
  - Contraception
  - Supplements
  - Side-effects: in polytherapy these, if possible, should include which drug is considered most likely to cause the side-effect reported.
  - VNS: the device needs to be checked and adjusted as appropriate
- Relevant life-style issues: these are diverse and include potential seizure triggers, driving, education, supervision, potential physical risk, employment, rehabilitation, and social integration. In women of reproductive age they include relation of seizures to monthly cycle, contraception, plans for pregnancy, and care of young children.
- Other comorbid conditions.
- Management plan: this needs to be very clearly stated to include the following:
  - Rationale for changes in drug therapy, doses recommended with changes guided by clinical response, suggested interim maximum doses, contact number if any concerns between appointments, situations where a newly introduced medication should be withdrawn promptly, etc.
  - If appropriate, investigations and consideration of surgery for epilepsy.
  - A record of information/advice given to patient or carers in clinic or of referrals to other services/members of team.
  - Options for future treatment.

awake / sleep
A = Aura: ... *provide brief description here*
O = Minor seizure: ... *provide brief description here*
X = Likely convulsion: ... *provide brief description here*

	Jan	Feb	Mar	Apr	May	Jun	Jul	Aug	Sep	Oct	Nov	Dec
1												
2												
3												
4												
5												
6												
7												
8												
9												
10												
11												
12												
13												
14												
15												
16												
17												
18												
19												
20												
21												
22												
23												
24												
25												
26												
27												
28												
29												
30												
31												

Fig. 4a.2 Example of a seizure chart.

Management of epilepsy in children

The most important aspect to the management of children with epilepsy is being confident in the diagnosis. Epilepsy is likely to be diagnosed after the second epileptic seizure although there needs to be confidence that events are epileptic in origin. Evidence from epidemiological studies suggest that further seizures are most likely to occur after two epileptic seizures; in 53% the second seizure will be within 6 months of the first. The recommendation as per NICE and SIGN is that diagnosis of epilepsy and any decision to treat should be made by a paediatrician with an interest in epilepsy—the definition of such however remains undeclared.

There is no question that the diagnosis of epilepsy should be made with certainty, and if there is any question review be undertaken. Once a child has been seen in casualty—even following a single seizure—an outpatient referral should be arranged with the paediatrician. A care pathway should be available within each district.

Thereafter a diagnosis of epilepsy may be made with security and a diagnosis of epilepsy syndrome where possible. A decision can then be made as to the most likely beneficial medication that should be used.

In some children treatment may not be imperative. Some children with infrequent seizures as part of idiopathic syndromes may not require immediate treatment although discussion with the family needs to be undertaken. The risk versus the benefit of the treatment requires careful discussion; in some, one or two seizures maybe all that occur—e.g. early onset benign epilepsy with occipital paroxysms. However such syndromes may also be highly responsive to AEDs and families may choose treatment over non-treatment.

Choosing the initial AED will depend on the seizure type, preferably the seizure syndrome. NICE have outlined first- and second-line medication, summarized in Table 4a.1. The final decision about initial medication should also take account of the adverse effect profiles and ultimate preference of the family and professional. In some instances, the formulation available will also need to be taken into consideration although most medications are now available in child friendly formulations. It is advisable to outline the most common side effects with the family, and offer a clear plan should this AED not work or should problems be encountered. Review at least 6-weekly in the first instance is recommended.

The advantage of syndrome diagnosis not only lies in being aware of the optimal AED, but also in outlining the prognosis. The likelihood of the epilepsy responding to a further appropriate and well tolerated AED after the initial two is small; managing expectations in the more difficult epilepsy syndromes is as important as treating seizures optimally. In addition, certain medications may aggravate seizures in certain syndromes, outlined in the third column of Table 4a.1. Such medications need to be avoided in these specific circumstances.

When children are controlled, medication review is required but may be as infrequently as annually. Regular blood tests are not required unless there is a suspicion of poor compliance or toxicity on the part of drug levels, or the child is unwell on the part of other tests. Should seizures continue, more regular review is required, perhaps with the aid of an epilepsy nurse. Discussion can be undertaken as to when AEDs may be discontinued. This again will most likely depend on the epilepsy syndrome—by carefully defining such, the likely duration of treatment can be estimated.

Referral onto to a tertiary service may be required in the event of ongoing seizures. Box 4a.5 outlines the indication for such a referral as declared by NICE. This does not indicate that all children should be seen within the tertiary service, but discussion with a tertiary paediatric neurologist may be indicated and discussion about further evaluation undertaken.

When to stop treatment

The prognosis with regard to seizure control will depend on the underlying cause of the epilepsy, in particular the epilepsy syndrome. Idiopathic epilepsy syndromes of onset in mid childhood have a good prognosis for seizure remission. Those of later onset are likely to require lifelong treatment although prognosis for seizure control is good. The symptomatic epilepsies are unlikely to remit; however medication should be kept to a minimum. A small number of the epileptic encephalopathies may show spontaneous remission. On balance, consideration to a trial weaning of medication should be given if a child remains seizure free for 2 years, considering the possible risk of further seizures according to syndrome. However such a wean should take place when the possibility of a seizure does not pose a major risk to quality of life—e.g. timing of exams, driving licence application.

Syndromes likely to remit:
- Benign epilepsy with occipital paroxysms—Panayiotopoulos Syndrome.
- Benign epilepsy with centrotemporal spikes—by 14 years.
- Childhood absence epilepsy.
- Syndrome of continuous spike wave of slow sleep.
- Landau–Kleffner syndrome.

Syndromes unlikely to remit:
- Juvenile absence epilepsy.
- Juvenile myoclonic epilepsy.
- Late onset occipital epilepsy—of Gastaut.
- Dravet's syndrome.
- Lennox–Gastaut syndrome.
- Myoclonic astatic epilepsy.

Table 4a.1 Choice of AED medication in children (adapted from NICE 2004)[3]*

Seizure type/ syndrome	First line	Second line	Drugs to avoid
Focal seizures	CBZ, LTG, OXC, TPM, VPA	CLB, GBP, LEV, PHT, TGB, ZON, PGN	
Generalized seizures			
Absence	ESM, LTG, VPA	CLB, CLN, TPM	CBZ, GBP, OXC, TGB, VGB
GTC	CBZ, LTG, VPA, TPM	CLB, LEV, OXC, ZON	TGB, VGB
Myoclonic	VPA, TPM	LTG, CLB, CLN, LEV piracetam	CBZ, GBP, OXC, TGB, VGB
Tonic	LTG, VPA,	CLB, CLN, LEV, TPM	CBZ, OXC
Atonic	LTG, VPA,	LEV, TPM CLB, CLN	CBZ, OXC, PHT
Childhood absence epilepsy	ESM, LTG, VPA	LEV, TOP	CBZ, OXC, PHT, TGB, VGB
Juvenile absence epilepsy	LTG, VPA	LEV, TPM	CBZ, OXC, PHT, TGB, VGB
Juvenile myoclonic epilepsy	LTG, VPA,	CLB, CLN, TPM, LEV	CBZ, OXC, PHT, TGB, VGB
BECTS	CBZ, LTG, OXC, VPA	LEV, TPM	
BCOS	CBZ, LTG, OXC, VPA	LEV, TPM	
Infantile spasms	VGB, steroids	CLB, CLN, VPA, TPM	CBZ, OXC
Dravets	VPA, TPM, CLB, CLN	LEV, stiripentol	CBZ, LTG, OXC, VGB
Lennox–Gastaut Syndrome	VPA, LTG, TPM	CLB, CLN, ESM, LEV, RUF	CBZ, OXC
Landau–Kleffner syndrome	Steroids, LTG, VPA	LEV, TPM	CBZ, OXC
CSWS	Steroids, CLB, CLN, VPA, LTG, ESM,	LEV, TPM	CBZ, OXC, VGB
Myoclonic astatic epilepsy	CLB, CLN, VPA, TPM,	LEV, LTG	CBZ, OXC

Abbreviations: CBZ: carbamazepine; LTG: lamotrigine, OXC: oxcarbazepine, VPA: sodium valproate, TPM: Topiramate, CLB: Clobazam, GBP: gabapentin, LEV: levetiracetam, PHT: phenytoin, TGM: tiagabine, ZON: zonisamide, PGN: pregabalin, ESM: ethosuximide, CLN: clonazepam, RUF: rufinamide, VGB: vigabatrin.

* This table has been adapted from Clinical Guideline, 20: the epilepsies. The diagnosis and management of the epilepsies in adults and children in primary and secondary care; published by the National Institute for Health and Clinical Excellence, October 2004 and is available from ⁀www.nice.org.uk Information on this table has been reproduced with permissions of NICE. NICE has not been involved in checking that the information been reproduced accurately.

Box 4a.5 When to refer to a tertiary service (NICE 2004)[3]

- Behavioural or developmental regression.
- Unidentifiable epilepsy syndrome.
- Younger than two years of age.
- Seizures not controlled within 2 years.
- Two AEDs have been unsuccessful
- Unacceptable medication side effects.
- Unilateral structural lesion.
- Psychiatric comorbidity.
- Diagnostic doubt.

The ketogenic diet

The ketogenic diet is not new; it is a high fat diet designed to mimic starvation by forcing the body to use fat as the main energy source with the resultant production of ketones. It has been used in the treatment of epilepsy for almost 100 years. However, it has recently gained further popularity with the recognition that not all children respond to antiepileptic medication.[1]

In the traditional ('classical') ketogenic diet the main fat source is long-chain fatty acids and is calculated on the basis of fat to carbohydrate (including protein) of 3 or 4:1. Concern arose, however, about possible side effects of the diet, as well as its palatability and what was perceived as a more palatable way of giving the diet was developed by use of a medium chain triglyceride supplement with each meal, while still maintaining low carbohydrate. Both diets are now widely used around the world. Although there may be regional and cultural differences as to which diet may be predominantly used, there is no evidence for any difference in efficacy between the two diets. Parental choice or needs of the child are more likely to determine which diet is used.

The ketogenic diet may be considered if a child fails to respond to AEDs. It cannot be seen to be a natural treatment as it still may have side effects, but some children who respond may be able to wean from medication. It requires a high degree of dietetic input, for meal calculation, as well as a high degree of commitments on behalf of the parents as well as the child. The limited dietetic resource available has to date been the chief determinant on extent of use in the UK. There is no clear evidence that any age group respond over and above others, although there is little experience in adults; it becomes very difficult to adhere to as a teenager in view of protein restriction. In addition there does not appear to be a greater response amongst some syndromes or seizure types over others, although anecdotal evidence suggests particular benefit in myoclonic astatic epilepsy, and reports in younger children suggest a particular benefit in infantile spasms.

The ketogenic diet cannot be undertaken lightly but with parental commitment is a realistic option for children who have not responded to medication. Further information can be gained from the parental support group Matthews Friends.[2]

References

1. www.matthewsfriends.org

2. Freeman JM, Kossoff EH, Freeman JB, et al. (2006). The Ketogenic Diet: A Treatment for Epilepsy in Children and Others, 4th edn. Demos, New York.

3. National Institute for Clinical Excellence (NICE) Clinical Guidelines, 20, October 2004. The epilepsies: diagnosis and management of the epilepsies in children and young people in primary and secondary care. www.nice.org.uk

Medical treatment of epilepsy

Neurochemistry of AED action

Pharmacodynamics is the discipline that studies the mechanisms of action of drugs through investigation of their biochemical and physiological effects. Much of what we know about the mechanisms of action of AEDs derives from preclinical studies.

Some comments on preclinical drug development

- The exact mechanism of action of most AEDs is largely unknown.
- The development of modern AEDs arises from empirical testing of some 20,000 chemical compounds in animals.
- The most commonly used animal models to test for potential AEDs are maximal electroshock (tonic extension seizures), subcutaneous pentylenetetrazol (clonic seizures), and the kindling model (focal seizures). The GABA-agonists picrotoxin and bicuculline are also used to precipitate seizures.
- In interpreting findings from preclinical drug development, it is often assumed that:
  - *Maximal electroshock* will identify compounds that can protect against generalized convulsive seizures. It is thought to identify compounds that prevent seizure spread.
  - *Subcutaneous pentylenetetrazol* will identify compounds that can protect against absence seizures. It is thought to identify compounds that prevent seizure initiation (elevate seizure threshold).
  - *The kindling model* will identify compounds that can protect against focal seizures.
  - *Post-tetanic potentiation* (transiently enhanced responsiveness to single stimuli following high-frequency electrical stimulation) is thought to facilitate local excitation and enhance seizure spread.
  - *Voltage-sensitive sodium channels* underlie neuronal action potentials. Prolonging the inactivation phase that follows firing prevents rapid burst firing.
  - *Low-threshold (T-type) calcium currents* in thalamic relay neurons induce low-threshold calcium spikes that are thought to be responsible for the repetitive thalamo-cortical loop firing that generates 3Hz spike-and-wave activity in absence seizures.

Actions of carbamazepine

- Effective against tonic seizures induced by electroshock and chemoconvulsants, suggesting that it limits seizure propagation.
- Effective against focal seizures in kindling models.
- Ineffective against clonic seizures induced by subcutaneous pentylenetetrazol or bicuculline.
- Effective against clonic seizures induced by picrotoxin.
- Effective in blocking post-tetanic potentiation, suggesting that it limits seizure spread.
- Reduces sustained repetitive firing of action potentials in neuron culture.
- Thought to prolong inactivation phase of voltage-sensitive sodium channels.

Actions of benzodiazepines and barbiturates

- Enhance inhibition by allosteric modulation $GABA_A$ receptor.
- Barbiturates increase mean duration of channel opening without changing ionic conductance or opening frequency.
- Phenobarbital at high doses inhibits N-type calcium currents.

Actions of ethosuximide

- Effective in protecting against seizures induced by subcutaneous pentylenetetrazol, picrotoxin, and bicuculline, suggesting that it raises seizure threshold.
- Ineffective against seizures induced by maximal electroshock.
- Reduces low-threshold (T-type) calcium currents in thalamic neurons. This is probably the mechanism of action for protecting against absence seizures.

Actions of felbamate

- Probably multiple mechanisms of action.
- Effective against seizures induced by kindling, maximal electroshock, NMDA, quisqualic acid, aluminium hydroxide, and other chemoconvulsants.
- Ineffective against pilocarpine-induced status epilepticus.
- Neuroprotective properties shown *in vivo* and *in vitro*. It reduces hypoxic injury in hippocampal slices and *in vivo*.
- Broad spectrum but use limited because of risk of aplastic anaemia and hepatic toxicity.
- Reduces neuronal sustained repetitive firing, suggesting inhibition of voltage-dependant sodium channels.
- Interacts with strychnine-insensitive glycine binding site of NMDA receptors.
- Inhibits NMDA-evoked ionic currents—a unique action among AEDs.
- Enhances GABA-evoked chloride currents via an unclear mechanism.

Actions of gabapentin and pregabalin

- Binds to the $\alpha 2\delta$ subunit of the voltage-gated calcium channels and reduces synaptic release of glutamate.
- Effective against tonic extension seizures induced by electrical and chemical stimuli.
- Effective in protecting against clonic seizures induced by subcutaneous pentylenetetrazol, but not by picrotoxin, bicuculline, or strychnine.
- Blocks audiogenic seizures in mice, and tonic and clonic seizures in gerbils.
- Reduces severity of kindled temporal seizures.
- Ineffective against absence-like spike-and-wave activity in Wistar rats.
- *In vivo*, there is substantial delay between peak plasma and brain concentrations.

Action of Lacosamide

- Enhances slow inactivation of sodium channels.
- Modulates CRMP-2 (collapse in response mediator protein-2).

Actions of lamotrigine

- Lamotrigine was developed as an AED because of its antifolate action, following the observation that phenytoin, phenobarbital, and primidone reduce folate levels, and that folate induces seizures in animals.
- Nevertheless, lamotrigine displays only weak anti-folate activity.
- Little correlation between anti-folate and AED actions.
- Actions similar to those of phenytoin and carbamazepine, even though, lamotrigine is more broad spectrum.
- Effective against tonic extension seizures induced by maximal electroshock, suggesting that it limits seizure propagation.
- Effective against focal seizures in kindling models.
- Ineffective against clonic seizures induced by subcutaneous pentylenetetrazol.
- Selectively blocks veratrine-evoked glutamate release. It does not affect KCl-induced release.
- Prolongs inactivation of voltage-dependent sodium channels and blocks sustained repetitive firing. This seems to be the *main mechanism of action*.
- It inhibits N-type calcium currents.
- Enhances I_h currents.

Actions of levetiracetam

Binds to a synaptic vesicular protein (SV2A), probably limiting excitatory transmission.

Actions of oxcarbazepine

- Structurally related to carbamazepine.
- *In vivo*, it is quickly and completely reduced to its active metabolite (10-11-dihydro-10-hydroxy-carbamazepine or HCBZ), which is responsible for the AED actions of oxcarbazepine.
- AED actions virtually identical to those of carbamazepine.
- Oxcarbazepine is considered to have fewer side effects than carbamazepine.
- Its active metabolite inhibits non-L-type high-voltage activated calcium channels (presumably P/O or N types).
- Prolonging inactivation of voltage-gated sodium channels also significant.

Actions of phenytoin

- Effective against tonic seizures induced by electroshock and chemoconvulsants, suggesting that they limit seizure propagation.
- Effective against focal seizures in kindling models.
- Ineffective against clonic seizures induced by subcutaneous pentylenetetrazol or bicuculline.
- Ineffective against clonic seizures induced by picrotoxin.
- Effective in blocking post-tetanic potentiation, again suggesting that they limit seizure spread.
- Reduces sustained repetitive firing of action potentials in neuron culture by prolonging inactivation of voltage-sensitive sodium channels.
- Blocks delayed rectifier potassium currents.

Actions of sodium valproate—valproic acid

- It protects against seizures induced by maximal electroshock, subcutaneous pentylenetetrazol, picrotoxin, and bicuculline, and kindling.
- It blocks repetitive firing in neuronal cultures.
- It inhibits voltage-sensitive sodium channels *in vitro*.
- It induces a modest reduction in T-type calcium currents.
- It modifies GABA metabolism and modestly increases brain GABA concentration in animals and humans.

Actions of tiagabine

- Enhances GABA-mediated synaptic transmission by inhibiting GABA uptake by neurons and glia, thus increasing the concentration and duration of action of GABA in the synaptic cleft.
- Effective against seizures induced by dimethoxyethyl-carboline carboxylate (DMCM), subcutaneous pentylenetetrazol, maximal electroshock (but only at high doses), audiogenic seizures in mice and rats, and by photic stimulation in photosensitive baboons.

Actions of topiramate

- Actions similar to those of phenytoin, carbamazepine, and lamotrigine.
- Effective against tonic extension seizures induced by maximal electroshock.
- Effective against focal seizures in kindling models.
- Ineffective against clonic seizures induced by subcutaneous pentylenetetrazol, picrotoxin, or bicuculline.
- Blocks voltage-dependent sodium channels and kainate-evoked currents.
- Enhances GABA-evoked chloride currents.
- Appears to decrease excitation and increase inhibition.
- It inhibits sustained repetitive firing, suggesting that it blocks voltage-dependent sodium channels.
- It reduces duration and frequency of actions potentials within spontaneous epileptiform bursts.
- Similarly to benzodiazepines, topiramate enhances $GABA_A$-evoked chloride currents, but this action is not reversed by flumazenil, a benzodiazepine antagonist.
- It inhibits N-type calcium currents.
- Weak carbonic anhydrase inhibitor.
- Multiple actions may be explained by a primary action on phosphorylation mechanisms.

Actions of vigabatrin

- Effective against strychnine-induced, audiogenic seizures, baboon photosensitive epilepsy and amydala kindling.
- Increases brain levels of GABA by irreversible inhibition of GABA transaminase, the enzyme responsible for metabolism of GABA.
- In a significant proportion of patients, it induces a visual field defect through a toxic action on retinal ganglion cells.

Actions of zonisamide
- Broad AED profile: protects against seizures induced by maximal electroshock, tonic extension seizures in spontaneous epileptic rats, audiogenic seizures in mice, focal seizures induced by kindling, cortical freezing, and application of tungstic acid.
- Reduces repetitive firing in neuron culture, suggesting inhibition of voltage-dependent sodium channels.
- Reduces voltage-dependent T type calcium currents.
- Decreases flunitrazepam binding to benzodiazepine receptors and muscinol binding to $GABA_A$ receptors, although electrophysiological studies have not demonstrated that zonisamide affect GABA induced ionic currents.
- Protects against myoclonic seizures.

Key reading

1. White HS (1997). Mechanisms of antiepileptic drugs. In *The Epilepsies 2*, Porter RJ and Chadwick D (eds). *Blue Books of Practical Neurology*, Butterworth-Heinemann, Boston pp. 1–30.

Principles of pharmacokinetics and therapeutic AED monitoring

In order to induce an effect, medication must be present in the appropriate concentration at the sites of action. This will depend on the extent and rate of absorption, distribution, binding, biotransformation, and excretion of the drug (Fig. 4b.1).

Absorption

- Drugs administered in aqueous solution are more rapidly absorbed than those given in oily solution or solid form (Box 4b.1).
- *Oral ingestion* is the most common method to administer medication because it is generally the safest, the most convenient, and the cheapest. Nevertheless, it cannot be used if the patient is frequently vomiting, if he/she is unconscious, or if the drug is destroyed by digestive enzymes or low gastric pH. It has the following *disadvantages*:
  - Absorption after oral ingestion depends on the presence of food or other medication in the GI tract.
  - Drugs are delivered by the portal vein directly to the liver, where they may undergo inactivation.
- *Parenteral injection*—intramuscular, subcutaneous, intravenous— guarantees a faster and more predictable absorption, and it can be used if the patient is unconscious, uncooperative, or unable to tolerate oral intake. Intramuscular and subcutaneous injections are less predictable than intravenous. Parenteral injection has the following *disadvantages*:
  - It can be painful.
  - Asepsis is required to prevent infection.
  - Intravascular injection may occur when it is not intended.
  - Self-medication may be difficult, dangerous or impossible.
  - With intravenous administration, unfavourable reactions can occur due to the high plasma concentration of the drug that can rapidly be achieved. Repeated administration depends on maintaining a vein available. Drugs with an oily vehicle should be avoided through this route because they can irritate the vein.
  - Many orally available drugs are not available in parenteral formulation.

Intravenous injection must be preformed slowly and constantly monitoring the patient's response and level of consciousness.

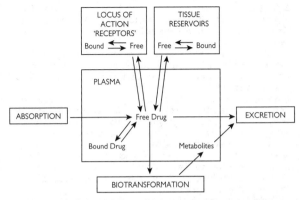

Fig. 4b.1. Representation of the interrelationship between absorption, distribution, binding, biotransformation, and excretion of a drug and its concentration at its locus of action. (Reproduced with permission from Goodman A, Goodman LS, and Gilman AG (1980). *Goodman and Gilman's The Pharmacological Basis of Therapeutics*, 6th edn. Macmillan Publishing Company, New York.)

Box 4b.1 Absorption of drugs in tablet form

The rate of absorption of drugs in tablets is in part dependent on the rate of dissolution of the tablet in the GI tract. This is the basis for the preparations called *slow-release, sustained-release, time-release,* or *pro-longed-action.* The tablets dissolve slowly so that the drug is released and absorbed during 8 hours or longer. This reduces the frequency of administration of the drug (possibly improving compliance), helps maintaining the therapeutic level overnight, and reduces the incidence of side effects by eliminating the sharp peaks in plasma concentration that can occur after administration via standard tablets.

- *Sublingual administration* through the oral mucosa. Absorption is fast and, since veins from the mouth drain to the superior vena cava, drugs absorbed in the mouth are protected from rapid inactivation by the liver.
- *Buccal:* provides greater surface area over which soluble agents can be administered. More socially acceptable than rectal route of administration in the event of patient being unconscious or unable to take oral medication.
- *Nasal:* nasally delivering of systemic therapy via solution or spray can be ideal for acute seizures because it is rapidly absorbed, it is socially acceptable and it avoids coughing or aspiration that can occur after sublingual or buccal administration in the unconcious patient.
- *Rectal administration:* often used when the patient is unconscious or when oral ingestion is precluded by frequent vomiting. The absorbed medication does not go directly to the liver. The *disadvantages* are that absorption can be irregular and incomplete, and some drugs can cause irritation of the rectal mucosa.
- *Bioavailability:* this term is often applied rather loosely. The expression 'differences in bioavailability' refers to differences in biological effects seen among pharmaceutical preparations that are chemically equivalent. More specifically, it often refers to the fact that similar preparations from different manufacturers, or different lots of identical preparation from the same manufacturer, may have a different degree of therapeutical and side effects.

Distribution of drugs

- After absorption into the bloodstream, drugs are distributed into the interstitial and cellular fluids.
- The rate of drug delivery to a tissue depends upon the blood flow (high for heart, liver, kidney, and brain; less for muscle, skin, and fat).
- Distribution is affected by drug binding to plasma proteins, particularly albumin. Most drugs travel in the bloodstream, either free in plasma or bound to proteins (Box 4b.2). Drug molecules strongly bound to plasma proteins:
  - Are not released to reach their sites of action in tissues or cells.
  - Are not metabolized.
  - Are not eliminated.
  - Consequently, at a particular moment in time, only the free plasma fraction of the drug can be considered biologically active. Since binding to plasma proteins is usually reversible, the fraction of the drug bound to proteins can be considered as a *drug reservoir*.
- Drugs might accumulate in certain tissues with a higher concentration than in others. Those tissues where a drug accumulates at a high concentration also behave as *drug reservoirs*.
- Drug accumulated in reservoirs can prolong drug action at the reservoir tissue as well as at distant sites.
- The distribution of drugs to the CNS is unique because of the *hematoencephalic barrier (blood–brain barrier)* surrounding the brain capillaries. *Drugs that reach most organs might not be able to reach brain cells.*

- If a drug stored in a drug reservoir is in equilibrium with that in plasma, the drug will be released into plasma when the plasma concentration declines slightly, maintaining plasma levels and drug action for as long as there is drug in the reservoir. Structures that frequently behave as drug reservoirs include:
  - Plasma proteins: mainly albumin. Protein binding is usually reversible. The extent of protein binding is specific for each drug.
  - Body fat: particularly for lipid-soluble drugs. In obese patients, fat content may be as much as 50% of body weight.
  - Muscle cells.
  - Bone.
  - Transcellular compartment: particularly the GI tract, into which drugs can be secreted and then reabsorbed.
- *Placental transport of drugs:* drugs that are transported across the placenta can cause congenital abnormalities and, if administered to the mother shortly before delivery, may have effects in the neonate. Drugs cross the placenta largely via simple diffusion. Lipid-soluble, non-ionized drugs cross more readily.

Box 4b.2 Concepts to keep in mind about protein binding

- Blood (plasma) levels determined by standard biochemical tests usually measure together the concentration of free drug and that of drug bound to proteins.
- However, only the free drug is responsible for drug action and side effects.
- Drops in protein plasma levels can increase side effects of drugs by increasing the concentration of free drug in plasma.
- Free drug levels should be monitored if protein levels are low—for instance, in liver or renal failure.
- If a drug binds to proteins, administration of a second drug that also binds to proteins can displace the initial drug from plasma proteins, significantly increasing its free drug level, thus increasing its biological action and side effects.
- Saliva levels of drugs run parallel to free drug levels, and can serve as an estimation of plasma free drug level without the need for bloodletting.

Biotransformation of drugs

- Drugs are often transformed into other molecules (metabolites) within the body, a process generically called *biotransformation*.
- Molecules, like many drugs, which are lipid soluble, weak acids or bases, are not easily eliminated—for instance, they are resborbed in the kidney.
- Metabolites are often less lipid-soluble and more polar than their mother drug, making them easier to eliminate.
- If metabolites are not biologically active, biotransformation results in inactivation of the drug.
- If metabolites are biologically active, their effects can be similar or different from those of the mother compound. Metabolites can be more toxic or have stronger therapeutic effects than the mother drug.
- Reactions involved in biotransformation can be classified into:
  - Non-synthetic: oxidation, reduction, hydrolysis.
  - Synthetic: conjugation—combining the drug or its metabolites with an endogenous compound, usually a carbohydrate, an amino acid, or a derivative of these such as acetic acid or sulphates.
- For the majority of drugs, hepatic microsomal enzymes are responsible for biotransformation. They are in the smooth endoplasmic reticulum of liver cells. They can inactivate significant amounts of drug after oral administration (*first-pass effect*).
- Microsomal enzymes also exist in other tissues such as in the epithelial cells in the digestive tract, in the plasma, kidney, and lung.
- Microsomal enzymes catalyze glucuronide conjugations and most of the oxidations (oxidase cytochrome P-450).
- Lipid solubility is required for drugs to penetrate the endoplasmic reticulum.
- Enzyme induction: activity of microsomal enzymes can be increased by a variety of drugs (for instance, phenobarbitone) and chemicals, a process that appears to be genetically determined.
- Since chronic administration of a drug can increase its own metabolism and that of others, interactions can occur between drugs simultaneously administered (co-medication).
- Non-microsomal enzymes are responsible for conjugations other than glucoronide formation, some oxidation, reduction and hydrolysis.
- Activity of hepatic microsomal and non-microsomal enzymes is reduced in the neonate, particularly if premature.

Excretion of drugs

- Drugs are excreted either unchanged or as metabolites.
- Excretion is more efficient for polar and non lipid-soluble compounds.
- The kidney is the most important excretory organ for drugs and metabolites.
- Compounds excreted in faeces are mainly non-absorbed orally ingested drugs, or metabolites excreted in bile and not absorbed in the intestine.
- Excretion of drugs in milk can induce unwanted effects in the breasfeeding neonate or infant.
- Metabolites of drugs formed in the liver are excreted with the bile into the GI tract. They can then be eliminated in the faeces or, more commonly, are reabsorbed into the bloodstream.
- Drugs excreted in saliva are usually swallowed and reabsorbed.

- The concentration of drugs in saliva parallels the concentration of the free drug in plasma.

Age-related considerations

- Various age-related factors change rate of elimination of medication with age.
- Overall rate of elimination is high in the infant and gradually reduces with age.
- This is related predominantly to increases in the capacity of the liver enzymes, although developmental changes in the distribution sites, renal function, and GI absorption also play a role.

Pharmacokinetic principles

- Pharmacokinetics studies the time variations of *drug concentration*, particularly in blood, serum and plasma, after drug administration. Drug concentrations in blood, serum, and plasma are largely determined by absorption, distribution, and excretion of the drug.
- *First-order kinetics:* elimination (or absorption) of the drug with time is assumed to follow an *exponential* curve because a constant *proportion* (fraction) of the drug is eliminated (or absorbed) per unit of time. This occurs when drug concentrations do not reach those levels required for saturation of the elimination process.
- *Zero-order kinetics:* elimination (or absorption) of the drug with time follows a *straight line* because a constant *amount* of the drug is eliminated (or absorbed) per unit of time.
- First-order kinetics can be characterized by the *constant rate* of elimination (often called k, defined as the fractional change per unit of time) or by the *half-life* (the time required to halve blood concentration). Both are independent of drug concentration and dose.
- *4 half-lives* are required for *nearly complete elimination* of a drug.
- The effects of a single dose of a drug are characterized by time to peak effect, its latency, amplitude of peak effect, and duration of effect (☐ see Fig. 4b.2).
- Doses repeated at intervals shorter than 4 half-lives will result in accumulation of the drug and steady increments in blood levels, often until a plateau is reached. If rapid effects are required (for instance in the treatment of status epilepticus) an initial larger dose (the loading dose) might be necessary.
- Some drugs, like phenytoin, show *dose-dependent elimination*. As drug concentration increases, so does the half-life. During the plateau phase, this behaviour results in increments in plasma concentration which are disproportionate to increases in dosage. They can be seen if the blood concentration approaches that required for saturation of elimination mechanisms.
- Dosage should be reduced in patients with impaired elimination (renal, hepatic or cardiac failure) to avoid excessive accumulation.
- *Monitoring blood levels:* these are essential for phenytoin use. They are helpful for some other AEDs. Free drug levels should be used in patients with low albumin levels—for instance, in renal, hepatic, or cardiac failure. Blood levels are useful to monitor or determine compliance. Compliance would often improve by the patient knowing that drug concentration is to be measured.

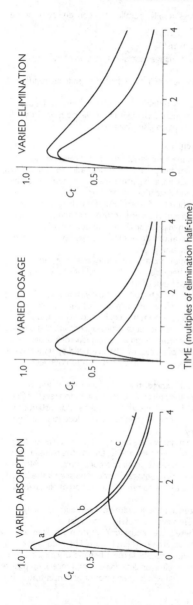

Fig. 4b.2 Fundamental pharmacokinetic relationships for single doses of drugs. *Varied absorption:* patterns to illustrate the influence of absorption (a) 100 times as rapid as, (b) 10 times as rapid as, and (c) equal to elimination. *Varied dosage:* patterns to illustrate the influence of a 2-fold difference in dosage (absorption 10 times as rapid as elimination). *Varied elimination:* patterns to illustrate the influence of a 2-fold difference in rate of elimination (lower curve, absorption:elimination = 10:1; upper curve, absorption:elimination = 100:5). (Reproduced with permission from Goodman A, Goodman LS, and Gilman AG (1980). *Goodman and Gilman's The Pharmacological Basis of Therapeutics*, 6th edn. Macmillan Publishing Company, New York.)

When to start treatment and overall prognosis with AED treatment

Treatment with AEDs is offered:
- When the diagnosis of epilepsy is highly probable or certain.
- In the event of unprovoked epileptic seizures.
- When the seizure severity or frequency justifies treatment.

This is influenced by individual circumstances. For example, a person may choose not to embark on long term AEDs if seizures are very mild (e.g. simple partial only) or rare and separated by many years. In addition to addressing risk of recurrence, the physician needs to discuss implications and consequences of continuing seizures. Examples include driving regulations, the possibility that more severe seizures may occur and potential associated risks, including risk of injury and to life.

Treatment is usually offered after a second epileptic seizure, but may be offered after a first seizure depending on:
- The underlying cause—e.g. structural progressive disease.
- Potential harmful consequences of seizures for the patient or dependent—e.g. infant.
- Patient requirements in relation to driving, employment, and social situations.

Observed recurrence rates after first (or early) seizures vary widely in different studies depending on whether those with prior seizures are excluded and on the time of assessment after the index seizure—the shorter the interval the higher the recurrence rate. Approximately 50% recur with some 50% of recurrences occurring within 6 months. Recurrence rates after a second seizure are higher at approximately 70% (📕 see Prognosis of epilepsy, pp.4–7).

Recurrence rates after a first seizure are higher with:
- Remote symptomatic epilepsy followed by idiopathic epilepsy.
- Abnormal EEG—generalized spike wave consistently reported, but many studies also show focal epileptiform EEG abnormalities to be a risk factor.
- Sleep-related seizures.

The inconvenience and potential side effects of long-term AEDs need to be balanced against the risks and consequences of uncontrolled seizures. The aim of treatment is to achieve seizure control with the least number of drugs, at the lowest effective doses, causing a minimum of adverse effects. The patient needs to be informed of the likelihood of medication controlling seizures.
- About 70% of those with newly-diagnosed epilepsy are controlled with treatment and about 50% enter long-term remission. Response to the first (suitable) AED is a good predictor of prognosis.
- There is debate as to whether seizures beget seizures and whether treatment should be given early. The main message from studies of early seizures is that early treatment reduces risk of recurrence but largely does not affect the likelihood of long-term remission (📕 see Box 4b.3). Nevertheless, a small minority may lose by delaying treatment because of consequences and complications of seizures. In general, however, in untreated populations, similar proportions respond even if the epilepsy is long-standing.
- While seizure control is achieved easily in the majority, a significant minority does not respond.

- In those who do not respond to the first 2–3 appropriate and tolerated AED regimens, the likelihood of responding to further AEDs or AED combinations, is significantly less.
- While improvements occur in a higher proportion, Seizure free rates in add-on drug trials in patients with refractory partial epilepsy are usually <10%.

Box 4b.3 The Multicentre trial for Early Epilepsy and Single Seizures (MESS) study

The MESS study addressed the relative risks and benefits of starting or withholding AED treatment *in a selected cohort of patients with few or infrequent seizures* in an unmasked, multicentre, randomized study. Outcomes included time to seizures as well as time to 2-year remission. Immediate treatment increased time to first and second seizure and to first tonic–clonic seizure. It also reduced the time to 2-year remission, however it did not affect long-term remission in this cohort. Further analysis showed number of seizures of all types at presentation, presence of a neurological disorder, and an abnormal EEG to be significant factors in indicating future seizures. 'Individuals with two or three seizures, a neurological disorder, or an abnormal EEG were identified as the medium-risk group, those with two of these features or more than three seizures as the high-risk group, and those with a single seizure only as the low-risk group.'[1]

Treatment response was analysed retrospectively in an unselected cohort of newly diagnosed adolescents and adults prescribed their first AED at the Western Infirmary in Glasgow, Scotland. Overall, nearly two-thirds of patients became seizure free for at least 12 months, of whom only 5.4% subsequently developed refractory epilepsy. Just over one-third were uncontrolled from the outset. Overall response rates (response to treatment was defined as achieving 12 months seizure freedom on an unchanged treatment schedule) with the first, second, and third treatment schedules were 50.4, 10.7, and 2.7% respectively. These figures are disappointing and may well be under-estimates, however, they are useful in reminding us that poor responders may be identified relatively early with subsequent treatment regimens associated with diminishing returns. Remission rates observed were highest in seniors at 85%, then in adolescents at 65%, with the remainder at 55%.[2]

More encouragingly, another study which looked at results of treatment changes in patients with apparently drug-resistant chronic epilepsy in one clinic reported that 16% of drug introductions resulted in seizure freedom for 12 months or more with a further 21% achieving a 50–99% seizure reduction.[3] While there are a number of factors that influence outcome in this study, it serves to remind us that skilled drug manipulation can be worthwhile in a significant proportion of patients with apparently drug resistant chronic epilepsy.

References

1. Marson A, Jacoby A, Johnson A, (2005). Immediate versus deferred antiepileptic drug treatment for early epilepsy and single seizures: a randomized controlled trial. Medical Research Council MESS Study Group. *Lancet*, **365**(9476), 2007–13.

2. Mohanraj R and Brodie MJ (2006). Diagnosing refractory epilepsy: response to sequential treatment schedules *European Journal of Neurology*, **13**(3), 277–82.

3. Luciano AL and Shorvon SD (2007). Results of treatment changes in patients with apparently drug-resistent chronic epilepsy. *Annals of Neurology*, 2007, **62**, 375–81.

What AED to start with

General considerations

The number of licensed AEDs has increased and this makes it difficult for the non-expert to choose the best medication for an individual. As post-marketing experience accumulates and new trial data become available, the relative positions of different AEDs change. This is thus a constantly evolving field. Taking an AED involves a significant investment of time and effort for the patient; it is thus an important step, which should be given due consideration. It is important to make an informed choice and if necessary seek advice from an expert and not select an AED at random. As a significant proportion respond to the first suitable AED for the syndrome, long-term side effects should be considered in selecting the first AED. Each prescribed medication is used in an optimal way to avoid the patient with intractable epilepsy wasting many months or more retrying it in the future. Although AEDs are licensed on the basis of proven efficacy in controlling seizures, there is no proof that they affect the underlying condition. Their use is hampered by the lack of guaranteed prediction of success at the start of treatment in the individual case, and the lack of early surrogate markers of efficacy. Therapeutic success takes time to ascertain and at present involves simply observing if there is improvement in seizure frequency. EEG follow-up, except in selected situations, is generally not an adequate surrogate marker of treatment success, although it is helpful in predicting likelihood of recurrence, particularly in younger patients. In time, pharmacogenetics may provide a more rational basis for AED selection in each individual. Methods assessing cortical excitability with the aim of predicting the likelihood of seizures occurring may help provide earlier measures of treatment success. For now, however, the choice of AED relies on matching patient and epilepsy characteristics with the profile of the drug. Once a medication is started, clinical response needs to be carefully monitored.

There are many factors influencing choice of AED and those who chose one drug for all should think again!

Factors influencing choice of AED—the epilepsy syndrome and seizure types

AEDs are not all broad spectrum. What helps one person's epilepsy may be ineffective, or worse still, can exacerbate seizures in another. In particular, narrow spectrum drugs, effective for partial epilepsy, can worsen generalized epilepsy syndromes. For example, carbamazepine can make absences, myoclonus, and sometimes GTCS in idiopathic generalized epilepsy (IGE) worse, with an adverse effect that can be dose-related.

Some AEDs only prevent certain seizure types. Ethosuximide mostly controls absences but not GTCS. Even where a medication is considered likely to be effective in a given syndrome, the patient's individual response should be monitored as this cannot be predicted with certainty. Always keep in mind the original pattern of the epilepsy. If previously infrequent seizures off treatment become frequent on treatment, in the absence of a competing explanation, consider that medication may be exacerbating the epilepsy.

In the young—including young adults—with unclassified epilepsy, choose a broad-spectrum AED as per generalized epilepsy.

Broad versus narrow spectrum medication

The more broad-spectrum drugs include sodium valproate, benzodiazepines, topiramate, and zonisamide. Phenobarbital is also reasonably broad spectrum as is to an intext levetiracetam. Lamotrigine is considered broad spectrum by some but is not as broad spectrum as some of the drugs already listed; in particular it can exacerbate myoclonus.

Carbamazepine, oxcarbazepine, gabapentin, pregabalin, vigabatrin, tiagabine, and phenytoin are considered narrow spectrum. Narrow spectrum drugs are not generally effective against, and may exacerbate certain seizure types such as absences or myoclonus. They may be effective against or exacerbate idiopathic GTCS, and sometimes the effect is dose-related, with exacerbations at higher doses. Caution is required in generalized epilepsies, where narrow spectrum drugs are usually best avoided.

Match the profile of the person with the profile of the medication!

Weight, gender, age, tolerance to medication, plans for pregnancy, other medical conditions, concomitant medication, and likely compliance are all important factors influencing choice of AED. To choose wisely, one needs to know well both the patient and the patient's epilepsy, in addition to being familiar with available AEDs.

Choosing an AED in IGE

It is easier to treat IGE in males! Sodium valproate is very effective at generally well-tolerated low-to-moderate doses in the majority of patients with IGE and for all seizure types. Important disadvantages include weight gain and the fact that its use is problematic in women of reproductive age. Compared to some other AEDs, it is reportedly associated with a greater risk of major malformations particularly with higher doses, and of increased educational needs amongst offspring. Lamotrigine is often used in women in this situation, as its profile in pregnancy is reasonable, with a low malformation risk reported by the Belfast pregnancy register at low to moderate doses. However, it is neither as effective as valproate in IGE nor as easy to use, and a subgroup may have more frequent seizures.

Other potentially effective medications in IGE include zonisamide, topiramate, levetiracetam, benzodiazepines, and phenobarbital, each with its own advantages and disadvantages. Phenobarbital is not preferred in pregnancy, and there is limited information in pregnancy for the others. Benzodiazepines can result in habituation, tolerance, and loss of efficacy. It remains to be determined how broad spectrum levetiracetam is, but it can be effective in IGE, particularly for myoclonus. Topiramate is not always well tolerated but it is broad spectrum and effective, but malformations have been reported in pregnancy. The role of zonisamide, which at the time of writing, has a licence for partial epilepsy, will become clearer with time, but it is very promising for young adults with IGE and is likely to be effective and broad spectrum, including for absences. In the 'generalized' arm of SANAD, a pragmatic large study comparing new and old AEDs in new onset cases, valproate was shown to be superior to lamotrigine and topiramate.[1a] Levetiracetam and zonisamide were not assessed.

Choosing an AED in partial epilepsy

Carbamazepine and lamotrigine are currently reasonable first choice medications in partial epilepsy (partial seizures with or without secondary GTCS). Lamotrigine has been shown to be better tolerated than carbamazepine in the 'partial' arm of the SANAD study, although carbamazepine may not have been used optimally.[1b] The study compared the carbamazepine arm with lamotrigine, topiramate, gabapentin, and oxcarbazepine, the latter added to the study belatedly with smaller numbers randomized. Levetiracetam, zonisamide, pregabalin, and clobazam were not included and a second SANAD study is under consideration.

For now, either lamotrigine or carbamazepine would be reasonable first choices, although both have limitations. For those who respond to carbamazepine at the expense of side effects, oxcarbazepine can be a good alternative, with similar good efficacy, but with increased risk of hyponatraemia. Both carbamazepine and lamotrigine have a reasonable profile in pregnancy. Clinical experience of the use of levetiracetam has demonstrated good efficacy and reasonable tolerability (despite occasional mood disturbances) and it is used increasingly early, including as first line, particularly as pharmacokinetic interactions are not a problem. Data in pregnancy is accumulating though still limited. There are many other medications licensed for partial epilepsy. These include gabapentin, pregabalin, tiagabine, topiramate, and zonisamide.

Phenytoin, phenobarbital, and primidone (partly metabolized to pheno-barbital) are older options. These have significant disadvantages. In partic-ular, phenytoin, which is still in frequent use, has major disadvantages, not least its side-effect profile and non-linear pharmacokinetics. Vigabatrin is associated with visual field defects and should not generally be prescribed de novo, except in West syndrome.

NICE and epilepsy

NICE addressed epilepsy in two very useful documents published in 2004:
- The NICE Technology Appraisal Guidance. Available at: 🖳 www.nice. org.uk/TA076 (Newer Drugs for Epilepsy in Adults) and www.nice.org. uk/TA0769 (Newer Drugs for Epilepsy in Children).
- Clinical Guidelines (an excellent wide-ranging document). Available at: 🖳 www.nice.org.uk/CG020

Specific AEDs—comparative efficacy and tolerability

Although there is overlap, there are differences in the mode of action of some AEDs which can result in a drug being effective when another has failed. In clinical practice, clear differences are observed overall in relative efficacy and tolerability between AEDs, although an individual's response is not possible to predict with any certainty.

Head-to-head comparisons between different AEDs are relatively limited and usually only powered to show lack of inferiority to the estab-lished AED. Overlapping confidence intervals in odds ratios in meta-anal-yses of published drug trials of new AEDs as add-on treatment generally failed to confirm differences in efficacy or tolerability between the dif-ferent AEDs. There were clear trends, however, which were interestingly, and not surprisingly, largely concordant with clinical impressions. It is likely that the differences were not significant because of lack of power and not because the drugs are equipotent or equally well tolerated. Unfortunately, some misunderstood this to be the case. Indeed, in the entirely different setting of SANAD, the pragmatic study already referred to, which com-pared efficacy and tolerability of (some) new AEDs versus valproate or carbamazepine in new onset epilepsy, clear differences in efficacy and tol-erability emerged.[1a,1b]

Head to head comparisons between drug AEDs have limitations

- The comparator drug may not be used optimally. An example is where a new AED is compared to carbamazepine, but with carbamazepine used sub-optimally (high escalation rates, high initial target does without slow release formulations).
- Studies are not usually powered to show superiority of one AED over another, but are often powered to demonstrate equivalence (judged by both upper and lower confidence intervals) or lack of inferiority(judged by lower confidence intervals). However, conclusions of lack of inferiority or equivalence may be flawed. These depend on how delta is defined, delta being the smallest important difference between the two treatments for a particular outcome. A delta of 20% for example, in a new onset cohort, where at least 50% are expected to respond, may be considered too high.

When should a newly licensed AED be used?

Caution here is indicated. Rare life-threatening drug side effects may not become apparent in clinical trials. This is because, at most, a few thousand people are involved in such trials and if infrequent, it is only after licensing that such side effects emerge. Epilepsy is a serious condition with an associated morbidity and excess mortality. For the most part treatment is indicated. With any medication, there is a risk of idiosyncratic life-threatening reactions, but these must be shown to be extremely rare indeed to justify prescribing a medication when there are alternatives. For example, felbamate, an effective and broad spectrum, AED, was found after licensing to be associated with a higher risk of aplastic anaemia and liver failure. This has resulted in very restricted use.

In general, until safe experience of hundreds of thousands of person-years of prescribing has accumulated, a new AED should be recommended for an individual patient only if:

• The severity of the epilepsy and its associated risks justifies it, and
• There are no better established alternatives.

In addition to being familiar with the data sheet, it is also advisable to seek advice from colleagues with experience in the use of a new AED, with regard to starting doses, side effects, and rates of introduction which are often slower than in the data sheet (Box 4b.4).

Drug data sheets and patient information leaflets can be found on Medicines.org.uk. Abbreviated information as well as lists of interactions are in the *British National Formulary*.[2]

Data sheets include important information on interactions, side effects, and use. They also include approved starting doses, rates of introduction, and maximum doses based on pre-licensing clinical trials. Starting doses and rates of introduction of AEDs, however, are in practice usually slower than advised in data sheets. Pre-licensing clinical studies are designed to demonstrate safety and efficacy of a new AED and not to establish optimal use. Following clinical experience, almost always, slower rates of introduction are adopted. The advice in this section, therefore, does not necessarily follow that stated in the data sheet. If there is clinical urgency, doses can be introduced faster than recommended here, but generally not faster than data sheet recommendations.

Box 4b.4 AEDs and delayed side effects—examples

Below are examples of some medium and long-term side effects associated with AEDs. Some require medication change, while others require management, monitoring or prevention. They should be considered when medication is first prescribed to avoid, if possible, later change in treatment when someone is already well controlled.

- Skin—e.g. acne, coarsening features, hypertrichosis with phenytoin.
- Soft tissue—association with Dupuytren's contracture and Peyronie's disease reported with older AEDs, such as phenytoin.
- Gums—hypertrophy, particularly with phenytoin.
- Hair loss—particularly valproate, regrowth may be curly, less commonly topiramate.
- Weight gain—e.g. valproate, gabapentin, pregabalin, and to a lesser extent carbamazepine.
- Weight loss—e.g. topiramate, zonisamide.
- Raised lipids—possible association with carbamazepine.
- Hyponatraemia—carbamazepine and oxcarbazepine.
- Folate deficiency, changes in blood count and effect on liver function—many AEDs.
- Low vitamin D levels, osteopaenia —usually but not exclusively enzyme-inducing AEDs.
- Effects on reproductive hormones, ovaries, menstrual cycle, fertility, and libido.
- Depression—e.g. levetiracetam, topiramate.
- Agitation irritability and other psychiatric disturbances—many AEDs.
- Effects on cognition—many AEDs.
- Decreased verbal fluency—topiramate.

Pre-licensing drug trials, prescription of unlicensed medication, or unlicensed use of a licensed drug

Pre-licensing clinical trials include 3 phases, preceded by extensive pre-clinical studies.

- *Phase I*: these are usually carried out with a small number of healthy volunteers in closely supervised conditions; they provide preliminary safety, pharmacokinetic, and dose-ranging data.
- *Phase II*: these extend phase I studies and test efficacy and tolerability in a group of patients.
- *Phase III*: these are randomized controlled trials in larger patient groups. Usually efficacy and tolerability is compared to standard treatment or placebo.

Once a medication is licensed, there is an on-going system of *post-marketing surveillance*.

Pre-licensing clinical trials are usually carried out using AEDs as add-on treatment in otherwise well adult patients with intractable partial epilepsy—excluding women who could become pregnant. Thus, initial licenses are usually granted for this category. One should not assume that the medication is narrow spectrum, not useful in children, and is not effective in monotherapy! With some medications, as trial data accumulates supporting other indications, the licence is gradually extended.

Sometimes, clinical experience supports an indication for a medication before a licence for that indication is issued. If there is clinical need, the medication may be prescribed outside licence. As drugs are almost always tested in adults before children, with paediatric licences often delayed, specialized paediatric units, often recommend new add-on AEDs, in intractable cases, outside licence. Those of any age who respond fully to an add-on drug may attempt withdrawal of other medications and end up on successful monotherapy. Some new medications show promise as broad-spectrum AEDs and may be offered to intractable patients with generalized epilepsy before there is a licence for this indication. This is acceptable clinical practice. It is important, however, that the patient is aware and is happy to take medication outside licence.

Prescription of unlicensed medication/unlicensed use

These medicines fall into two categories:
- Medicines that are unlicensed, and
- Medicines that are licensed but are being used outside of their product licence.

Prescribing in either of these categories is not generally recommended. However it is recognized that in some circumstances this may be appropriate.

Points for consideration in the UK[3]

- Prescribers have a duty in common law to take reasonable care and to act in a way consistent with the practice of a responsible body of peers of similar professional standing.
- Legal responsibility for prescribing falls to the practitioner who signs the prescription, or in primary care, the practitioner whose stamp is detailed on the FP10.
- Responsibility must also be taken for overseeing the patient's care, monitoring, and any follow up treatment or arranging for another doctor to do so.
- In situations following a recommendation by a consultant specialist, the prescriber is unlikely to be found negligent if they have taken steps to become familiar with the drug, are able to monitor the drug completely, and have access to effective consultant support.
- When an unlicensed medicine or an unlicensed use of a medicine is prescribed, the prescriber is professionally accountable for his/her judgement in doing so, and may be called upon to justify his/her actions.

Some common errors in AED management

The correct action in one setting may be an error in another!
- Not listening to the patient's preferences.
- Aiming for too high a dose too early—the lowest dose that controls attacks is not established.
- Introducing AED too slowly—e.g. with frequent seizures and no side effects.
- Not going high enough—if there has been improvement with a modest dose, it is worth going higher to the maximum tolerated dose.
- Not exploring each medication to its maximum potential.
- Not changing medication in time—if a good dose of an AED has made no difference whatsoever, sometimes it is best to cut your losses.

- Increasing the dose when there are side effects—they will only get worse.
- Increasing the dose when seizures are controlled—what is the point?
- Under-treating if infrequent seizures—patient loses time before control is achieved.
- Using wrong increments, decrements, and rate of change. This can be too fast or too slow. Consider half-life of AED (and interactions), specific drug, seizure control, previous patient experience, and priorities/tolerance of the individual patient before advising in each specific case. Allow the patient to adjust where appropriate.
- Not being aware that AEDs may exacerbate seizures—compare with seizure frequency before AED was started.
- Not being aware of interactions—check and check again both when withdrawing and adding an AED.
- Not reducing the dose if control is no better on a higher dose—this adds to the total drug load and side effects and reduces the likelihood of tolerating add-on AEDs.
- Reducing the old drug before the efficacy and tolerability of the added AED is established for that patient; this is particularly relevant for those on monotherapy, if there has been a good response to the first drug—patient can be left exposed with no cover.
- Making too many changes together—this makes it difficult to attribute cause in case of an adverse outcome. One (preferably) or two (at a most) changes at a time are generally advised.
- Adding and adding AEDs while forgetting to withdraw.
- Advising changes, if there is no clinical urgency, before getting to know the patient and the previous history well.
- Forgetting to ask about triggers before making treatment decisions— e.g. there is no point increasing the dose, or changing medication if the reason for the seizure was forgetting dose.
- Not keeping a good record of treatment.
- Not asking for a record of seizures or documenting seizures in the notes.
- Not reviewing the diagnosis if seizures are uncontrolled.

References

1a. Marson et al. (2007) The SANAD study of effectiveness of valproate, lamotigene, or topiramate for generalised and unclassifiable epilepsy: an unblinded randomised controlled trial. *Lancet* March 24;369(9566): 1016–26

1b. Marson et al. (2007)The SANAD study of effectiveness of carbamazepine, gabapentin, lamotingine, oxcarbaxepine, or topiramate for treatment of partial epilepsy: an unblinded randomised controlled trial. *Lancet* March 24;369(9566): 1000–15

2. *British National Formulary*. Available at: ⌂ http://www.bnf.org/bnf

3. GMC (2008) Good Practice in Prescribing Medicines. Available at: ⌂ www.gmc-uk.org/guidance/current/library/prescriptions_faqs.asp

How to use AEDs

Basic principles

Here is some general advice on how to prescribe AEDs. Attention to detail and some subtlety in prescribing can make the difference between success and failure.

- Document the baseline frequency and severity of seizures before commencing AEDs.
- Throughout treatment document medications taken including: starting doses, dose escalation, maximum doses, effect on seizures, side effects, duration of treatment, and reason for discontinuation.

Some always work up to the same target dose irrespective of patient age, response, or tolerance. A target dose, corresponding to what is usually a low average maintenance dose, is reasonable as an initial dose to build up to, if tolerated and if seizures are very infrequent. Where seizures are frequent, the target is not the dose but the desired effect, namely seizure prevention on the lowest dose—with minimum side effects. 📖 See Box 4b.5 for terminology used in relation to side effects.

Introducing an AED

- Ensure that the patient or carer understands basic principles as appropriate to the individual case.
- Encourage the patient or carer to keep a seizure chart.
- Unless there is clinical urgency, start on low doses and build up gradually to minimize dropout from transient side effects. Start with even lower doses in the elderly or in those generally intolerant or wary of medication such as many patients with learning difficulties. This makes it easier to achieve maintenance on the lowest effective dose for the individual.
- Do not increase the dose—and inform the patient likewise—if there are significant side effects likely to be attributed to the medication, as these will predictably worsen.
- Inform the patient which possible side effects are likely to be transient and which require cessation of treatment such as allergic reactions.
- In someone with frequent seizures, a so-called target dose is not useful. The target should be seizure control. There is no need to increase the dose beyond that needed to achieve this.
- In someone with infrequent seizures, the concept of a target dose is helpful; but remember that most patients are controlled on low-to-moderate doses (📖 see Tables 4b.1a and 4b.1b).
- If seizures continue to be uncontrolled, and assuming no side effects, continue escalating the dose and do not allow months to pass on low ineffective doses. To achieve this, follow-up arrangements need to be in place with the GP, epilepsy nurse, or in epilepsy clinics neurology.
- If someone improves on medication on a particular dose, but higher doses do not confer additional benefit, gradually reduce back to the lowest dose that showed maximum benefit.
- Give the informed patient flexibility within a pre-defined dose range and time-scale without insisting on rigid adherence to a dose escalation, irrespective of response and side effects.

Box 4b.5 Terminology currently in use in relation to frequency of side effects in drug data sheets

- *Very common:* >1 in 10
- *Common:* between 1 in 100 and 1 in 10
- *Uncommon:* between 1 in 1000 and 1 in 100
- *Rare:* between 1 in 10,000 and 1 in 1000
- *Very rare:* <1 in 10,000

What next?

What next? Patient is still experiencing fits, how high do I go before considering an alternative?

There is no point increasing the prescribed dose if the patient has side effects or does not adhere to the treatment regimen. Patients sometimes do not take medication because they do not feel well on it, not only because of general reluctance or difficulty with adherence due to lifestyle, routine, or discipline. Gently probe about side effects and adherence to treatment before making decisions.

If unprovoked seizures continue despite good tolerance and adherence to treatment, the dose is gradually titrated up, unless seizure frequency is increasing for no apparent reason with the increase in dose. Keep in mind that an AED may infrequently *exacerbate* epilepsy. This is uncommon but is encountered sufficiently regularly for us to caution about it. If the seizure chart suggests that this may be the case, then the choice of AED needs to be reconsidered even if the maximum tolerated dose has not been reached.

If there is no increase in seizures, and no side effects, and the epilepsy is still uncontrolled, the dose should be increased until the maximum tolerated or maximum licensed dose is reached. Although only successful in a proportion, this should, nevertheless, be attempted. It is not efficient in the long term to change medications too early, without trying higher doses, as the patient may later end up wasting time and effort revisiting the same drug if the initial dose tried is considered inadequate. If the medication is well tolerated but there is no improvement by the maximum licensed dose, there is usually little point going higher. If there is excellent improvement by the maximum licensed dose with no side effects, but the patient is still not seizure free, consideration may be given to higher than licensed doses, with the patient's consent.

Table 4b.1a Incremental benefit in complete seizure control for patients with newly treated epilepsy when increasing the daily dose to higher and maximum tolerated doses. (Reproduced from Deckers et al. Epilepsy Research, **53**: 1–17, © 2003, with permission from Elsevier.)

Author	Low (mg per day)	Seizure-free (%)	Average (mg per day)	Seizure-free (%)	High (mg per day)	Seizure-free (%)	Maximum tolerated (mg per day)	Seizure-free (%)
Kwan and Brodie (2001)	200–300 CBZ	4.3	400–600 CBZ	30.8	700–800 CBZ	3.8	900–1600 CBZ	2.8
Kwan and Brodie (2001)	200–500 VPA	7.9	600–1000 VPA	36.5	1100–1500 VPA	7.8	1600–2500 VPA	4.9
Kwan and Brodie (2001)	50–100 LTG	12.9	125–200 LTG	38.6	225–300 LTG	6.4	325–600 LTG	3.8
Brodie et al. (2002)	1200 GBP	3.5	1800 GBP	56.3	2400 GBP	13.2	3600 GBP	2.8
Brodie et al. (2002)	100 LTG	3.9	150 LTG	50.9	200 LTG	14.7	300 LTG	6.9
Chawick et al. (1999)[a]	50 TPM	39	>50–100 TPM	10	>100–200 TPM	0	>200–500 TPM	10
All AEDs	Low	11.9	Average	37.2	High	7.7	Maximum	5.2

The data show the limited utility of increasing to above average daily doses in patients with newly treated patients still reporting seizure. Abbreviations CBZ: carbamazepine, GBP: gabapentin, LTG: lamotrigine, TPM: topiramate.

[a] The seizure-free period was either 12 or 6 months.

Table 4b.1b Incremental benefit in responder rate (50% or more seizure reduction versus baseline) for patients with refractory partial epilepsy when increasing the daily dose to higher and maximum tolerated doses. (Reproduced from Deckers CLP, Genton P, Sills GJ, et al. (2003). Current limitations of antiepileptic drug therapy: a conference review. *Epilepsy Research*, **53**, 1–17 with permission from Elsevier).

Author	Low (mg per day)	Responder rate (%)	Average (mg per day)	Responder rate (%)	High/and maximum (mg per day)	Responder rate (%)
Abou-Khalil (2000)	>200 TPM	47	200–400 TPM	9	>400 TPM	0
Barcs et al. (2000)	600 OXC	26.8	1200 OXC	14.4	2400 OXC	8.8
US Gabapentin Study Group (1993)	1200 GBP	17.6	1800 GBP	8.8	n.a.	n.a.
Shorvon and Rijckevorsel (2002)	1000 LEV	28	2000 LEV	4	3000 LEV	9
All AEDs	Low	29.9	Average	9.1	High	5.9

The data show the limited utility of increasing to above average daily doses in patients with refractory epilepsy still reporting seizures at average daily doses. Abbreviations: GBP: gabapentin, LEV: levetiracetam, OXC: oxcarbazepine, TPM: topiramate.

What next? Medication is well-tolerated but is not sufficiently effective as monotherapy: add-on therapy or sequential monotherapy?

- Sequential monotherapy is generally recommended but it may not be appropriate for everyone. If someone has responded with say an 80% reduction in seizures, or an abolition of the more severe seizures, has no side effects with the first medication, and is *not a woman of childbearing age*, then a small dose of an add-on medication is a perfectly reasonable, often effective, option.

- In someone who has not responded to a significant extent to the first medication, and in women of childbearing age, sequential monotherapy is more appropriate.
  - However, unless the patient is worse on the first medication, do not withdraw the first medication until you have established that the patient tolerates the second medication, appears to be improving with the second medication, and/or has reached an average maintenance dose. Otherwise, it may be the second medication that is withdrawn! Early 'cross-over' is not appropriate in someone on monotherapy unless side effects necessitate prompt withdrawal of the first drug.
  - Remember, or look up, pharmacokinetic and pharmacodynamic interactions between the two medications.
  - Consider that someone at the threshold of tolerance of one medication may not tolerate the second as well without a small reduction in the first. An example is when lamotrigine is added to high-dose carbamazepine.
  - Recommend contraception during the change-over period where appropriate.

What next? Sequential monotherapy of 2–4 appropriate medications is unsuccessful

- Continue on one medication as baseline; choose the most effective and tolerated of the monotherapy medications tried at an optimum dose (maximum benefit for minimum side effects); this may be below the maximum dose reached.
- Consider add-on medication appropriate to the syndrome.
- Some combinations have been considered synergistic, but evidence is limited.
- Introduce add-on medication and if necessary increase the dose.
  - If seizure-free, maintain a long period of stability without seizures before considering any changes. The patient may later wish to consider gradually reducing or withdrawing the first medication, but understandably, may not wish to take the risk of relapse in doing so.
  - If ineffective gradually withdraw the less effective or less well-tolerated of the two medications and consider an alternative.
- Always consider interactions when medications are withdrawn or added.

Combination therapy may be effective where monotherapy fails!

How to add another AED in someone on polytherapy?
- One change at a time is usually recommended as, if there is a clinical change, causality is easier to ascribe.
- Keep the most effective and best-tolerated as the baseline medication.
- If possible, simplify regimen by withdrawing the least effective medication(s) first, usually sequentially if more than one, before adding another. Always consider interactions when planning medication withdrawal. If withdrawal is not possible or unsuccessful, or if there is clinical urgency, cross-over, with one medication introduced and another add-on medication withdrawn is reasonable, so long as effective baseline medication is maintained. Remember that some medications especially if taken long-term cannot be withdrawn quickly because of risk of rebound seizures/status.

How to withdraw an AED?
There are many different scenarios as per these examples:

Withdrawing an AED in someone with serious allergic reactions or potentially life-threatening side effects.
This has to be done promptly and quickly with careful observation. Clobazam may be used if necessary to cover the period of risk or until another medication is established.

Withdrawing an AED in a poorly controlled patient on polythrapy
Uncontrolled patients can end up on many drugs. A small proportion need and benefit from a complicated polytherapy regimen. Many, however, do not. They risk more side effects and interactions. They are uncertain of the contribution of different medications to seizure control or side effects and are still experiencing seizures. Before recommending a change on the basis of continuing seizures, however, consider whether severe seizure types or status episodes/admissions are controlled even though seizures still occur.

This is a difficult situation without easy solutions. The following may be considered when the patient is in agreement:
- Try and avoid complicating treatment further—or this situation in the first place—by always withdrawing the last medication added if it has not clearly helped.
- If possible, simplify treatment, by attempting to withdraw medications perceived to be least effective by both the patient and the physician. Review all previous clinic letters and notes as this will significantly aid the decision-making process. If there is more than one, they are usually withdrawn sequentially, while continuing with medications considered effective. Always consider interactions when medications are withdrawn. Removing an enzyme inhibitor may result in reduced levels of the remaining drug with loss of efficacy. Removing an enzyme inducer may result in increase in side effects, although the total drug load is reduced, because levels of a remaining medication rise; dose adjustments of remaining medications may be needed before recommencing the withdrawal process. Temporary, minor worsening in seizure control may occur as a drug is withdrawn. If it settles spontaneously or with rescue medication, there is no automatic

need to reverse the reduction. If there is a sustained increase in seizures on the other hand then it may be necessary to reverse the reduction back to the last dose associated with stable seizures and reconsider the strategy.

Withdrawing one AED in a well-controlled patient on polytherapy

Consider why you wish to consider withdrawal of any AED as the risk of loosing control may not be worth taking for the individual. Discuss the advantages and disadvantages of doing so carefully with the patient. It may be that side effects are present that could be improved by AED load reduction. On the other hand, the patient may have had great difficulty achieving good control and may not wish to jeopardize the situation, in which case leave well alone unless clear benefit is expected in making the change and the patient is in agreement.

Withdrawing AEDs in a patient in remission

Withdrawal can be considered, but not necessarily attempted, in adult patients who have been seizure-free for a minimum of 2 years, preferably 5 years.

- Enquire first if they really are seizure-free. Not infrequently patients omit to mention minor attacks that they do not consider significant but which nevertheless indicate that the epilepsy is active.
- Considering withdrawal should not be equated with advising withdrawal. A decision to withdraw is one the informed patient and not the physician makes.
- The risk of relapse is lower the longer the period of seizure freedom, however, some syndromes often need lifelong treatment. Even in patients seizure-free for several years, there is a risk of relapse of between 20–40%, and patients may find this risk unacceptable. Risk of relapse can be individualized using the MRC AED withdrawal study formula (📖 see Table 4b.2).
- Patients should be reminded of the physical and social risks associated with seizures before embarking on withdrawal, including a very small risk to life.
- Patients need to be informed of social and legal implications of possible seizure recurrence when driving (📖 see Lifestyle, pp.533–534)
- Withdrawal should be gradual. Abrupt withdrawal can precipitate severe rebound seizures with certain medications. Patients on several AEDs usually have one withdrawn at a time, but look out for the effect of interactions—removing an enzyme-inducing AED may result in toxicity from a remaining drug. Removing an enzyme inhibitor may result in reduced levels of the remaining drug with loss of efficacy. Dose adjustments of the remaining drug may be needed.

How useful are drug levels?

📖 This is addressed as appropriate in sections dealing with specific medications. Phenytoin levels are essential to guide dosage, because of its saturation kinetics. For other medications, levels can be useful in a number of circumstances including adherence to treatment, assessment of possible side effects, interactions, and pregnancy.

How useful are blood tests in general?

Physicians vary in their use of these. Blood tests can be helpful in monitoring for haematological or biochemical side effects that may not be clinically apparent but may limit dose escalation or require supplements. Examples include neutropenia (e.g with carbamazepine), thrombocytopenia (e.g. valproate), hyponatraemia (e.g. carbamazepine and oxcarbazepine), raised cholesterol (e.g. carbamazepine), low folate (e.g. phenytoin), and low calcium/vitamin D (enzyme-inducing AEDs). More rare idiosyncratic reactions such as acute aplastic anaemia, severe allergies, multi-organ or liver failure are more likely to present clinically than to be picked up by routine blood tests in asymptomatic individuals. It is often wise to carry out baseline investigation prior to commencing any AED medication, and to screen for the above changes at suitable intervals but not essential to routinely perform on a regular basis unless clinically warranted.

Reference ranges for drug levels are shown in Table 4b.3.

Table 4b.2 Prognostic index for recurrence of seizures within 1 and 2 years after continuing AED treatment or starting slow withdrawal. (Reproduced with permission from Medical Research Council antiepileptic drug withdrawal study group (1993). Prognostic index for recurrence of seizures after remission of epilepsy. *British Medical Journal*, **306**, 1374–8.)

Starting score (all patients)	−175
Age 16 years or older	add 45
Taking more than one antiepileptic drug	add 50
Seizures after start of antiepileptic drug treatment	add 35
History of primary or secondarily generalized tonic–clonic seizures	add 35
History of myoclonic seizures	add 50
Electroencephalogram in past year:	
Not available	add 15
Abnormal	add 20
Period free from seizures (Number of years)	add $\dfrac{200}{t}$
Total score	T
Divide total score by 100 and exponentiate	$z = e^{T/100}$
Probability of recurrence of seizures:	
Continued treatment	
By one year	$1 - 0.89^z$
By two years	$1 - 0.79^z$
Slow withdrawal	
By one year	$1 - 0.69^z$
By two years	$1 - 0.60^z$

Table 4b.3 Reference ranges for drug levels

Drug	Metabolite	Units	Ref. range	Ref. range metabolite
Acetazolamide		mg/L	2–12	
carbamazepine	Carbamazepine-10,11-epoxide	mg/L	1.5–9	
Carbamazepine (free)		mg/L	0.5–3	
Clobazam	Desmethylclobazam	mcg/L	<200	<2000
Clonazepam		mcg/L	25–85	
Desmethylmethsuximide		mg/L	10–40	
Diazepam	Nordiazepam	mg/L	<1.0	<1.5
Ethosuximide		mg/L	40–80	
Felbamate		mg/L	20–60	
Gabapentin		mg/L	2–20	
Oxcarbazepine	10-hydroxy Carbamazepine	mg/L		15–35
Lamotrigine		mg/L	1–15	
Levetiracetam		mg/L	6–20	
Nitrazepam		mcg/L	50–150	
Phenobarbital		mg/L	5–30	
Phenytoin		mg/L	7–20	
Phenytoin (free)		mg/L	0.7–2	
Pregabalin		mg/L	*	
Primidone	Phenobarbital	mg/L	<13	5–30
Stiripentol		mg/L	*	
Sulthiame		mg/L	2–12	
Tiagabine		mcg/L	20–100	
Topiramate		mg/L	5–20	
Valproate		mg/L	50–100	
Valproate (free)		mg/L	4–11	
Vigabatrin		mg/L	5–35	
Zonisamide		mg/L	15–40	

* Still in development—we do give an advisory at the moment. (Kindly provided by Dr David Berry, Guys Hospital, London.)

Pharmacological interactions

This section refers to general principles. Please refer to Table 4b.5 and individual drug sections. The article by Patsalos and Perucca, from which much of this section is sourced, is particularly useful.[1]

Interactions are pharmacodynamic or pharmacokinetic.

Pharmacodynamic

This refers to modification of the pharmacological effect at the site of action, which is not due to changes in drug levels. They can be additive, synergistic, or antagonistic. They may result in enhanced efficacy or greater risk of toxicity. Such interactions, though likely to be important, are difficult to study or prove and difficult to discern in clinical practice with complex polytherapy.

Pharmacokinetic

These affect absorption, distribution, and elimination and affect drug levels.

Absorption

Food may affect rate of absorption of AEDs without reducing bioavailability and without significant clinical effects. Much less commonly, oral constituents may bind medication reducing bioavailability (e.g. phenytoin and certain nasogastric feeding formulas). Transporters involved in drug absorption may show saturation and may be induced or inhibited by concomitant medication, with uncertain clinical significance.

Distribution

Displacement from plasma binding proteins can occur when medications are highly protein bound and in significant concentrations. More of the active free fraction usually results in greater clearance and lower total levels without an important clinical change. There is a potentially important interaction between phenytoin and valproate, both highly protein bound. Valproate may inhibit phenytoin metabolism as well as displacing phenytoin. To avoid phenytoin toxicity, avoid total levels in the upper end of the usual 'therapeutic range' with concomitant use.

Elimination:

- Enzyme induction:
  - Enzyme induction of an isoenzyme results in reduced levels of a medication which is a substrate for the isoenzyme, by increasing its elimination. This may result in loss of efficacy. It may also result in an increased level of an active metabolite with increased toxicity.
  - The clinical effect of enzyme induction is a gradual dose-dependent process influenced by the rate of enzyme synthesis and degradation as well as time to steady-state. This applies when an enzyme-inducing drug is added or withdrawn. The time course is usually of the order of weeks.
  - Examples of potent inducers include carbamazepine, phenobarbital, phenytoin, and primidone.
- Enzyme inhibition:
  - This results in decreased rate of metabolism of a medication through blocking the activity of a metabolizing enzyme. The usual result is higher blood levels with risk of toxicity. It could also result in lower levels of an active metabolite.

- The effect is immediate and is seen as soon as the blocking drug is added with maximum effect depending on the (new) half-life of the medication and time to steady state.
- An example of a potent inhibitor is sodium valproate (e.g of lamotrigine metabolism).

Important isoenzyme families (☐ see Table 4b.4)

Both CYP mediated reactions and UGT mediated glucuronidation are susceptible to inhibition and induction.

- Four CYP isoenzymes (CYP3A4, CYP2D6, CYP2C9, and CYP1A2) have a role in the metabolism of 95% of all drugs, with 50–70% of all drugs substrates of CYP3A4. CYP2C9, CYP2C19, and CYP3A4 are particularly important in AED interactions.
- Uridine glucuronyl transferases (UGTs) catalyse glucuronidation with two distinct families, UGT1 and UGT2.

Box 4b.6 AED interactions: key messages

- AED interactions are clinically important.
- Interactions need to be considered both when medication is added or withdrawn.
- Check sources regularly including BNF, data sheet, and local pharmacists.
- The effect of enzyme induction is seen within a few weeks while the effect of enzyme inhibition is immediate with maximum effect depending on half-life and time to reach steady state.
- Important examples of interactions include:
  - Reduced efficacy of oral contraceptive pill and of steroids with enzyme inducing AEDs.
  - Effect on warfarin (if possible, choose AED without this interaction: if not possible check whether AED enhances or reduces warfarin efficacy and monitor prothombin time (INR, international normalized ratio) frequently when AED is introduced.
  - Effect of AEDs on each other. Enzyme-inducing drugs reduce the half-life (and thus efficacy and duration of action per dose) of other AEDs if metabolized by the liver. Valproate may prolong the half-life of some AEDs and this increases the potential for toxicity (☐ see Table 4b.5).

Table 4b.4 Substrates, inhibitors, and inducers of the major (CYP) isoenzymes involved in drug metabolism. (Reproduced from Patsalos PN and Perucca E (2003). Clinically important drug interactions in epilepsy: General features and interactions between antiepileptic drugs. *The Lancet Neurology*, **2**, 347–56 with permission from Elsevier)

Isoenzymes	Substrates	Inhibitors	Inducers
CYP1A2	Psychotropic drugs: amitriptyline, clozapine, clomipramine, fluvoxamine, haloperidol, imipramine, mirtazapine, olanzapine Miscellaneous: caffeine, theophylline, paracetamol, tacrine, tamoxifen, R-warfarin	Ciprofloxacin Clarithromycin Fluvoxamine Furafylline	Carbamazepine Phenobarbital Phenytoin Primidone Cigarette smoke Charcoal-grilled meat Rifampicin
CYP2C9	AEDs: phenobarbital, phenytoin, valproic acid Non-steroidal anti-inflammatory drugs: celecoxib, diclofenac, ibuprofen, naproxen, piroxicam Miscellaneous: fluvastatin, losartan, tolbutamide, torasemide, S-warfarin, zidovudine	Valproic acid Amiodarone Chloramphenicol Fluconazole Fluoxetine Fluvoxamine Miconazole Sulfaphenazole	Carbamazepine Phenobarbital Phenytoin Primidone Rifampicin

(Continued)

Table 4b.4 Substrates, inhibitors, and inducers of the major (CYP) isoenzymes involved in drug metabolism. (Reproduced from Patsalos PN and Perucca E (2003). Clinically important drug interactions in epilepsy: General features and interactions between antiepileptic drugs. *The Lancet Neurology*, **2**, 347–56 with permission from Elsevier) (*continued*)

Isoenzymes	Substrates	Inhibitors	Inducers
CYP2C19	AEDs: diazepam, S-mephenytoin, methylphenobarbital, phenytoin, Psychotropic drugs: amitriptyline, clomipramine, imipramine, citalopram, moclobemide Miscellaneous: omeprazole, propranolol, proguanil, R-warfarin	Felbamate Oxcarbazepine(weak) Topiramate(weak) Cimetidine Fluvoxamine Omeprazole Ticlopidine	Carbamazepine Phenobarbital Phenytoin Primidone Rifampicin
CYP2D6	Psychotropic drugs: amitriptyline, citalopram, chlorpromazine, clomipramine, clozapine, imipramine, desipramine, fluoxetine, fluphenazine, fluvoxamine, haloperidol, mianserin, mirtazapine, nortriptyline, olanzapine, paroxetine, perphenazine, risperidone, thioridazine, venlafaxine, zuclopenthixol Cardiovascular drugs: alprenolol, bufuralol, encainide, flecainide, metoprolol, propafenone, propranolol, timolol, pindolol Miscellaneous: codeine, debrisoquine, dextromethorphan, phenformin, tramadol	Cimetidine Fluoxetine Haloperidol Paroxetine Perphenazine Propafenone Quinidine Thioridazine	No inducer known

	Substrates	Inhibitors	Inducers
CYP2E1	AEDs: felbamate, phenobarbital Miscellaneous: dapsone, ethanol, halothane, isoniazid, chlorzoxazone	Disulfiram	Alcohol Isoniazid
CYP3A4	AEDs: carbamazepine, ethosuximide, tiagabine, zonisamide, some, benzodiazepines (eg. alprazolam, midazolam, trizolam) Psychotropic drugs: amitriptyline, clomipramine, clozapine, haloperidol, imipramine, sertraline, nefazodone, mirtazapine, risperidone, ziprasidone, olanzapine Cardiovascular drugs: amiodarone, atorvastatin, diltiazem. felodipine, lovastatin, nimodipine, nifedipine, quinidine, simvastatin, verapamil Miscellaneous: alfentanil, astemizole, cisapride, clarithromycin, ciclosporin A, cyclophosphamide, erythromycin, fentanyl, glucocorticoids, itraconazole, ketoconazole, indinavir, oral contraceptive steroids, sildenafil, tacrolimus, tamoxifen, terfenadine	Cimetidine Ciclosporin A Diltiazem Erythromycin Flucoxamine Grapefruit juice Indinavir Itraconazole Ketoconazole Nefazodone Dextropropoxyphene Ritonavir Troleandomycin Verapamil	Carbamazepine Phenobarbital Phenytoin Primidone Oxcarbazepine[†] Topiramate[†] Felbamate[†] Glucocorticoids[†] St John's Wort Rifabutin Rifampicin

*This list is intended for guidance only and should not be regarded as exhaustive. Prediction of drug interactions based on this table should be with caution, because enzyme induction and inhibition may coexist and because many other factors (Panel) are involved in determining whether a clinically significant drug interaction will or will not occur.

[†]These inducers are weaker or may induce CYP3A4 isoenzymes only in certain tissues.

Table 4b.5 Expected changes in plasma concentrations when an AED is added to a pre-existing regimen. (Reproduced from Patsalos PN and Perucca E (2003). Clinically important drug interactions in epilepsy: General features and interactions between antiepileptic drugs. *The Lancet Neurology*, **2**, 347–56 with permission from Elsevier)

AED added	Pre-existing AED														
	PB	PHT	PRM	ETS	CBZ	VPA	OXC	LTG	GBP	TPM	TGB	LEV	ZNS	VGB	FBM
PB	..	PHT↑↓	NCCP	ETS⇊	CBZ⇊	VPA⇊	H-OXC↓	LTG⇊	↔	TPM⇊	TGB⇊	↔	ZNS⇊	↔	FBM⇊
PHT	PB↑	..	PRM↓ PB↑	ETS⇊	CBZ⇊	VPA⇊	H-OXC↓	LTG⇊	↔	TPM⇊	TGB⇊	↔	ZNS⇊	↔	FBM⇊
PRM	NCCP	PHT↑↑	..	ETS⇊	CBZ⇊	VPA↓	?	LTG⇊	↔	TPM⇊	TGB⇊	↔	ZNS⇊	↔	FBM⇊
ETS	↔	↔	NE	..	↔	VPA↑	NE	NE	NE	NE	NE	NE	NE	NE	NE
CBZ	↔	PHT↑↑	PRM↓ PB↑	ETS⇊	..	VPA⇊	H-OXC↓	LTG⇊	↔	TPM⇊	TGB⇊	↔	ZNS⇊	NE	FBM⇊
VPA	PB⇑	PHT↓*	PB⇑	ETS↑↓	CBZ-E↑	..	↔	LTG⇑	↔	TPM↓	↔	↔	↔	NE	↔
OXC	PB↑	PHT↑	?	?	CBZ↓	↔	..	LTG↓	NE	?	?	NE	↔	NE	NE
LTG	↔	↔	NE	NE	↔	↔	NE	..	NE	NE	NE	↔	NE	NE	NE
GBP	↔	↔	NE	NE	↔	↔	NE	NE	..	NE	NE	↔	NE	NE	NE

TPM	↕	↕	PHT⇑	NE	↕	VPA↓	?	NE	?	NE	?	NE
TGB	↕	↕	↕	NE	↕	↕	NE	NE	∷	NE	?	NE
LEV	↕	↕	↕	NE	↕	↕	NE	NE	NE	NE	NE	NE
ZNS	↕	↕	NE	NE	CBZ↑↕	↕	?	NE	NE	NE	∷	NE
VGB	PB↓	PHT↕	PRM↓ PB↓	NE	CBZ↑	↕	NE	NE	NE	NE	NE	∷
FBM	PB⇑	PHT⇑	?	NE	CBZ↓ CBZ-E↑	VPA⇑	↕	?	NE	NE	?	∷

PB = phenobarbital: PHT = phenytoin: PRM = primidone: ETS = ethosuximide: CBZ = carbamazepine: VPA = valproic acid: OXC = oxcarbazepine: LTG = lamotrigine
GBP = gabapentin: TPM = topiramate: TGB = tiagabine: LEV = levetiracetam: ZNS = zonisamide: VGB = vigabatrin: FBM = felbamate: H-OXO = 10-hydroxy-oxcarbazepine (active metabolite of OXC): CBZ-E=carbamazepine-10,11-epoxide. NE=none expected: *free (pharmacologically active) concentration may increase; NCCP = not commonly coprescribed; ↓ = a minor (or inconsistent) decrease in plasma concentration: ⇓ = a clinically significant decrease in plasma concentration: ↑ = a minor (or inconsistent) increase in plasma concentration: ⇑ = a clinically significant increase in plasma concentration
↔ = No change: ↓ = a minor (or inconsistent) decrease in plasma concentration: ⇓ = a clinically significant decrease in plasma concentration: ↑ = a minor (or inconsistent) increase in plasma concentration: ⇑ = a clinically significant increase in plasma concentration

Genetic predisposition, ethnicity, and drug metabolism

- Drug responsiveness and drug-related toxicity are influenced by genetic determinants. This is also referred to in relation to drug hypersensitivity syndromes discussed in the next section.
- In addition to genetic predisposition to the epilepsy and AED target, which can influence drug response, we need to consider drug transporters and drug metabolizing enzymes.
- Many of the known drug transporters have broad specificity and can influence AEDs and other medications. They have been particularly studied in oncology. They may provide one of the explanations for pharmaco-resistant epilepsy.
- Recent advances in pharmacogenomic research have led to a greater understanding of inter-individual differences in drug-induced adverse reactions, toxicity, and therapeutic response. Ethnicity is an important variable in drug metabolism and response and encompasses both genetic and environmental factors.
- Some drugs are excreted unchanged by the kidneys. Others are metabolized in the liver (phase I: oxidized, hydroxylated, or reduced), conjugated (phase II: usually by glucuronidation), then excreted.
- Pharmacogenetic differences exist for a number of phase 1 enzymes including cytochrome P450 isoenzymes. As cytochrome P450 (CYP450) enzymes are implicated in the metabolism of many antiepileptic medications, inter-individual variability of these enzymes is likely to have a clinically significant effect. Patients can be referred to as extensive, intermediate, or poor metabolizers. Adverse effects and toxicity are more common in poor metabolizers. However, the opposite is the case where the toxicity is due to the metabolite and not the parent drug.
- Genetic variations can result in toxicity to an AED at standard doses.

Example

Phenytoin is metabolized by cytochrome P450 isozymes with significant genetic polymorphisms (CYP2C9, CYP2C19). CYP2C9 accounts for much of the metabolism of phenytoin. Variants may be associated with impaired metabolism, significant reductions in daily dose requirements, and toxicity at similar doses. The frequency of poor CYP2C9 metabolizers is estimated at 6–8% of Caucasians. Poor CYP2C19 metabolizers are present more frequently in Asians than in Africans or Caucasians.

References

1. Patsalos PN and Perucca E (2003). Clinically important drug interactions in epilepsy: General features and interactions between antiepileptic drugs. *The Lancet Neurology*, **2**, 347–56.

Allergic hypersensitivity reactions to AEDs

Allergic hypersensitivity to AEDS is well recognized. In addition to common urticarial eruptions usually associated with mild morbidity, AEDs are also associated with widespread maculopapular rash, AED hypersensitivity syndrome (AHS), Stevens–Johnson syndrome (SJS), toxic epidermal necrosis (Lyell syndrome/TEN) and erythema multiform (EM). Such reactions occur more frequently, but not exclusively with aromatic AEDs.

Cross-reactivity can occur between the aromatic AEDs carbamazepine, phenytoin, phenobarbital, and oxcarbazepine. Furthermore, in a study of 1890 adult patients on AEDS, the rash rate was approximately 5 times greater in patients with another AED drug rash than those without. The rate of rash in this subgroup was 8.8%, versus 1.7% in those without another AED rash.[1]

The same study quoted an average rate of AED rash of 2.8%. Higher rash rates were seen with phenytoin (5.9%, p = 0.0008; 25.0% in those with another AED rash, p = 0.001), LTG (4.8%, p = 0.00095; 14.4%, p = 0.025), and CBZ (3.7%, not significant; 16.5%, p = 0.01). Significantly lower rates were seen with levetiracetam (0.6%), gabapentin (0.3%), and valproate (0.7%) and lower rates were also observed with felbamate, primidone, topiramate, and vigabatrin (<1%, not significant). There were 4 cases of SJS with 4 AEDs.

Reliable incidence figures for hypersensitivity reactions are difficult to ascertain. They vary with genetic susceptibility and have been shown to be reduced by a slower rate of introduction for some medication. This is generally advised unless there is clinical urgency. Quoted figures on the incidence of *severe* skin reactions from some AEDs are:

- Phenytoin: 9/10,000.
- Carbamazepine: 6.2/10,000.
- Lamotrigine: 0.5–1/100 (adults >12 years). The risk is higher in younger children, in those also on valproate, which inhibits glucuronidation of lamotrigine and prolongs its half-life, and with rapid dose escalation.

While severe skin reactions may be the cutaneous manifestation of AHS, this is not usually the case.

AHS is a potentially fatal drug-induced, multiorgan syndrome usually presenting within the first 8 weeks of initiation of therapy with fever followed by a cutaneous reaction. Internal organ involvement most commonly affects the liver, but can also be haematologic, pulmonary, or renal. AHS has been reported as fatal in approximately 10% of cases. AHS is associated with aromatic AEDs (e.g. phenytoin, carbamazepine, phenobarbital, and primidone) and with non-aromatic AEDs (e.g. lamotrigine, sodium valproate). The true incidence of AHS is unknown, given the variability in clinical presentation, likely under-reporting and lack of diagnostic criteria. Estimated frequency for aromatic drugs is between 0.1–1/1000 exposures.

It is essential in all allergic hypersensitivity reactions that early symptoms are recognized and the medication withdrawn as soon as possible.

The mechanism of hypersensitivity reactions is unknown but it is thought, with aromatic amines, that induction of cytochrome P450 enzymes leads

Carbamazepine (Table 4b.8)

Overview

Carbamazepine has deservedly been and continues to be a first-line medication in adults and children for many years and has served us well. With the availability of many new AEDs, its position is being evaluated. It is by no means clear if and which medication will replace it as first line in the long-term.

Carbamazepine's main *advantages* are:
- It is very effective.
- It is reasonably safe including in pregnancy.
- It has mood stabilizing properties.

Its *disadvantages* are:
- It is not broad spectrum
- It is often not tolerated if introduced quickly
- Even with slow introduction, a proportion feel cognitively impaired on it
- As an enzyme-inducing AED it has important interactions; it also affects bone metabolism and is associated with raised lipid levels.
- Among other side effects, potentially serious allergic reactions may occur, including SJS.
- Rarely there is an effect on cardiac conduction in those at risk.
- Its tolerability is limited in the elderly.

Where **not** to choose, or use with caution?
- Do not recommend it for people with a history of myoclonus or absences. It may well make these seizure types worse particularly with higher doses.
- Do not select it where the epilepsy diagnosis is likely to be idiopathic primary generalized epilepsy. Although it can be effective, it is less likely to be successful than broad spectrum medication and can worsen the epilepsy, sometimes more so with higher doses.
- Do not select as your standard first choice in the elderly who may have a propensity to heart block, who generally do not tolerate it well, and who are more likely to be taking concomitant medication.

Dosing strategies
- We recommend slow introduction and gradual titration in routine practice. This is more likely to be tolerated and therefore successful. Auto-induction lowers levels in the few weeks after starting. The elimination half life of carbamazepine and its epoxide metabolite drops significantly in the first 3 weeks.
- The long-acting preparation (Retard®/low release) is preferred. The smaller scored Retard® tablets of 200mg make it easy to start on 100mg. While breaking the slow release tablet in half is acceptable, chewing or crushing it is not.
- We suggest starting with half a tablet (100mg) nocte and increasing by 100mg increments once/week (or slower depending on tolerance), until 200mg twice/day. This is a reasonable initial dose to work up to and can be increased later as appropriate. Even this low dose, however, is not always tolerated. If patients have frequent attacks, they can be asked to build up to the minimum dose needed to prevent seizures.

There is no point taking more. Many patients achieve full control with detectable and effective blood levels on low doses. Levels below the usual quoted therapeutic range can be effective.

- *In children*, starting dose should be 2.5mg/kg/day, increasing by such increments weekly to 10mg/kg/day, to be reviewed thereafter.
- For those who experience very infrequent seizures and who are very keen to achieve full control as quickly as possible (for example, to resume driving or for over-riding reasons of safety), it is reasonable to work up to a target level without waiting for the next seizure to occur. Assuming no significant side effects, in these circumstances, we recommend slowly titrating up in the first instance to a trough (pre-dose) level around the lower end of the 'therapeutic' range.
- Patients are advised that, if they are feeling drowsy or tired on any dose, then they should not increase the dose until, and unless, side effects subside.
- It is important to advise the patient to stop the medication in the event of a drug rash, mucosal ulcers, or rare idiosyncratic drug reaction occurring in the first few weeks after introduction. Hypersensitivity reactions may be less likely with slower titration.
- For those people who remain subdued or cognitively affected on it after the initial few weeks, consider an alternative

There is a *difference in bioavailability* between carbamazepine ordinary preparation and the retard/controlled release preparation. They cannot be swapped mg per mg. The dose of the controlled release preparation needs to be a little higher to achieve the same effect. When changing from one to the other, and as a rough guide, approximately 100mg of ordinary carbamazepine is equivalent to about 120–125mg of controlled release. Calculate the equivalent dose, then round up or down depending on total dose and whether the patient is over or under treated, then adjust depending on clinical response once a steady state has been reached.

Table 4b.8 Carbamazepine

UK trade names	**Tegretol®, Tegretol Retard® amongst others**
Mode of action	Blockade of sodium channels
Usual preparations	Tablets: 100, 200, 400mg Chewtabs: 100, 200mg Slow release (Carbamazepine Retard®): 200, 400mg Liquid: 100mg/5mL Suppositories: 125, 250mg (125mg suppository is equivalent to 100mg tablet)
Maximum licensed dose	2000mg
Typical daily dose in adults	400–600mg/day, suggested stating dose is 100mg
Typical daily dose in children	Up to 20mg/kg/day (higher doses tolerated in the very young owing to greater clearance rates): • <1 year: 100–200mg/day • 1–5 years: 200–400mg/day • 5–10 years: 400–600mg/day • 10–15 years: 600–1000mg/day
Dosage intervals	Ordinary: 2–3 doses per day Slow release: 1–2 doses per day, usually 2
Quoted range for pre-dose blood levels	4–12mg/liter (4–12mcg/mL) ~ (17–50micro mol/L). Carbamazepine epoxide about 30% of carbamazepine levels
Protein binding	70–80%
Oral bioavailability	85–100 % may vary with formulation
Time to peak levels	4–8 hours
Metabolism and excretion	Almost completely metabolized—hepatic epoxidation (Cytochrome P450 3A4) and conjugation
Elimination half-life in adults	9–27 hours (longer after single dose)
Elimination half-life in children	In neonates: 8–28 hours In older children: 14–27 hours
Other	Autoinduction of carbamazepine and epoxide metabolite (complete within 20–30days). Elimination half life falls by ~50%
Active metabolites	Carbamazepine epoxide
Main interactions	Enzyme inducing AED; interacts with other AEDs, warfarin, and oral contraceptive pill. See text, data sheet, and BNF
Main indications	Partial and generalized tonic–clonic seizures

Dose ranges

- In a recent prospective study comparing controlled-release carbamazepine and levetiracetam monotherapy as first treatment in newly diagnosed epilepsy, of all patients achieving 6-month (1-year) remission, 80.1% (86.0%) in the levetiracetam group and 85.4% (89.3%) in the carbamazepine group did so at doses of 500mg twice/day of levetiracetam or 200mg twice/day of slow released carbamazepine. The authors concluded that this trial 'has confirmed in a randomized, double-blind setting previously uncontrolled observations that most people with epilepsy will respond to their first-ever AED at low dosage'.[1] 📖 See Table 4b.1 for response rates in relation to dose with different AEDs.
- Although most people who respond do so at relatively low doses of around 400mg–600mg, there is marked inter-individual variability, some patients requiring less or much more. Doses are guided by tolerability and response.
- For those who appear to be responding, with no side effects, the dose can be increased if seizures continue, usually by 100mg or 200mg increments, as clinically indicated. Allow sufficient time between increments to assess response. Some achieve better control with higher doses and a few are® comfortable even on as much as 1000mg twice a day of the Retard® preparation. Many, however, do not tolerate higher doses. Common dose-related side effects include diplopia, difficulty in focusing, dizziness, tiredness, cognitive impairment, and occasionally diarrhoea. If side effects considered likely to be medication-related emerge, then, irrespective of dose or indeed level, the dose should be reduced gradually until side effects resolve. In some patients a high level of the epoxide metabolite results in side effects despite the carbamazepine level being reasonable.
- If seizure control improves with medication but further dose increases do not confer additional benefit, then gradually reduce back to the lowest dose providing maximum benefit. Add-on medications are likely to be better tolerated in the future.

What else?

- Patients should be warned about the possibility of hypersensitivity reactions that requires discontinuation
- Women who are on or may be prescribed the oral contraceptive pill (OCP) or other hormone treatment must be told about the need for a higher dose of the OCP and its reduced efficacy.
- Women of childbearing age must also be told about potential teratogenicity and the need to take folic acid prior to conception. Carbamazepine has a good profile in pregnancy, and while it is associated with a low of risk of malformations the risk is lower than that associated with valproate and comparable to lower doses of lamotrigine. As with other enzyme inducing AEDs, oral vitamin K1 supplementation to the mother is advised in the last 4 weeks of pregnancy, in addition to vitamin K given to the newborn at birth.
- Weight gain can occur with carbamazepine but this is a major concern in a minority only as the average weight gain is low.

- It is sensible to give general advice about bone protection and mention possible interactions with other medications, where appropriate.
- Carbamazepine may have interactions with other drugs. There is also an interaction with grapefruit juice (□ see Grapefruit juice and AEDs p.375)
- Alcohol tolerance may be reduced as with other AEDs.
- There is some evidence that cholesterol levels may rise in those susceptible.

How useful are carbamazepine levels?

Dosing is primarily guided by clinical response, not plasma levels!

However, plasma levels can be useful in a number of circumstances, as per the examples below:

- To check adherence to treatment. For example, if carbamazepine is reportedly ineffective, check levels before changing to another AED: there may be none detected!
- Levels can guide dosing in selected cases e.g., as already discussed above, in individuals with very infrequent seizures.
- Levels can provide objective evidence for the inter-individual variation in clearance and half-life, and aid interpretation of clinical response or side effects. Checking the epoxide level (rare indication) may help explain side effects in those with low levels.
- In controlled patients, knowing the level at which control is achieved can help management in changing situations such as pregnancy or withdrawal of other potentially interacting drugs. For this to be useful, levels need to be taken at similar times in relation to the dose, for example trough or pre-dose.
- Levels can help avoid escalating dose to levels above the usual quoted range, associated with more risk of toxicity.

Do not dismiss a dose as 'homeopathic' just because it is lower than the quoted range. Such doses can be protective.

References

1. Brodie MJ, Perucca E, Ryvlin P, et al. (2007). Comparison of levetiracetam and controlled-release carbamazepine in newly diagnosed epilepsy. *Neurology*, **68**, 402–8.

Clobazam (Table 4b.9)

Overview

Clobazam is a very effective, broad spectrum, well-tolerated anti-epileptic agent, also licensed for short-term treatment of severe anxiety. It is less sedating than some other benzodiazepines. There is a risk of tolerance developing with regular use although the likelihood of this occurring is uncertain, reportedly ranging from 0–77% of cases. Tolerance may develop within a few weeks, but is also observed over months. While tolerance undoubtedly occurs, this should not preclude the use of clobazam in epilepsy, not only as intermittent treatment but also regularly in some cases.

How to use?

Intermittent treatment

Clobazam 'as required' can be helpful in many situations such as aborting a cluster of seizures, prevention of seizures on important/vulnerable days, during other AED withdrawal, or for the control of catamenial exacerbation of seizures.

The individual may wish to establish a tolerated effective dose to use in these circumstances, usually by taking the first 10mg tablet (or half a tablet or 5mg in those known generally intolerant of medication) on an evening to establish tolerability. If well tolerated, 10mg may be taken on special occasions, at the beginning of a cluster, or when vulnerable, with further doses given if needed.

If 10mg is ineffective, then 20mg is given at the beginning of the next cluster, with a further 10mg dose given as appropriate. Where cover is needed for a few days, as in catamenial epilepsy, 10mg once or twice/day for a few days may be given to cover the time of greatest risk depending on the individual case. Future doses are then adjusted as necessary. Frequency of use is monitored.

Regular treatment

The patient is informed that while clobazam is very likely to be effective initially in the majority, duration of benefit in an individual is unknown. It may be long-term or wane with time. Ten (10mg) at night is a reasonable starting dose which can be increased gradually, as necessary. Withdrawal must be gradual following chronic treatment because of habituation.

Prescribing

Clobazam in the UK is 'black listed' for indications other than epilepsy. Endorse non-private prescriptions with 'SLS' (Selected List Scheme).

Main side effects

Clobazam, a 1,5-diazepine, was synthesized from 1,4-diazepines. It is associated with less sedation and cognitive impairment than the parent structure. Side effects are to some extent dose related. They are also more likely with polytherapy, possibly partly due to complex interactions. Irritability, disinhibition, depression, and behavioural change may occur in those with epilepsy associated with other handicap, but are infrequent in other groups, where it is generally well tolerated and easy to use.

Table 4b.11 Ethosuximide

UK trade names	Zarontin®, Emeside®
Mode of action	Decrease burst firing of thalamocortical neurons through reduction of thalamic T-type calcium currents. Mechanisms not fully elucidated.
Usual preparations	• Capsules: 250mg • Syrup: 250mg/5mL
Maximum licensed dose	2000mg/day
Typical daily dose in adults	500mg–1000mg
Typical daily dose in children	• <6 years: 250mg/day • >6 years: 500–1000mg/day or 25 mg/kg/day
Dosage intervals	2–3 doses per day
Quoted range for blood levels	40–100mcg/mL(a few require higher levels)
Protein binding	0% (saliva and CSF levels approximate to plasma)
Oral bioavailability	Nearly completely absorbed
Time to peak levels	1–7 hours
Metabolism and excretion	Extensively metabolized to inactive metabolites by hepatic oxidation and then conjugation
Elimination half-life in adults	40–60 hours (reduced with enzyme-inducing agents)
Elimination half-life in children	~30 hours
Active metabolites	None
Main interactions	See text
Main indications	Absence seizures

Gabapentin (Table 4b.12)

Overview

- This is a narrow-spectrum medication licensed for partial epilepsy as an add-on drug and as monotherapy (>12 years). It is also licensed for neuropathic pain, where it has been widely used. It is generally safe and well tolerated. Its low interaction potential makes it easy to use, but it is not the most potent of AEDs. Some respond, so it is still worth considering, although the similar AED pregabalin is considered more potent.

- Gabapentin is an amino acid that crosses several membrane barriers in the body via a specific amino acid transporter competing with leucine, isoleucine, valine, and phenylalanine. A saturable amino acid transport system applies to the blood–brain barrier. Absorption of gabapentin is limited by saturable, active, dose-dependent transport in the GI tract.

- Gabapentin can exacerbate seizures, particularly myoclonus and absences. Attempts to withdraw concomitant AEDs in treatment refractory patients on polytherapy, to reach gabapentin monotherapy have a low success rate.

- Gabapentin can be used safely in porphyria. 📖 See AEDs and porphyrias, pp.374–375

Side effects

Somnolence, dizziness, ataxia, fatigue, and weight gain are relatively common side effects. GI symptoms and oedema and are also reported, amongst other side effects. Its propensity to cause allergic reactions is low. Pancreatitis has been rarely reported.

Dosing schedule

In general it is preferable to start on low doses, e.g. 300mg nocte, and if tolerated, increasing at weekly intervals. It is usually given 2 or 3 times/day. Low doses have a low response rate. If there is some benefit with average doses, it may be worth going up to 3600mg pd, if seizures continue and there are no side effects. Some have tried higher doses up to 4800mg, which can be given in 4 divided doses, but the yield at this stage is not likely to be high. See data sheet for those with renal impairment.

Profile in pregnancy (📖 see also AEDs and breastfeeding, pp.370–372)

Limited information is available and major malformation rates in humans cannot be quoted.

Table 4b.12 Gabapentin

UK trade name	Neurontin®
Mode of action	Reduce glutaminergic action by binding to alpha2-delta subunit of voltage-gated calcium channels
Usual preparations	• Capsules: 100, 300, 400 400mg • Film-coated tablets: 600, 800mg
Maximum licensed dose	4800mg
Typical daily dose in adults	600–3600mg/day
Typical daily dose in children	>12 years: 300–900mg/day or 30–50mg/kg/day
Dosage intervals	(2) usually 3 doses per day
Quoted range for blood levels	Not usually performed (2–20mcg/mL)
Protein binding	0%
Oral bioavailability	Absorbed via small intestine L-amino acid transport system with saturable absorption which decreases with increasing dose, is generally unaffected by food, but may be enhanced by some food. Bioavailability: 60% of 300mg capsule; 35% or less for doses >3600mg.
Time to peak levels	2–3 hours
Metabolism and excretion	Renal excretion unmetabolized—independent of dose
Elimination half-life in adults	5–7 hours
Active metabolites	None
Main interactions	Co-administration with aluminium and magnesium antacids reduces bioavailability; pretreatment with morphine increases absorption of gabapentin
Main indications	Focal epilepsies, neuropathic pain

Lacosamide

Overview

Lacosamide has only recently been licensed as adjunctive treatment for partial epilepsy with secondary generalization in those 16 years old or over. It is said to be well tolerated. Clarification of its role, optimal dosing regime and safety profile awaits further post-marketing experience.

Summary

- It enhances slow inactivation of sodium channels and modulates CRMP-2 (collapsin response mediator protein-2).
- The following formulations are available: tablets; 50mg, 100mg, 150mg, 200mg; Syrup; 15mg/ml = 200ml; i.v.; 10mg/ml. 1 vial = 20ml (bioequivalence of tablets, syrup and iv formulation).

- It is advisable as with any medication to start on a low dose. The maximum licensed dose is 400mg/day, given twice daily. Protein binding is less than 15% and oral bioavailability ~ 100%. Time to peak levels is between 0.5 to 4 hours after oral administration. It is not extensively metabolized; 95% of the dose is excreted in urine (40% unchanged). Elimination half-life in adults is ~13 hours and time to steady state is 3 days.
- Plasma concentrations of lacosamide may be slightly decreased by concomitant treatment with carbamazepine, phenytoin, and phenobarbital.

Lamotrigine (Table 4b.13)

Overview

Since lamotrigine was licensed in the UK, with successful advertising, it is now widely used and considered a first-line treatment. It was marketed as an effective 'broad' spectrum AED without adverse cosmetic effects and with a good profile in women of childbearing age, the latter implied by an advertising campaign even before supporting data regarding safety in pregnancy was available.

Lamotrigine performed well in comparison with carbamazepine in partial epilepsy in the SANAD study, comparing new versus old AEDs in new-onset cases, where it was better tolerated with reportedly comparable efficacy. While this may be the case in this setting, in general it is considered less effective than carbamazepine. It performed less well than valproate, in terms of efficacy, in primary generalized epilepsy. It is a useful medication but has limitations.

Main advantages

- Good tolerability with generally low adverse effects on mood or cognition.
- It can have a mood-stabilizing effect.
- It has a reasonable profile in pregnancy in terms of low teratogenicity at low to moderate doses.
- It is considerd more broad spectrum than carbamazepine.

Some disadvantages/limitations

- It is not as broad spectrum and is clearly less effective than valproate in IGE, including JME. Although it can be effective in IGE it has the potential to worsen the epilepsy, particularly myoclonus.
- It is not very potent as add-on treatment in intractable partial epilepsy.
- Because its potential to cause serious allergic reactions is minimized by slow titration, an effective dose takes time to achieve. It is therefore not first choice where a prompt effect is needed.
- It has clinically relevant pharmacokinetic disadvantages, namely:
  - Clinically relevant reduction of LMT levels by the OCP and in pregnancy.
  - Its half-life is significantly reduced by enzyme-inducing AEDs and prolonged by valproate.
  - There is a large inter-individual difference in its metabolism; this along with the interactions above results in an effective therapeutic dose which varies greatly.

Who not to give it to

Certain myoclonic epilepsy syndromes.

Table 4b.13 Lamotrigine

UK trade name	Lamictal®
Mode of action	Blocks voltage gated sodium channels, inhibits pathological release of glutamate and glutamate-evoked action potentials
Usual preparations	• Tablets: 25, 50, 100, 200mg • Dispersible: 2, 5, 25, 100mg • Not available as chewtabs
Maximum licensed dose	See text
Typical daily dose in adults	Wide range: 50–500mg/day depending on individual and concomitant Rx
Typical daily dose in children	• Without sodium valproate: 2.5–7.5mg/kg/day twice daily • With sodium valproate: 1–5mg/kg/day
Dosage intervals	Usually 2/day. Occasionally 1. Rarely 3
Quoted target range for blood levels	1–3mcg/mL (1–15mg/L)
Protein binding	55%
Oral bioavailability	100%
Time to peak levels	Variable: ~ 2.5 hours. Range 1–3 hours or longer with a wider range in children (slightly delayed after food)
Metabolism and excretion	Hepatic glucuronidation (without phase I reaction)
Elimination half-life in adults	This shows large inter-individual variability: • Steady state mean half-life in adults ~30 hours (± 14) • With enzyme inducers: mean 14 hours • With sodium valproate: mean 70 hours • Clearance reduced in Gilbert's syndrome and to a small extent in the elderly • Clearance increased in children <12, especially <5 years
Elimination half-life in children	Mean half-lives are shorter in children <12 years of age, particularly <5 years
Active metabolites	None
Main interactions	Lamotrigine has major interactions: see text, tables, BNF, and data sheet
Main indications	Focal and generalized epilepsies
Other	• Modest dose related auto induction • Weak inhibitor of dihydrofolate reductase

Dosing strategies

1) Slow titration is associated with less allergic reactions. Start on a low dose:

- As monotherapy: 25mg/day.
- As add-on to valproate 25mg every other day (or 12.5mg daily) for 2 weeks then 25mg/day.
- As add-on to some enzyme inducing drugs without valproate, can start on 50mg, although 25mg is comonly used.
- *In children* on sodium valproate, starting dose is 0.1mg/kg/day, increasing over 6 weeks to 0.5mg/kg/day. In children not on sodium valpoate the starting dose is 0.5mg/kg/day increasing over 6 weeks to 2mg/kg/day.

2) Build up gradually increasing no faster than fortnightly.

3) It can be prescribed in a once or twice daily regimen in monotherapy, but remember the variability in half-life. Twice/day is advisable in someone on an enzyme inducing AED. In someone also on valproate without an enzyme-inducing AED, once/day is sufficient because of the long half-life. If there are peak dose side effects or pre-dose break-through seizures, 3/day can be considered for those on higher doses or concomitant enzyme-inducing AEDs.

4) In those with frequent seizures, advise the patient to increase by increments of 25mg (or 25–50mg if on enzyme-inducing AED and not on valpo-rate) at intervals of 2 weeks or longer, depending on the clinical situation, and assuming no side effects, until seizures are controlled. The dose range is wide and seizure control is the aim rather than a particular target dose! If seizures are infrequent, a reasonable initial maintenance dose of 50mg/day of lamotrigine in someone on valproate, or 50–75mg twice/day in monotherapy is reasonable. The dose is increased further if seizures continue, assuming no side effects. Of note is that there appears to be synergy with valproate in some generalized epilepsy syndromes and often an add on maintenance dose of 25mg is sufficient. 📖 see Table 4b.1, pp.275–279 for response rates in relation to dose with different AEDs.

5) Maximum doses quoted in the data sheet are 500mg on monotherapy, 200mg on valproate, and 700mg on enzyme-inducing drugs. Higher doses can be given in a minority if tolerated.

What else should I tell the patient in addition to information on dose?

- Warn the patient of the possibility of rash and other allergic reactions which necessitate prompt withdrawal.
- Generally, lamotrigine is well tolerated.
- Dose-related side effects include dizziness and difficulty focusing/double vision experienced at peak level. These usually necessitate a small dose reduction; changing to thrice daily regimen may help in those on concomitant enzyme-inducing AEDs, but these side effects usually indicate that the maximum tolerated dose has been reached. In someone on maximum tolerated dose of carbamazepine, a small reduction in carbamazepine usually helps when lamotrigine is added in minimizing side effects.

- Insomnia and headache may occur as can behavioural or neuropsychiatric side effects which may limit use. Insomnia may be helped by giving the larger dose in the morning and bringing forward the second dose of the day to early evening or late afternoon. Alternatively, in some on monotherapy (or if also on valproate), lamotrigine can be given only in the morning where appropriate.
- The female patient needs to be informed that starting and stopping the OCP will affect lamotrigine levels with potentially clinically significant effects. On coming off the OCP, a rise in levels may be associated with emergent side effects and on starting the OCP a drop in levels may be associated with loss of efficacy. Lamotrigine levels can also drop in pregnancy rising post-partum, and this too can have a clinically significant effect. Depending on the case, doses often need to be increased significantly during pregnancy and decreased again post-partum period. Lamotrigine is also present in breast milk.
- If someone restarts lamotrigine after an interval off it, the dose is increased gradually as though initiating therapy.

How useful are levels?

Lamotrigine levels are available but samples are often sent to reference laboratories with slow turn around times. As with other AEDs, levels are very helpful if non-adherence to treatment is considered. Effective levels vary widely, with some controlled on very low levels and others at levels above the usual quoted range. Levels above the range are more likely to be associated with side effects. Levels may also be helpful in certain clinical situations, such as in those where high doses are contemplated, in pregnancy when levels decrease, or where interacting medications are being added or removed. Decisions regarding dosing are often made without waiting for the result of the level to become available, although the level may inform future decisions. For example if seizures occur in pregnancy, the dose is usually increased. Sometimes the dose is increased pre-emptively.

Other blood tests are not required routinely

Pregnancy

Lamotrigine has a reasonable profile regarding teratogenicity in pregnancy at low to moderate doses. Give folic acid 5mg/day prior to conception. Decreased lamotrigine levels can occur in early pregnancy with further reductions throughout pregnancy. Levels rise again quickly after delivery. Lamotrigine doses usually need to be increased in pregnancy and decreased after depending on the individual case.

Interactions

As already indicated, lamotrigine has important interactions as discussed below. Please refer to interaction 🕮 Tables 4b.4, p.290 and 4b.5, p.291 and look up every concomitant drug before introducing or withdrawing.

Principles
- UDP-glucuronyl transferases metabolize lamotrigine.
- AED inducers—phenytoin, carbamazepine, phenobarbital and primidone, but not oxcarbazepine—induce lamotrigine glucuronidation and increase dose requirements.
- Lamotrigine does not itself significantly induce or inhibit hepatic oxidative drug-metabolizing enzymes. An effect of lamotrigine on drugs metabolized by cytochrome P450 enzymes are unlikely.
- Lamotrigine only has modest autoinduction without significant clinical consequence.
- Sodium valproate inhibits lamotrigine glucuronidation increasing mean half life of lamotrigine nearly 2-fold.
- Lamotrigine does not displace other AEDs from protein binding sites.
- Oral contraceptive pill reduces the level of lamotrigine.

What do I do when other interacting treatment is withdrawn or added?
Enzyme-inducing AEDs

Enzyme-inducing AEDs reduce lamotrigine levels by ~40% (up to 55% with phenytoin). Thus, if enzyme-inducing medications are withdrawn, this will result in a significantly higher level of lamotrigine. In those already at maximum tolerated dose of lamotrigine, this will result in toxicity and reduction in lamotrigine dose is needed, until side effects resolve. The opposite is the case if such treatment is added, when lamotrigine dose may need to be increased to maintain efficacy.

OCP

If the OCP is withdrawn, this will result in a significantly higher level of lamotrigine (on average 2-fold higher if not on concomitant enzyme inducers). The dose may need adjustment depending on clinical state. The opposite is the case if the OCP is added, when lamotrigine dose may need to be increased to maintain seizure control.

Valproate:

Valproate prolongs the half-life of lamotrigine. The effect of valproate on lamotrigine half-life is initially dose related, with an effect demonstrated even when very low valproate doses are used. Most of the effect is probably already there by 500mg of valproate/day. There is likely to be individual variability in metabolism and half life, which is also affected by other concomitant medication. The guidance given next will therefore need to be adjusted to the individual clinical situation.

Valproate withdrawal

If valproate is withdrawn, this will result in a shorter half-life of lamotrigine and a lower level. If the aim is to maintain the same level (depending on the clinical situation) lamotrigine dose needs to be increased. As a rough guide, someone on 50mg twice/day of lamotrigine and 600mg/day of valproate, on withdrawing valproate, may need to end up on ~lamotrigine 100mg twice/day to maintain similar blood levels of lamotrigine, the process of reduction of one and increase of the other gradually carried out and adjusted according to clinical need.

The opposite is the case if valproate is added when lamotrigine levels rise significantly. Possible approaches are discussed next; no doubt there are others. Whichever regimen is followed, we advise against sudden rises in lamotrigine levels to avoid adverse reactions.

- If lamotrigine has not been effective consider withdrawing it before adding valproate if appropriate in the individual case.
- If the person is on a very small dose of lamotrigine and a controlled rise in its level is desired, then, if there is no clinical urgency, valproate can be added at a small dose of 100mg, and increased at increments of 100mg every 2 weeks until 500mg of valproate is reached. This will result in a controlled slow rise in lamotrigine level; further rises with higher doses of valproate cannot be excluded but lamotrigine levels will be largely stable. A faster introduction of valproate can be carried out in this situation, if clinically indicated. For example, if someone is on 50mg of lamotrigine and 500mg of valproate is added, it would take approximately 5 half lives of a gradual increase in lamotrigine concentrations before a new steady state is reached—roughly equivalent to double the original dose of lamotrigine, which in this case is likely to be acceptable. This approach would not give an acceptable rate of rise with high doses of lamotrigine.
- If, on the other hand, lamotrigine dose is already moderate or high, and if the aim is to keep its levels broadly unchanged, then lamotrigine dose must be reduced significantly and early on when valporate is added. A gradual change over a long period can be achieved with a small starting dose of valproate of 100mg, with decrements in lamotrigine dose but still aiming eventually for about half the original dose by the time valproate has reached 500mg, adjusted according to clinical state. If a quicker change is planned, valproate can be added at a dose of 500mg/day at night, this dose chosen as one with close to maximum inhibition. Lamotrigine dose needs to be reduced from the next dose after valproate is added, aiming over 2–3 days for approximately half the original lamotrigine dose, again adjusted depending on clinical state. This can introduce some instability and needs to be carried out cautiously keeping in mind, individual variability, likely half-life of lamotrigine on valproate, individual tolerance, and dose of lamotrigine.

Levetiracetam (Table 4b.14)

Overview

Although only licensed in 2000, levetiracetam has deservedly and very quickly become a widely used add-on AED, superseding some other 'new' AEDS licensed before it. It is also increasingly used as first line in mono-therapy. It is effective, reasonably well tolerated, and broad spectrum.

In a head-to-head comparison in new onset partial epilepsy, equivalent seizure freedom rates (📖 see Box 4b.7) with carbamazepine were observed. Levetiracetam is also used in generalized epilepsy. It is particularly effective in myoclonus, but is also effective in absences and GTCS, although it may exacerbate the latter. The introduction of an intravenous preparation also widens possibilities for use, and although outside licence, its successful use in status epilepticus has been reported. There are reports of its use in porphyria (📖 see Antiepileptics drugs and porphyries, pp.374–375). The lack of enzyme-inducing effect is an advantage, for example, with HIV combination treatment.

Levetiracetam is now licensed for:
- *Monotherapy* for partial seizures with or without secondary generalization from 16 years of age with newly diagnosed epilepsy.
- *As add-on therapy*:
  - For partial seizures with or without secondary generalization from 4 years of age.
  - In the treatment of myoclonic seizures in JME from 12 years of age.
  - In the treatment of primary GTCS in IGE in adults and adolescents from 12 years of age.

The concentrate is licensed for intravenous solution when oral administration is not feasible.

Main advantages
- Efficacious.
- Reasonably well tolerated.
- Reasonably broad spectrum.
- Pharmacokinetic interactions are not a problem.

Some disadvantages/limitations
- Associated with neuro psychiatric side effects including depression and irritability.
- Can cause behavioural problems in patients with learning difficulty.
- Information is limited in pregnancy.
- Less broad spectrum than valproate in generalized epilepsies.
- A proportion seem to respond but the benefit is lost with/despite dose increases. It is not clear if this is due to a therapeutic window or lack of sustained effect in a subgroup.
- In patient with chronic refractory epilepsy who respond to levetiracetam, it remains to be seen how successful withdrawal of concomitant AEDs will be.

Table 4b.14 Levetiracetam

UK trade name	Keppra®
Mode of action	Binds selectively with high affinity to synaptic vesicle protein SV2A, involved with exocytosis and presynaptic neurotransmitter release
Usual preparations	• Tablets: 250, 500, 750, 1000mg • Oral solution: 100mg/mL • Concentrate: 100mg/mL for solution for infusion
Maximum licensed dose	3000mg
Typical daily dose in adults	1000–3000mg (some studies have used higher doses)
Typical daily dose in children	20–40mg/kg/day (up to 60mg/kg/day)
Dosage intervals	2 doses per day
Quoted range for blood levels	6–20mg/L There is low intra and inter subject variability and plasma levels can be predicted from the oral dose of levetiracetam as mg/kg bodyweight reducing need for monitoring levels
Protein binding	<10%
Oral bioavailability	Close to 100%; food slows absorption but not extent
Time to peak levels	1.3 hours
Metabolism and excretion	About 1/4 dose is hydrolysed in blood to an inactive metabolite. Both levetiracetam and its main metabolite are renally excreted; the rate correlates with creatinine clearance.
Elimination half-life in adults	7 hours increased in elderly to ~10 hours
Elimination half-life in children	6 hours (5 in those with epilepsy)
Active metabolites	None
Main interactions	Few
Main indications	Focal seizures and generalized seizures (see text)
Other	Linear kinetics (500–5000mg)

Box 4b.7 Levetiracetam versus carbamazepine

In a new-onset partial epilepsy, double-blind, non-inferiority trial in adults, patients were assigned to levetiracetam (500mg twice daily, if necessary titrated up to 1500mg twice/day, n = 288) or controlled-release carbamazepine (200mg twice daily, up to 600mg twice/day, n = 291). The primary endpoint was 6-month seizure freedom, with a further 6-month maintenance period. Of patients randomized to levetiracetam 73.0% (56.6%) were seizure free compared to 72.8% (58.5%) receiving controlled-release carbamazepine. Withdrawal rates for adverse events were 14.4% with levetiracetam and 19.2% with carbamazepine. A useful, but not altogether surprising, observation is that of patients achieving 6-month (1-year) remission, *80.1% (86.0%) in the levetiracetam group and 85.4% (89.3%) in the carbamazepine group did so at the lowest dose level (500mg twice/day of levetiracetam and 200mg twice/day of controlled-release carbamazepine).*

The authors conclude that the study supports previous clinical observations that most people with epilepsy will respond to their first-ever AED at low dosage.[1]

When and how to use and dosing strategies

Levetiracetam may be used as monotherapy or as add-on therapy.

As monotherapy

- Of note are the results of the comparative study in new onset partial epilepsy with the majority of patients responding to the starting dose of 500mg twice/day (📖 see Box 4b.7). Thus, a reasonable maximum initial 'target' dose is 500mg twice/day, however some patients may respond to less, and slow titration allows for the minimum effective dose.
- Although studies have been carried out successfully introducing levetiracetam at 2000mg/day or even 4000mg/day, introduction at high dose is not advised routinely as tolerability is reduced.
- In an average adult outpatient in monotherapy, introduce at 250mg nocte, and increase to twice daily, assuming no side effects and continuing seizures at intervals of 2 weeks or more. In those with frequent seizures, the dose is guided by response. In others, a reasonable initial target dose is between 250mg twice/day and 500mg twice/day depending on tolerance. Those who are too tired on 250mg, can take 125mg until they are used to it.
- The dose is built up gradually if seizures continue; the dose at which a response occurs can be as low as the starting dose, particularly as add-on therapy. The dose can be gradually increased to the maximum licensed dose. Doses beyond the licensed dose, up to 4000mg/day, may be used/tried by a small minority with no side effects and an excellent response, if not seizure free. Sometimes, an early good response is lost with dose escalation, and occasionally this is regained with careful dose reduction. While some patients gain additional benefit with escalating doses, more is not always better, and clinical experience raises the possibility of a therapeutic window.
- In those where it is used as add-on therapy, assess response to the initial 250mg dose before increasing further. Some may become seizure free without much dose escalation. If the aim is to try for monotherapy,

however, in the majority the dose of levetiracetam will need increasing, if tolerated, to allow reduction of other medication.

• A starting dose of 62.5mg or 125mg is advised in the elderly, who have reduced tolerance to medication in general as well as reduced creatinine clearance. In addition to smaller dose increments, intervals between dose increments may also need to be increased.

• If insomnia occurs, change the timing of the dose. Tiredness is a common early side effect but it is often transient although this may take a few weeks. Early marked neuropsychiatric disturbances are an indication for withdrawal as are hypersensitivity reactions. Neuropsychiatric disturbances, such as depression, behavioural change, aggression and irritability, can also occur with chronic treatment and can limit the use of this AED.

When to use with caution

• While it is used in this situation, caution is required in those with learning difficulty/behavioural problems, as it can significantly exacerbate behavioural problems.

• Depression can be both an early and late side effect.

• Caution is required with reduced renal clearance.

• In those with IGE with minor seizures only (e.g. myoclonus or absences), GTCS have been observed after its introduction, though infrequently.

What else do I need to know or tell the patient where appropriate?

Tiredness is often transient and although it may last weeks it is worth persevering. In most patients there is no weight change although both weight gain and loss have been reported. A tremor may occur which is dose related, sometimes in association with valproate. Mood disturbances (irritability/depression)should be looked out for. Warn about the possibility of allergic reactions which are infrequent. As with any treatement, advise patient to report any seizure exacerbation.

Profile in women and pregnancy

Information is still limited regarding teratogenicity. Early information from the Belfast Pregnancy Register is encouraging in relation to major malformations, but it should not be assumed to be safe until it has been shown to be so. Pregnancy outcomes in relation to whether there are more subtle effects on behaviour and educational needs will take years to establish.

What else do I monitor?

There is no specific indication for routine monitoring.

Interactions

Elimination half-life reportedly slightly reduced in children with epilepsy and other AEDs but one study did not show a significant interaction.

References

1. Brodie MJ, Perucca E, Ryvlin P, et al. (2007). Comparison of levetiracetam and controlled-release carbamazepine in newly diagnosed epilepsy. *Neurology*, **68**, 402–8.

Oxcarbazepine (Table 4b.15)

Overview

Oxcarbazepine is an effective AED against partial seizures with secondary generalization, probably equipotent to carbamazepine. Although it was not licensed in the UK until 2000, it was licensed in Denmark in 1990. It has some similarities with carbamazepine and is reportedly better tolerated. However, hyponatraemia appears more common. Its half-life is short but it has an active metabolite with a long half-life of about 9 hours. Autoinduction has not been observed. Although it reportedly has fewer interactions than carbamazepine, it nevertheless has significant drug interactions.

Rash can occur with oxcarbazepine but less commonly than with carbamazepine. There is a 25% cross-sensitivity (rash) with carbamazepine. *Therefore, if there is history of a rash with carbamazepine, consider an alternative AED.* It costs more than carbamazepine but less than other 'new' AEDs.

Consider oxcarbazepine in partial epilepsy particularly:
• Where carbamazepine is effective, but not well tolerated.
• To avoid some interactions with carbamazepine.
• For quicker loading as it has a better tolerability to rapid titration.

Dosing strategies

Oxcarbazepine may be started at 150mg/day given at night and increased soon after to 150mg twice/day, with the dose gradually increased depending on clinical need. Oxcarbazepine can be introduced more quickly than carbamazepine and it is possible to start on 300mg twice/day

Pregnancy

Limited information is available and major malformation rates in humans cannot be quoted. Oral vitamin K_1 supplementation to the mother is advised in the last 4 weeks of pregnancy, in addition to vitamin K given to the newborn at birth. Oxcarbazepine level decrease significantly in pregnancy, and dose adjustments are often needed.

Some important interactions

• Oxcarbazepine has important interactions. 📖 see Tables 4b.4, pp.290–291, and look up every concomitant drug before introducing or withdrawing.
• Oxcarbazepine and its pharmacologically active metabolite (MHD, monohydroxyderivative) are weak inducers of the cytochrome P450 enzymes including CYP3A4 and of UDP-glucuronyl transferases.

Table 4b.15 Oxcarbazepine

UK trade name	Trileptal®
Mode of action	Blockade of sodium channels
Usual preparations	Tablets: 150, 300, 600mg Oral suspension 60mg/mL
Maximum licensed dose	2400mg
Typical daily dose in adults	600–2400mg/day
Typical daily dose in children	6-12 years: 4–5mg/kg twice daily increased to usal maintenance of 15mg /kg twice daily (max 23mg/kg twice daily) 12–18 years: usual maintenance 0.3–1.2g twice daily
Dosage intervals	2 doses per day
Quoted range for blood levels	Blood levels not usually measured
Protein binding	40% for active metabolite monohydroxy derivative, MHD
Oral bioavailability	>95%
Time to peak levels	Of active metabolite 4–5 hours
Metabolism and excretion	Hydroxylation and then conjugation with renal elimination of metabolites
Elimination half-life in adults	~1 hour but 9 hours for MHD
Elimination half-life in children	5–8 hours for MHD (approximately two-thirds of the adult clearance)
Active metabolites	MHD
Main interactions	See text
Main indications	Focal seizures
Kinetics	Linear
Other	No auto-induction; can be introduced more quickly than carbamazepine

- It may result in reduced levels/efficacy of some medications, including carbamazepine (0–22% decrease but 30% increase of epoxide) and the OCP.
- Oxcarbazepine and MHD inhibit CYP2C19, which metabolizes phenytoin and phenobarbital the levels of which may be significantly increased with higher oxcarbazepine doses (phenytoin 0–40% increase, phenobarbital 14–15% increase).
- Unlike carbamazepine, oxcarbazepine reportedly does not interact with warfarin, cimetidine, erythromycin, or dextropropoxyphene.
- Oxcarbazepine and MHD levels are reduced (by 29–40%) by strong inducers of cytochrome P450 enzymes (carbamazepine, phenytoin, and phenobarbital).
- As with carbamazepine, concomitant therapy with lamotrigine may result in adverse effects requiring dose reduction. Lamotrigine levels have been shown to be modestly reduced by oxcarbazepine. The clinical relevance of this has not yet been fully determined nor the effect of lamotrigine on increasing MHD levels.

> **Box 4b.8 How to substitute oxcarbazepine for carbamazepine**
>
> *Usual ratio of 1.5 oxcarbazepine to 1 ordinary carbamazepine*
> - Overnight substitution only if carbamazepine dose is low or for exceptional indications, otherwise gradual substitution is recommended.
> - The approximate equivalent doses are: 100mg *ordinary* carbamazepine = 150mg oxcarbazepine.
> - Keep generally within the maximum licensed dose of oxcarbazepine in planning the switch.
> - Work out desired dose of oxcarbazepine, and round up or down to nearest tablet size depending on desired effect based on whether the patient is over or under treated:
>   - Is the patient on low/moderate doses/levels of ordinary carbamazepine and is the patient generally under-treated? If so use ratios of ~100mg carbamazepine = 150mg oxcarbazepine.
>   - Use ratio of 100mg carbamazepine = 125mg of oxcarbazepine if the patient is on modified release carbamazepine; if the patient is also over-treated, and on a modified release formulation of carbamazepine, a ratio of 1:1 may also be considered in selected cases.
> - Replace on a weekly or fortnightly basis 200mg of carbamazepine with the appropriate (higher) dose of oxcarbazepine.
> - Adjust the dose, based on clinical response.
> - Monitor sodium and FBC, particularly the former.

Phenobarbital (phenobarbitone) (Table 4b.16)

Overview

- The use of phenobarbital in epilepsy dates back to around 1912.
- It is an effective, inexpensive, broad-spectrum AED still widely used in countries where cost is the major consideration.
- It can be effective in many seizure types and syndromes including GTCS, primary or secondarily generalized, absences, myoclonus, and partial seizures. There is some evidence to suggest that carbamazepine is more likely to control partial seizures than phenobarbital.
- It also has a role in neonatal seizures.
- It is effective in status epilepticus.
- It should be considered as an option in intractable patients.
- It is not recommended as a first-line or second-line AED unless economic considerations are paramount. Disadvantages include:
  - It is sedating, habituating, and enzyme inducing. It has also been associated with behavioural problems and hyperkinetic behaviour in children and insomnia in the elderly.
  - It is an aromatic AED associated with hypersensitivity reactions with cross-reaction with other aromatic AEDs.
  - Other disadvantages include drug interactions, teratogenicity, secretion in breast milk, cognitive and educational adverse effects, and soft tissue fibrosis with long-term use (e.g. palmar (Dupuytren's) or planter nodules/contractures and Peyronie's disease). Because of its effect on vitamin K_1 metabolism, oral vitamin K_1 should be given to the mother in the last 4 weeks of pregnancy and the neonate given vitamin K_1 at birth. It also has an effect on bone metabolism and its use is associated with osteopenia, osteoporosis, and osteomalacia. Proactive measures to prevent osteopenia, including prevention of vitamin D deficiency, are advised.
- Phenobarbital has a very long half-life. Like phenytoin, for a quick effect, loading is required as discussed in the section on status epilepticus. where phenobarbital intravenously is effective with a reasonable side-effect profile. It can also be given intramuscularly where, in adults, its absorption kinetics are similar to the oral route.
- 📖 see Tables 4b.4, pp.290–291 for AED interactions. Due to its enzyme inducing effects, it has major pharmacokinetic interactions with many other agents. It increases the clearance of medications metabolized by the liver, thus shortening half-life and generally reducing efficacy. Increased adverse effects may occur if the metabolism of concomitant medication to toxic metabolites is induced. As it is metabolized by the liver, its own metabolism is altered by enzyme inducing agents. Furthermore, a number of drugs inhibit its metabolism, notably valproate. *If valproate is added to phenobarbital, this can precipitate toxicity and encephalopathy.* Depending on phenobarbital dose, dose adjustments are needed in the majority. There may also be pharmacodynamic interactions with benzodiazepines.

- To minimize withdrawal from acute toxicity on introduction, a dose of 30mg/day is suggested in adults in the outpatient setting. Dose increments should take into account the long-half life and be guided by clinical considerations.
- Maintenance doses are between 45–120mg/day. Higher doses can be given as tolerated and are rarely ≥240mg/day.
- Control of GTCS is more often reported on lower serum levels that control of partial seizures.
- Monitoring should include bone parameters and folate levels.
- It should not be withdrawn without good reason or careful reflection in those who have been on it for years with good tolerability and efficacy. If it is withdrawn in such circumstances, this is done extremely slowly over prolonged periods. Some have used decrements of 30mg every 4 weeks. This is probably too fast except where the maintenance dose is high, when this may be reasonable to start with. We suggest smaller decrements at longer intervals, particularly in those on lower doses and on long-term therapy: by 7.5–15mg every 2–3 months or so depending on the starting dose, duration of treatment and concomitant medication. Caution is required because of habituation. Consideration of effect of drug withdrawal on concomitant medication is also needed.

Phenobarbital prescription requirements in the UK

- Phenobarbital is a schedule 3 controlled drug.
- Prescriptions are valid for 28 days only.
- Address of prescriber must be in the UK.
- Repeats are not allowed.
- Prescriptions must be written so as to be indelible and must be signed and dated.
- Prescriptions must include:
  - Dose—the use of 'as directed' is not sufficient.
  - Form.
  - Strength.
  - Total quantity of the preparation in both words and figures.

Table 4b.16 Phenobarbital (phenobarbitone)

UK trade names	Generic
Mode of action	Main action: enhancement of GABA$_A$ inhibition—📖 for other actions, see Neurochemistry of antiepileptic drug action, p.252
Usual preparations	• Tablets: 15, 30, 60mg • Elixir: 15mg/5mL (NB contains 38% alcohol and should not be used in children) • Mixture 15mg/5mL (extemporaneously prepared and thus unlicensed) • Injection: 200mg/mL, 15mg/mL, 30mg/mL, 60mg/mL
Maximum licensed dose	Doses ≥ 240mg/day are rarely used in adults
Typical daily dose in adults	60–180mg/day
Typical daily dose in children	• 1 month–12 years: initially 1–1.5mg/kg twice daily, increased by 2mg/kg daily as required to a usual maintenacnce of 2.5–4mg/kg once or twice daily. • 12–18 years as per adults
Dosage intervals	1/day
Quoted range for blood levels	10–40mcg/mL (modified by development of tolerance)
Protein binding	40–60%
Oral bioavailability	80–100%
Time to peak levels	Variable: 1–3 hours
Metabolism and excretion	Hepatic oxidation, glucosidation, and hydroxylation, and then conjugation
Elimination half-life in adults	75–136 hours (shorter with enzyme-inducing agents)
Elimination half-life in children	37–73 hours
Active metabolites	None
Main interactions	Has major interactions: see texts
Main indications	Very broad: see text
Other	Linear pharmacokinetics

Phenytoin and fosphenytoin (Table 4b.17)

Overview

- Although phenytoin is still one of the widely used AEDS, we do not recommend it as first line because of the disadvantages outlined here, except in the acute situation.

- Phenytoin can be effective in preventing partial seizures although levels required for controlling these are higher than those required for controlling GTCS. It is very effective in secondarily GTCS and often in primary GTCS. However it is not effective for absences or myoclonus. Aggravation of these seizure types is probably less common than with carbamazepine although it has been reported. Phenytoin can also aggravate epilepsy at toxic levels.

- Specifically, phenytoin should not be given in Unverricht–Lundborg disease where it can aggravate the epilepsy and underlying disorder.

- Phenytoin can be given orally in tablet or liquid form as well as intravenously. The intravenous preparation is very alkaline and is toxic to veins and soft tissues, and care is needed in following recommendations for administration and for monitoring. Phenytoin must not be given intramuscularly as absorption is very slow and inconsistent. The prodrug fosphenytoin can be given intravenously and intramuscularly. It is less alkaline with fewer local side effects. Although it is administered more quickly, as it is a prodrug, the onset of action is no faster than phenytoin.

- Phenytoin is particularly helpful where there is clinical urgency. This is because it is possible to load phenytoin in the acute situation relatively quickly and achieve a therapeutic level. It is widely used in convulsive status epilepticus. However, it has been shown to be less effective in status, if used alone, than other agents against which it has been tested; it is usually used in conjunction with benzodiazepines.

- Non-linear pharmacokinetics: Fig. 4b.3 demonstrates how initial linear kinetics become non-linear as the dose is increased, a change which occurs at different doses in different people. At higher levels, moderate dose changes can result in major changes in blood levels with consequent loss of efficacy or toxicity.

- It has major drug interactions and is enzyme inducing. It undergoes hepatic metabolism (mainly CYP2C9) and other agents/medication can affect this process. Given phenytoin's pharmacokinetics, this can have clinical consequences.

- It has significant long-term side effects—e.g. hirsutism, gum disease, coarse features, connective tissue change, lymphadenopathy, osteopenia, neuropathy, nystagmus, ataxia, cerebellar damage in those susceptible and mood disturbances. Movement disorders may also occur (tremor, dyskinesias, chorea) and can be dose related.

Table 4b.17 Phenytoin and fosphenytoin

UK trade names	Epanutin® (phenytoin); Pro-Epanutin® (fosphenytoin)
Mode of action	Blockade of sodium channels
Usual preparations	**Phenytoin:** • Capsules: 25, 50, 100, 300mg • Chewtabs: 50mg • Liquid suspension: 30mg/5mL[1] • Injection: 250mg/5mL **Fosphenytoin: 10mL vials:** 1mL contains 75mg of fosphenytoin (equivalent to 50mg of phenytoin), referred to as 50mg PE (phenytoin equivalent). Each 10mL vial contains 750mg of fosphenytoin (equivalent to 500mg of phenytoin) referred to as 500mg PE.
Maximum licensed dose	500mg, exceptionally above (doses must be guided by serum levels, see text)
Typical daily dose in adults	200–400mg/day (guided by drug levels)
Typical daily dose in children	2.5–5mg/kg/day (higher in neonates)
Dosage intervals	1–2 doses per day
Quoted range for blood levels	10–20mg/L (mcg/mL) or 40–80 micromoles/L. See text for discussion of range. Note that measures are needed. There is a non-linear relation between dose and serum level
Protein binding	69–96% (usually 90% in adults)
Oral bioavailability	95% although may vary with formulation
Time to peak levels	4–12 hours
Metabolism and excretion	Hepatic oxydation and hydroxylation, and then conjugation.
Elimination half-life in adults	Average 22 hours, range 7–42 hours; steady state is achieved in 7–10 days
Elimination half-life in children	• In neonates: 10–60 hours • In older children: 5–14 hours
Active metabolites	None
Main interactions	Many interactions; see text, interaction 📖 Tables 4b.4 and 4b.5, and SPC
Main indications	• Focal and generalized seizures (excluding myoclonus and absence seizures) • Status epilepticus
Other	Non-linear pharmacokinetics

[1]Suspension of phenytoin 90mg in 15mL may be considered to be approximately equivalent in therapeutic effect to capsules or tablets containing phenytoin sodium 100mg.

- Although there may be a genetic predisposition to some of these side effects, some are more likely if the level is maintained at the upper end of the 'therapeutic range' of up to 20mg/L. With this in mind some reasonably favour an upper range up to 16mg/L. This is probably optimal for many, but it should noted that a proportion benefit and tolerate levels around and slightly above 20mg/L. It has been argued that a range of 7–25mg/L is more appropriate. Whatever range is quoted, it should be remembered that higher levels are associated with a higher risk of short- and long-term side effects some of which are serious and irreversible.

- Hypersensitivity reactions occur as with other aromatic AEDs and are an indication for prompt withdrawal with cover provided with an alternative AED.

- Phenytoin must not be stopped abruptly in chronic therapy. This can precipitate severe convulsive seizures or status epilepticus. For those who have been on it for many years, slow withdrawal is advised. Particular caution is needed with initial dose decrements, as these may result in a large change in blood level.

- Phenytoin and valproate are both protein bound. Valproate, displaces phenytoin, increases phenytoin free fraction, increases phenytoin clearance, and reduces total phenytoin levels. In this situation, total levels may mislead. Higher free levels may be present for a given total level with a greater incidence of toxicity.

- Similarly, where protein levels are low, total phenytoin levels reflect higher free phenytoin levels and therefore a therapeutic effect is expected at lower total levels than usual. Toxicity may occur at levels within the 'therapeutic range'. Corrected levels of phenytoin may be calculated for given albumin levels, but at least one formula used does not give an accurate indication. Free phenytoin levels from a salivary sample, if available, may be helpful in this situation.

- Slow metabolizers have higher levels and incidence of toxicity for a given dose. As with some other AEDs, dosage should be individualized as there is wide inter-patient variability in phenytoin serum levels for a given dose with variable elimination amongst different subjects.

- Weight can give some guidance to dose in adults as well as children (📖 see Fig 4b.3). In the non-acute setting, aim for 200–300mg/day (3–4mg/kg/day for an adult, higher in children) and 100mg/day in the elderly. Adjust dose depending on blood levels taken after 7–10 days, the time it can take to achieve a steady state. A therapeutic effect is less likely at levels below 5mg/L. Benefit can be observed with control of GTCS at levels below the so called 'therapeutic range' of 10–20mg/L while partial seizures may require levels within the therapeutic range. If appropriate, the dose is increased. Dose increments depend on measured levels, target level and clinical need. As an approximate guide, if the level is well below 5mg/L, increase dose by 50mg or more, depending on target level. If the level is between 5–8mg/L, increase dose by 25–50mg. If level is 9mg/L, increase dose by 25mg. Some recommend larger increments and these will need to be guided by clinical priorities (quick control vs minimum dose to control seizures).

- It takes up to 8 days for a steady state to be reached after a change in dose.
- Some patients achieve control on levels below the usual therapeutic range. A small number of patients require and tolerate levels above the therapeutic range as discussed above.
- Check levels more frequently if there is any relevant change in concomitant medication.
- Check biochemical screen, FBC, folate, calcium, and vitamin D levels and replace if deficient. Phenytoin may affect glucose metabaolism.
- Teratogenicity including the occurrence of cleft lip/palate and heart malformations may occur in children of women receiving phenytoin. Vitamin K should be given to the mother for the last 4 weeks to pregnancy and to the neonate at birth.

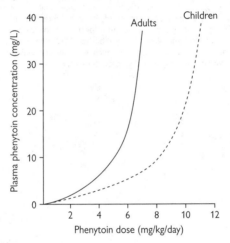

Fig. 4b.3 Plot of mean steady-state plasma phenytoin concentration against drug dose in adults (N = 21) and children younger than 15 years (N = 15). (Reproduced with permission from Shorvon SD, Perucca E, Fish DR et al. (eds.) (2004). *The Treatment of Epilepsy*, 2nd edn, Blackwell Science, Oxford.)

Piracetam (Table 4b.18)

Piracetam was first developed in the 1960s as a cyclic derivative of GABA. Although piracetam does not have a licence as a cognition enhancer in the UK, its trade name reflects its nootropic effect. It was noted early on to improve memory in rodents before an anti-seizure effects was shown. It has also been investigated for use in protecting against the effects of injury as well as in Raynaud's phenomenon. It inhibits platelet function, reduces blood and plasma viscosity through an increase in cell membrane deformability, and reduces plasma concentrations of fibrinogen and von Willebrand's factor; these properties should be kept in mind should someone taking piracetam require major surgery.

Piracetam's licence in the UK is for myoclonus, for which it needs to be taken in large quantities. Its indications are limited. It can be used in any form of epileptic myoclonus including Unverrich–Lundborg—where levetiracetam can also be used. Its mode of action is still reportedly unknown, although the mode of action of its more potent analogues levetiracetam, discovered in 1992 and already an established AED with broader efficacy than piracetam, and brivaracetam, which is undergoing clinical trials, is through binding synaptic vesicle glycoprotein SV2A.

Table 4b.18 Piracetam

UK trade names	Nootropil®
Mode of action	Unclear
Usual preparations	Tablets (scored): 800, 1200mg Solution: 333mg/mL
Maximum licensed dose	20g per day
Typical daily dose in adults	Very variable; can be 35g per day
Dosage intervals	2–3 doses per day
Quoted range for blood levels	Undetermined
Protein binding	0%
Oral bioavailability	<100%
Time to peak levels	30–40min
Metabolism and excretion	Renal excretion, unmetabolized. Dose to be adjusted in renal failure as per product information
Elimination half-life in adults	5–6 hours
Elimination half-life in children	
Active metabolites	None
Main interactions	Limited information: mostly negative
Main indications	Myoclonus: not licensed in children

Primidone (Table 4b.19)

Brief summary

- Acute initial toxicity (sedation, dizziness, nausea) even with small doses may occur and result in treatment withdrawal but tolerance develops quickly. Introduction at very low doses (62.5mg/day) is advised.
- Primidone is an effective AED which shares many properties with phenobarbital to which it is partly metabolized, along with a third active agent phenylethylmalonamide. Primidone and phenobarbital are broad-spectrum medications. Either can be considered in intractable patients, where appropriate, including in JME. It is not clear however, if there is any advantage of primidone over phenobarbital.
- Comparative trial data suggests similar clinical efficacy with phenobarbital.
- On average, a quarter of primidone is converted to phenobarbital. The dose of primidone needed to achieve the same level of phenobarbital is approximately 5 times higher than the dose of phenobarbital. More is converted to phenobarbital with some concomitant treatment with other enzyme inducing AEDs.
- Primidone is enzyme inducing and has important interactions—including with the OCP.
- Primidone can affect bone metabolism. It shares this and other side effects including potential teratogenicity with phenobarbital. It is excreted in breast milk.
- Primidone is habituating and should not be stopped suddenly (📖 see Phenobarbital p.326). There was concern a few years ago when its supply was not assured, but it now seems to be readily available.
- Primidone is also licensed for essential tremor.
- Primidone is readily available in tablet formulation. The liquid suspension was discontinued a few years ago.

Table 4b.19 Primidone

UK trade name	Mysoline®
Mode of action	Similar to phenobarbital. The action of primidone is due to 3 active agents: primidone and two major metabolites, phenobarbital and phenylethylmalonamide
Usual preparations	• Tablets: 250mg • Oral suspension: oral suspension has been discontinued in the UK and is now only available as a named patient medication sourced internationally 125mg/5mL (Liscandia, Germany).
Maximum licensed dose	Data sheet lists 1.5g/day adults; 1g children
Typical daily dose in adults	500–750mg/day
Typical daily dose in children	• <2 years: 125–250mg twice daily • 2–5 years: 250–375mg twice daily • 5–9 years: 375–500mg twice daily • 9–18 years: up to 750mg twice daily
Dosage intervals	2 doses per day
Quoted range for blood levels	As phenobarbital (into which it is metabolized)
Protein binding	• Low for primidone and phenylethylmalonamide • Phenobarbital ~50%
Oral bioavailability	90–100%
Time to peak levels	3 hours
Metabolism and excretion	Metabolized to phenobarbital and phenylmethylmalonamide. 40% excreted unchanged in urine
Elimination half-life in adults	Very variable 6–18 hours, longer for the two active metabolites
Elimination half-life in children	5–11 hours
Active metabolites	Phenobarbital and phenylmethylmalonamide
Main interactions	Enzyme inducing so has important interactions
Main indications	Broad spectrum: focal and generalized seizures (including absence and myoclonus)

Rufinamide (Table 4b.20)

Overview

This newly licensed AED is in the unusual situation of being licensed in the UK for use as add-on treatment for seizures only for those with Lennox–Gastaut syndrome above the age of 4 years, where it appears to be particularly effective in reducing drop attacks (tonic or atonic seizures). Studies have also shown efficacy in partial seizures and no doubt it will be used in focal epilepsy where other medications have failed. While post licensing experience is limited, its use should be restricted to specialists. It has significant interactions as described below and the potential to exacerbate seizures and precipitate status. Other side effects are listed next and include vomiting and gait disturbances. Abrupt withdrawal is not recommended. It interacts with the OCP. There is no experience of nufinamide use in pregnancy.

Adverse events

- Exacerbation of epilepsy and status epilepticus leading to discontinuation in 20% cases according to the product data sheet.
- Dizziness, somnolence, ataxia, gait disturbances, vomiting, anorexia, weight loss, headache, anxiety, insomnia, hyperactivity, diplopia, and blurred vision.
- Hypersensitivity syndromes.
- Decrease in QTc interval proportional to concentration, of uncertain clinical significance.

Interactions

- Rufinamide concentrations may be decreased by carbamazepine, phenobarbital, phenytoin, primidone, or vigabatrin (the latter having the smallest effect on rufinamide concentrations).
- Valproate significantly increases rufinamide plasma concentrations especially in those with low body weight (<30kg). Consider dose reduction of rufinamide in those <30kg when valproate is added, and an increase in dose if valproate is withdrawn.
- Rufinamide may decrease phenytoin clearance and increase levels. Consider reducing the dose of phenytoin if rufinamide is added as appropriate.
- Rufinamide at 800mg twice a day reduced both ethinylestradiol and norethisterone in a combined oral contraceptive (ethinylestradiol 35mcg and norethisterone 1mg). Women of child-bearing potential using hormonal contraceptives should be advised to use an additional safe and effective contraceptive method.
- Rufinamide does not significantly inhibit cytochrome P450 enzymes, but it induces the cytochrome P450 enzyme CYP3A4. It may therefore reduce levels of drug metabolized by this enzyme; the effect is described as modest-to-moderate.
- Close monitoring and dose adjustments where needed is recommended with drugs with a narrow therapeutic window such as warfarin and digoxin if rufinamide is added.

Table 4b.20 Rufinamide

UK trade name	Inovelon®
Mode of action	Modulates sodium channels prolonging their inactive state
Usual preparations	100mg, 200mg, and 400mg scored tablets
Maximum licensed dose	Dependant on weight for adults children>4: <ul><li>30–50kg: max. 1800mg</li><li>>50–70kg: max. 2400mg</li><li>>70kg: max. 3200mg</li></ul>
Typical daily dose in adults	To be established
Typical daily dose in children	To be established; Doses are lower in those with low body weight and on valproate
Dosage intervals	Twice/day taken with water—if necessary crushed and administered in half a glass of water. Usually taken with food
Quoted range for blood levels	
Protein binding	34%
Oral bioavailability	Bioavailability dependent on dose. As dose increases, bioavailability decreases. Food increases bioavailability and peak plasma concentrations
Time to peak levels	6 hours
Metabolism and excretion	Metabolized by hydrolysis to inactive metabolite
Elimination half-life in adults	6–10 hours
Elimination half-life in children	Lower clearance in children related to size (surface area)
Active metabolites	–
Main interactions	Rufinamide has clinically significant interactions as described in text–including with valproate
Main indications	Lennox–Gastaut (drop attacks) and partial seizures (current licence only for the former)

Sodium valproate (Table 4b.21)

Overview

Sodium valproate is a broad-spectrum AED, arguably the most broad spectrum available; effective in both generalized and partial epilepsies, as well as different seizure types, including absences and myoclonus. It is very effective in IGE often at low-to-moderate well-tolerated doses. It is therefore the standard AED against which efficacy of new AEDs in IGE should be compared. In partial epilepsy, higher doses are more often required with more side effects. In our view, it is therefore not a first choice AED in partial epilepsy, although it can be effective. While it is usually well tolerated at low-to-moderate doses, it is less well tolerated with higher doses, often because of weight gain, tremor, sedation, and hair loss.

Main advantages

- Broad spectrum covering many seizure types.
- Particularly effective in IGE compared to other AEDs.
- Good early tolerability.
- Low propensity to exacerbate seizures.

Some disadvantages/limitations

- Dose-related side effects of weight gain, postural tremor, sedation and hair loss—re-growth may be curly.
- Higher doses associated with motor or cognitive slowing, unsteadiness, or extrapyramidal features in those susceptible.
- Reported association of polycystic ovary syndrome in those susceptible, usually with weight gain.
- Enzyme inhibitor with clinically significant drug interactions including with lamotrigine and phenobarbital.
- Higher rate of teratogenicity and increased educational needs amongst offspring of women taking valproate in mono- or polytherapy with a dose-related effect.
- Reportedly associated with osteopenia despite not being enzyme inducing.
- Life-threatening side effects include risk of pancreatitis and liver failure (very rare in adults) and in susceptible groups (e.g. mitochondrial disease, a contraindication).
- Thrombocytopaenia.

When and how to use and dosing strategies

Valproate is a first-choice AED in generalized epilepsies in men and in women not of childbearing age. The same applies to younger onset unclassified cases, a significant proportion of whom have IGE. Many with IGE respond to low moderate doses. Clinical experience suggests that there may be an early and delayed effect when it is introduced and the same applies to when it is withdrawn, when loss of effect may not all be immediate. The mechanism for this is unknown. Fig. 4b.4 shows maintenance doses in a retrospective analysis of valproate treatment in a large cohort of IGE cases.

Table 4b.21 Sodium valproate

UK trade names	Epilim® (Epilim Chrono®), Depakote®, Episenta®, Orlept®
Mode of action	• Not fully elucidated. • Enhances GABA inhibition (increases GABA synthesis and inhibits GABA catabolism, inhibits excitatory neurotransmission, modulates voltage dependent sodium currents.
Usual preparations	• Crushable tablets: 100mg • Enteric-coated tablets: 200mg, 500mg • Modified release tablets (Epilim Chrono®): 200mg, 300mg, 500mg • Prolonged release (Episenta®): 150mg, 300mg, 500mg, and 1000mg • Oral solution: 200mg/5mL • Liquid (Epilim®—sugar free): 200mg/5mL • Syrup (Epilim®): 200mg/5mL • Intravenous (Epilim®): 400mg/4mL • Intravenous (generic): 300mg/3mL
Dose range	300–3000mg/day—max. quoted in Epilim® data sheet 2500mg/day
Typical daily dose in adults	600–1000mg in IGE, higher in focal epilepsy.
Typical daily dose in children	• 1 month–12 years: 12.5–15mg/kg twice daily • 12–18 years: 0.5–1g twice daily
Dosage intervals	• Ordinary: 2–3 doses per day • Long-acting: 1–2 doses per day
Quoted range for blood levels	Ranges quoted are 40–100mg/L (mcg/mL) (or 300–700 micromol/L). However, levels are generally not helpful except for compliance. Diurnal variation in blood levels without consistent relationship with clinical effect.
Protein binding	High 80–95%. More unbound drug in the elderly
Oral bioavailability	<100% food may slow down but not decrease extend of absorption
Time to peak levels	1–10 hours
Metabolism and excretion	Hepatic oxidation and then conjugation
Elimination half-life in adults	6–15 hours (slightly longer in elderly)
Elimination half-life in children	8–15 hours (longer in neonates)

(Continued)

Table 4b.21 Sodium valproate *(continued)*

Kinetics	Linear, except for free levels at high doses
Active metabolites	None
Main interactions	These are important. Valproate is an enzyme inhibitor and prolongs the half life of some other medication. It can also displace other highly protein bound medications. See text
Main licensed indications	Generalized and partial epilepsy

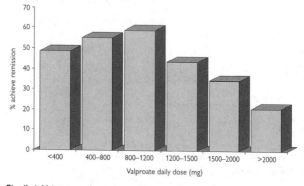

Fig. 4b.4 Maintenance doses observed in a retrospective analyses of valproate treatment in a large cohort of idiopathic generalized epilepsy cases. (Reproduced with permission from Dr Andrew Nicolson, Consultant Neurologist, Walton Centre, Liverpool.)

- Long acting preparations are generally better tolerated especially at higher doses. These can be given once or twice a day depending on dose and formulation.
- A reasonable initial dose for adults is 300–600mg in 24 hours increased as tolerated and as necessary. Some (usually IGE) respond to low doses but most require a dose of 500mg/day and above. The higher the dose the more likely the side effects. In general, side effects are more prominent above 1000mg although there is a large inter-individual variability, a few benefiting from and tolerating high doses of up to 3000mg/day.
- Look up interactions with concomitant medications before prescribing.
- Prescribing valproate in women of childbearing age should be through specialist advice with other treatment options explored first and the woman counselled on associated risks. If prescribed in this setting, the total dose, wherever possible, is kept below 1000mg/24 hours and split in divided doses to avoid high peak levels. Long-acting preparations are advised.

When not to choose?

- Consider an alternative first choice for those with symptomatic/lesional partial epilepsy—other treatments are likely to be effective at lower equivalent doses
- In women with IGE of childbearing age, and although valproate is likely to be the most effective AED, consider other treatment options with better profile in pregnancy first
- Where possible, do not select valproate as first choice in someone with tremor, motor slowing or with a tendency to weight gain as it is may well exacerbate these.
- Avoid in those with possible metabolic defects/mitochondrial disease which could predispose to liver failure.
- The following contra-indications are listed in the Epilim® 'data sheet': a) active liver disease; b) personal or family history of severe hepatic dysfunction, especially drug related; c) hypersensitivity to sodium valproate; and d) porphyria.

What else?

- Warn the patient about the possibility of weight gain, as, although not universal, it happens often enough for this to be a consideration.
- Inform patients and carers how to recognize rare, potentially serious reactions.
- Inform women about teratogenicity and possible increased educational needs amongst offspring.
- Inform about the possibility of hair loss, often a dose-related side-effect. This is usually reversible although re-growth may be curly.
- Valproate is generally well tolerated early.
- Sedation may occur and can be transient.
- GI side effects are often transient and are less likely if taken with or after food and with coated preparations.
- It is used as a mood stabilizer and as prophylaxis for migraine.
- A small proportion complain of headache or irritability—the latter more common in children with hyperactivity and behavioural problems.

- Anaemia, leucopenia, or pancytopenia are rare and usually reversible. Not infrequently, a dose-related asymptomatic mild decrease in platelet count is observed. However, valproate has an inhibitory effect on platelet aggregation and there can be an increase in bleeding time, usually aymptomatic, or, rarely, reduction of fibrinogen, particularly with high doses. It is advisable to screen for this before major procedures particularly in those on high doses.
- Other adverse events include hypersensitivity reactions which are rare, hirsutism, acne, peripheral oedema, and gynaecomastia.
- Life-threatening side effects are very rare in adults.
  - Encephalopathy with increased seizure frequency may occur, necessitating withdrawal. Sometimes there is no other cause. However, consider drug interactions, e.g. if concomitant treatment with phenobarbital for example. Also consider hyperammonaemia, although this is relatively common and asymptomatic at mild or moderate levels. In selected cases, withdrawal and investigation for possible underlying metabolic disorders, such as urea cycle enzyme deficiency, is required.
  - Reversible dementia with reversible cerebral atrophy has been rarely reported.
  - Very rare cases of haemorrhagic syndrome related to low fibrinogen have been reported in neonates whose mothers were on valproate.
  - Pancreatitis rarely occurs, as an idiosyncratic reaction, more commonly in younger age groups.
  - Liver failure: risk factors include polytherapy with AEDs, infants and young children <3 years, those with severe epilepsy, organic brain disease, psychomotor retardation, metabolic, mitochondrial, or degenerative diseases. Any symptoms compatible with this, even if non-specific, should be assessed promptly particularly in susceptible populations.
  - Bone marrow suppression and thrombocytopaenia.

What next if there is a very good response on the optimal dose for the patient with no side effects, but the patient still experiences unprovoked seizures?

There are a number of options:
- Alternative monotherapy as previously discussed.
- Possible options for add-on therapy include:
  - Introducing a small dose of lamotrigine in a male patient or woman not of childbearing age. As valproate and lamotrigine appear to be synergistic, the combination is often successful even with low doses. Start with 25mg every other day and build up slowly, no faster than fortnightly. Often 25mg or 50mg/day of add-on lamotrigine is sufficient. This combination is not recommended in women of childbearing age, pending information on teratogenicity.
  - In someone overweight, add-on treatment with topiramate or zonisamide may counteract the weight problem.
  - Add-on levetiracetam may also be successful, again sometimes with a low dose.

Profile in women and pregnancy

Other than weight gain, there is a reported association with polycystic ovary syndrome although the risk is difficult to assess, as this syndrome is relatively common in the general population. One view is that valproate probably exacerbates a pre-existing tendency in those susceptible.

Importantly, both major malformations and increased behavioural problems/educational needs appear to be increased overall in offspring if the mother is on valproate during pregnancy either as monotherapy (with a greater risk with higher doses) or polytherapy. Those with increased educational needs may have associated craniofacial features. Major malformations observed include neural tube defects such as myelomeningocele and spina bifida with an estimated incidence of 1–2%, craniofacial and limb defects, cardiovascular malformations, hypospadias, and multiple anomalies.

Of note is that the risk of major malformations with low dose valproate is relatively low.

Interactions

Summary: there are important clinically relevant interactions between valproate and a number of medications. As it has no enzyme inducing effect, it does not reduce the efficacy of the oral contraceptive pill. It displaces other drugs from plasma protein and inhibits hepatic metabolism, thus enhancing efficacy/toxicity of some other medications. Valproate levels are reduced by enzyme inducing drugs, and valproate free level is enhanced by protein binding medications.

Look up potential interactions with valproate with any concomitant prescribing. *Some* important interactions are highlighted below.

- Other AEDs: 📖 see Table 4b.5 pp.290–291.
    - Caution and dose adjustments are particularly needed if valproate is added to other medication the metabolism of which is inhibited by valproate. For example, its interaction with lamotrigine (📖 see pp.316–317) and phenobarbital or primidone results in clinically significant increased levels of the other medication with potentially adverse consequences. A corresponding drop in their levels with loss of efficacy occurs if valproate is withdrawn.
    - Valproate decreases total plasma phenytoin concentration and increases free phenytoin levels. It displaces phenytoin from plasma protein binding sites and reduces hepatic catabolism. Short and long-term side effects are more likely for a given total phenytoin level. If this combination, which is not ideal, is used, and where free phenytoin levels are not available, it is advisable to aim for the lowest effective dose of phenytoin, to avoid total levels in the upper half of the quoted therapeutic range and to monitor for side effects.
    - Valproate can also potentiate the effect of carbamazepine and dose adjustments may be needed as clinically indicated.
- Other interactions include valproate raising zidovudine levels with potential toxicity. Interactions may also occur with anti-psychotics and anti-depressants.
- Adjustment of valproate dose may be needed if enzyme-inducing treatment is added or withdrawn to avoid loss of efficacy or side effects.
- Valproate levels can also be affected by other medication. Highly protein bound agents, such as aspirin, may increase free valproate levels. Cimetidine and erythromycin may increase valproate levels through reduced hepatic metabolism. Carbapenem antibiotics such as imipenem, panipenem, and meropenem may decrease valproate levels. Colestyramine may decrease the absorption of valproate.
- For oral anticoagulants 📖 see Antiepileptic medication and warfarin, p.358.

How useful are levels?

These are available but, although useful for assessment of recent compliance, they are not useful to guide dosing, which is better guided by clinical response. There is diurnal variation in levels and no good relationship between levels, side effects, or clinical response.

What else could be monitored and what other effects have been observed?
Monitor FBC (including platelets), biochemical profile including liver function tests, weight and bone density, the latter if other risk factors are present. Transiently increased liver enzymes may occur at the beginning of therapy. With long-term use, liver function tests are often normal. Check bleeding time and coagulation if clinically indicated or prior to major procedures. Other effects of valproate on investigations include normalized EEG in IGE and positive urine tests for ketones. Mild-to-moderate rise in ammonia levels is relatively frequent and usually, but not aways asymptomatic.

Tiagabine (Table 4b.22)

Overview

This is a narrow-spectrum, reasonably tolerated AED with efficacy in partial epilepsy. It is licensed as an adjunctive therapy only.

Who not to give to?

It should not be prescribed to those with possible generalized epilepsy syndromes including those with generalized spike wave on EEG, myoclonus or absences.

How to use

Start with 5mg/day taken at the end of a meal. If tolerated, increase weekly by 5mg until 15mg/day in two or 3 divided doses.

- In patients on enzyme inducing AEDs, and given the markedly reduced half-life of tiagabine, increase gradually to 10mg, 3 times/day if tolerated.
- Consider further increase as clinically indicated.

Dose ranges: mean doses are higher in those on enzyme inducing AEDs than those not induced. Most patients will require/tolerate <60mg/day in divided doses. A small proportion in open label trials have taken higher doses.

Other: CNS side effects including dizziness, tiredness, nervousness, tremor, concentration difficulty, emotional lability, slowness of speech and depressed mood may occur. Early side effects such as dizziness and tiredness can be transient. Caution is suggested with slow introduction and supervision in those with a history of depression or behavioural problems. Cases of nonconvulsive status epilepticus have been reported. Tiagabine should be avoided in those with unclassified or generalized epilepsy syndromes. De novo seizures have been reported in patients with no history of epilepsy prescribed tiagabine for other indications.

Profile in pregnancy: unknown

Interactions

Tiagabine half-life is reduced from 5–9 hours to 2–3 hours in those on enzyme–inducing medications, with higher tiagabine dose requirements and reduced plasma concentration by a factor of 1.5. Tiagabine does not have any clinically significant effect on warfarin, digoxin, OCP, or, generally, other AEDs.

Table 4b.22 Tiagabine

UK trade names	Gabitril®
Mode of action	Increases synaptic GABA availability through selective inhibition of GABA reuptake by presynaptic membrane
Usual preparations	Tablets: 5, 10,15mg
Maximum licensed dose	Not clear: in open label trials doses of around 100mg have been used in a small subgroup.
Typical daily doses in adults	15–60mg/day (those on enzyme inducing AEDs require higher doses than those not on enzyme inducing AEDs)
Typical daily dose in children	0.25–0.75mg/kg/day
Dosage intervals	2–3 doses per day
Quoted range for blood levels	Uncertain, as blood levels vary considerably during the day
Protein binding	96%
Oral bioavailability	89%
Time to peak levels	Mean ~1 hour, delayed by food to mean of ~2.6. Given short half-life, it is advisable to take tiagabine at the end of a meal to reduce fluctuations in levels.
Metabolism and excretion	Hepatic oxidation and conjugation
Elimination half-life in adults	7–9 hours (2–3 hours in induced patients)
Elimination half-life in children	3.2 hours (3 to 10 years old) 5.7 hours in children on valproate
Active metabolites	None
Main interactions	Half life reduced and dose requirements increased with enzyme inducing AEDs
Main indications	Focal seizures with or without secondary generalization (licensed as adjunctive therapy in those aged 12 years and over)

Topiramate (Table 4b.23)

Overview

Topiramate was first licensed in the UK in 1995. It is a useful, effective, broad-spectrum AED licensed as add-on treatment and as monotherapy. It is also licensed for migraine. Other potential effects are being explored in painful neuropathies, obesity, alcohol and other dependence as well as neuroprotection.

It is not, however, well tolerated in a significant proportion, especially when used as add-on treatment and with higher doses. Side effects include weight loss, mood and behavioural change with an increase in suicide-related events, reduced verbal fluency with increasing doses, a small risk of kidney stones (<2%), metabolic acidosis, and, very rarely, acute angle closure glaucoma. Gastrointestinal side effects and alopecia have also been reported infrequently. Paraesethesia is a relatively frequent side-effect. Adverse effects are often dose-related and topiramate is better tolerated with lower doses and monotherapy. Information in pregnancy is limited but it has teratogenic potential.

It is a very useful medication. It is undoubtedly potent and broad spectrum, with efficacy in generalized and partial seizures and syndromes, both as add-on treatment and in monotherapy. However, in view of its profile, it is not a first-line drug. It should also generally not be an early choice adjunctive treatment in partial epilepsy. In generalized epilepsies choice is more limited. Primarily because of lower tolerability, it did not perform as well as other medications in either the 'generalized' or 'partial' arm of the SANAD study (📖 see p.274, references 1a and 1b). It still has a very useful role in intractable epilepsy, with its administration best supervised by a specialist. Because of limited data being available on concomitant use, it is best avoided with medications that also inhibit carbonic anhydrase such as zonisamide or acetazolamide.

How to use topiramate

- Exclude a personal or family history of kidney stones and advise good hydration.
- Inform the patient that it does not suit all and may have to be withdrawn, but that it is an effective drug and thus taking it may prove worthwhile.
- Weigh the patient and monitor weight. If significant weight loss occurs stop increasing the dose and observe closely. Dose may need to be reduced if weight loss is significant or the medication withdrawn depending on extent.
- Warn the patient of:
  - The potential for mood or behavioural disturbances and monitor for this (reduce dose or withdraw)
  - Angle closure glaucoma (this is very rare at < 1/10,000 per patient year of estimated exposure) and usually occurs early in treatment; emergency ophthalmic assessment and prompt treatment is needed. Topiramate withdrawal is advised with adequate management to avoid seizures.
  - Reduced verbal fluency (reduce dose until it resolves).

Table 4b.23 Topiramate

UK trade name	Topamax®
Mode of action	• Blockade of sodium channels • Marked enhancement of GABAA inhibition • Weak inhibition of (excitatory) AMPA-Kainate glutamate receptors • Very weak carbonic anhydrase activity - not its mode of action
Usual preparations	• Tablets: 25, 50, 100, 200mg • Sprinkle: 15, 25, 50mg
Maximum licensed dose	400mg max recommended as initial therapy (max 800mg as adjunctive therapy—☐ see text)
Typical daily dose in adults	100–400mg/day
Typical daily dose in children	**Monotherapy:** • 6–16 years: 1.5–6mg/kg twice daily • 16–18 years: 50mg twice daily to max. 200mg twice daily **Adjunctive:** • 2–16yrs: 2.5–4.5mg/kg twice daily • 16–18yrs: 100–200 twice daily to max. 400mg twice daily
Dosage intervals	2 doses per day
Quoted range for blood levels	Not usually measured. Some quote 9–12mg/L
Protein binding	15–41%
Oral bioavailability	<100% (>80%)—delayed but not reduced by food
Time to peak levels	1.5–4 hours—delayed by food
Metabolism and excretion	80% renal excretion unmetabolized; up to 50% metabolized in those on enzyme inducing AEDs
Elimination half-life in adults	• Mean 21 hours; 12–15 hours with enzyme inducing AEDs • Low intersubject variability
Time to steady state in adults	4–8 days (longer if renal impairment)
Elimination half-life in children	• 10–15 hours • In presence of enzyme-inducing drugs: 6–8 hours
Active metabolites	None
Main interactions	See text: topiramate levels are lowered by enzyme-inducing AEDS. Topiramate at higher doses reduces oestrogen levels in OCP. It may also inhibit metabolism of phenytoin in some
Main indications	Partial and generalized seizures; migraine

- Monitor patient regularly for side effects. Weight loss, speech and cognitive side effects can slowly develop and result in treatment failure if the dose is not reduced until side effects resolve. The other concern is that such side effects may occur and affect the patient's quality of life who, nevertheless, may not report them.

Doses

In an average adult, start on 25mg/day only. A very small proportion responds to this dose. In the majority, higher doses are required. Increase, usually no faster than fortnightly, to 25mg twice/day, then by 25mg increments either morning or evening. Increase only if seizures continue and there are no side effects. Reasonable initial target doses in someone not on enzyme inducing AEDs is 50–100mg/day (□ see Tables 4b.1a and 4b.1b, pp.278–279).

Doses can be increased further following review if no side effects are observed. Most maintenance doses are between 100–400mg, doses being on average greater in those on enzyme-inducing AEDS. Although some patients are maintained on doses outside this range, most patients do not tolerate high doses. Furthermore, dose ranging studies suggest no increase in efficacy with much higher doses, and the maximum dose of 800mg/day, mentioned in the data sheet as adjunctive therapy, is not usually used and would not be tolerated by most.

Interactions

□ see BNF, datasheet; Tables 4b.4, and 4b.5, pp.290–291; Pharmacological interactions.

- Up to 50% of topiramate is metabolized if given with enzyme-inducing AEDs compared to 20% without.
- Topiramate concentrations are reduced by enzyme-inducing AEDS. Carbamazepine, for example, reduces topiramate levels by about 40%. If such AEDS are withdrawn, this may result in emergent side effects and necessitate reduction in topiramate dose until side effects resolve.
- Topiramate is a mild enzyme inducer. It increases the oral clearance of ethinylestradiol mostly at higher doses.
- Topiramate inhibits P450 isoenzyme CYP2C19, responsible for 20% of phenytoin metabolism. Thus in a proportion, this may result in an increase in levels

Pregnancy

There is insufficient human pregnancy outcome to define risk but topiramate has teratogenic potential.

Vigabatrin (Table 4b.24)

Overview and summary

- Vigabatrin is a designer drug, an analogue of GABA, a major inhibitory neurotransmitter. It acts as a substrate for GABA transaminase which it inactivates by irreversible binding, thus inhibiting the metabolism of GABA.
- Vigabatrin was licensed as an add-on treatment in partial epilepsy ushering in an era of newly licensed AEDs. Despite neuropsychiatric side effects, it seemed initially to be very promising, with low pharmacokinetic interactions and very good efficacy as add-on medication. It was later shown not to be as effective as carbamazepine in a head-to-head monotherapy trial in new onset epilepsy. With the emergence of a serious, common, and often irreversible side effect, it has not lived up to its promise. The use of vigabatrin is now known to result in a retinopathy with progressive reduction in visual fields in about one-third of those using it.
- Vigabatrin is currently a first-line drug in West syndrome only, especially those with an underlying diagnosis of tuberous sclerosis. (see Neurocutaneous syndromes, pp.470–477). In other situations, it should be avoided and only rarely considered. Patients already on vigabatrin are informed of this risk and offered gradual withdrawal. Those with previously intractable epilepsy, who have responded dramatically to vigabatrin, may choose to remain on it if a) they are aware of the potential risk; b) have normal visual fields; and c) undergo specialist assessment and regular monitoring of visual fields. Others still experiencing significant seizures should be advised to gradually withdraw. Those in whom visual fields cannot be monitored are also advised to attempt withdrawal, while taking the epilepsy into consideration.
- Anecdotally, tolerance with loss of efficacy can develop. Withdrawal often needs to be very gradual. Cover with short-term clobazam if necessary.
- Other side effects include neuropsychiatric adverse effects (e.g. depression, hyperactivity, agitation, psychosis, stupor, confusion) weight gain, diarrhoea, drowsiness, insomnia, ataxia, tremor.
- As a narrow spectrum medication it can worsen absences, myoclonic jerks, and precipitate non-convulsive status
- *Interactions*: vigabatrin is not metabolized, not protein bound and does not induce hepatic cytochrome P450 enzymes and has a low interaction rate. It can reduce phenytoin concentrations gradually (mechanism unknown).
- *Pregnancy*: data limited but suggest teratogenic potential. The data sheet quotes congenital anomalies reported in 14.5% of exposed pregnancies, of which 64.3% were major malformations, with spontaneous abortion reported in 10.9%. The presence of concomitant AED treatment complicates assessment.

Table 4b.24 Vigabatrin

UK trade name	Sabril®
Mode of action	Increases GABA through inhibition of GABA aminotransaminase
Usual preparations	• Tablets: 500mg • Powder sachet: 500mg
Maximum licensed dose	3 g/day
Typical daily dose in adults	1000–3000mg/day
Typical daily dose in children	• 1 month–12 years: 40–75mg/kg twice daily • 12–18 years: 1–1.5g twice daily
Dosage intervals	• 1–2 doses per day. • 2 doses per day in children with infantile spasms.
Quoted range for blood levels	Considerable inter-individual variation in plasma levels is observed
Protein binding	0%
Oral bioavailability	Almost 100%
Time to peak levels	0.5–2 hours
Metabolism and excretion	Renal excretion unmetabolized
Elimination half-life in adults	5–8 hours
Active metabolites	None
Main interactions	May gradually reduce phenytoin levels (mechanism unknown)
Main indications	West Syndrome. 📖 See text—effective in focal epilepsies but with serious side effects

Zonisamide (Table 4b.25)

Overview

Zonisamide was licensed in the UK in 2005. It is not, however, so new as it has been used widely in Japan since 1989, and in the US since 2000. Although its UK license is only as adjunctive therapy for partial epilepsy, it is effective in monotherapy and is broad spectrum with reports of efficacy in generalized seizures including absences and myoclonus. Like topiramate it is associated with a risk of kidney stones and weight loss; the latter appears to be less marked. It is also very rarely associated with aplastic anaemia. Its position in relation to other AEDs is still to be defined, but despite limitations, it has promise both in relation to good efficacy and reasonable tolerability. Anecdotally, it is better tolerated than topiramate. Interestingly, there have been reports of its successful use in progressive myoclonic epilepsies (Unverricht–Lundborg and Lafora body disease). Information in pregnancy is lacking.

How to use

- Exclude a personal or close family history of renal stones.
- Advise adequate hydration.
- Record and monitor weight in view of possible associated weight loss.
- Warn about the possibility of hypersensitivity reactions. As zonisamide is a sulphonamide derivative, hypersensitivity to sulphonamides is a contraindication.
- Start on 25mg twice/day (data sheet recommends 50mg twice/day). Some start at 25mg/day. Zonisamide has a long half-life of about 60 hours if taken without concomitant enzyme-inducing AEDs, and takes longer than predicted (~13 days) to reach a steady state. Where a quick effect is needed, the dose can be increased weekly. Otherwise, slow escalation, every 3–4 weeks, allows for individual tolerability per dose to be established and, in those with frequent seizures, the minimum effective dose for the individual to be used. If taken with enzyme inducing drugs, titration can be faster and doses generally needed are higher.
- Titrate the dose until seizures improve or side effects emerge. In those with frequent seizures, there is no need to increase if seizures improve on low doses. In those with very infrequent seizures or on enzyme-inducing AEDs, titrate in the first instance, if tolerated, to 75–100mg twice/day, otherwise to 50mg twice/day. Individual requirements vary. The dose can be further increased as needed.
- After the titration phase, zonisamide can be given once/day.

Table 4b.25 Zonisamide

UK trade name	Zonegran®
Mode of action	Not fully elucidated; acts on sodium and calcium channels and has a modulatory effect on GABA neuronal inhibition. Carbonic anhydrase inhibitor but this is not thought to be the main mode of action
Usual preparations	25mg, 50mg and 100mg capsules
Maximum licensed dose	Data sheet refers to 500mg—higher doses have been used
Typical daily dose in adults	100–400mg (the higher doses if on enzyme inducing AEDs)
Typical daily dose in children	100–400mg/day
Dosage intervals	Twice/day initially during titration later can given once/day
Quoted range for blood levels	20–30mcg/mL
Protein binding	40–50%
Oral bioavailability	Approximately 100%. Oral bioavailability is not affected by food, although peak plasma and serum concentrations may be delayed.
Time to peak levels	2–5 hours
Metabolism and excretion	Reductive cleavage of benzisoxazole ring by CYP3A4 to form 2-sulphamoylacetylphenol (SMAP) and by N-acetylation. Drug and inactive metabolites can be glucuronidated. Both renally excreted. No autoinduction.
Elimination half-life in adults	60 hours; reduced in the presence of enzyme-inducing drugs:
Elimination half-life in children	Adolescents (12–18 years): limited data indicate that pharmacokinetics in adolescents dosed to steady state at 1, 7, or 12mg/kg daily, in divided doses, are similar to those observed in adults, after adjustment for bodyweight.
Active metabolites	None
Main interactions	See text
Main indications	Although the current UK licence is for adjunctive treatment in partial epilepsy, zonisamide can be used more widely, is broad spectrum and has been used in monotherapy

Interactions
- As zonisamide has little or no effect on liver enzymes, it generally does not affect the pharmacokinetics of other medications. It does not affect the OCP or levels of other AEDs to a significant extent.
- Enzyme-inducing AEDs, such as phenytoin, carbamazepine, and phenobarbital reduce the half-life of zonisamide, and therefore its blood levels.
- There is no data on safety or pharmacodynamic interactions if used with other carbonic anhydrase inhibitors, topiramate, or acetazolamide. Avoid co-administration if possible. If not, keep overlap short-term. Avoid use with other agents that may also predispose to kidney stones.

Pregnancy and breast feeding
There is insufficient human data on use in pregnancy and teratogenic risk is unknown. Teratogenicity has been observed in animal studies. Breast-feeding is not recommended during zonisamide treatment or for 1 month after.

Adverse events
These include—amongst others—anorexia, weight loss, abdominal pain, hypersensitivity reactions including SJS, nephrolithiasis, cognitive and neuropsychiatric side effects, decreased sweating/hyperthermia, and an effect on blood count including aplastic anaemia.

AEDs in special situations

Bone health and AEDS

Background

There is an association between an increased risk of fracture and long-term use of AEDs in epilepsy. Possible reasons for this include:

- Increased risk of injury and fracture from seizures in epilepsy.
- Increased risk of falls from AEDs and associated handicap.
- Increased risk of osteopenia from reduced mobility due to associated disability.
- Despite conflicting data, there is evidence for a direct effect of some AEDs on bone health with increased risk of osteomalacia and osteoporosis. The effect of individual drugs is difficult to ascertain given the direction involved, polytherapy, changes in treatment, and other confounding variables. The effect may be partly related to the enzyme-inducing effect of some AEDs, such as phenobarbital, phenytoin, primidone, or carbamazepine. Other poorly understood mechanisms operate. Valproate, for example, is not enzyme-inducing but was also reported as associated with a decrease in bone density. With enzyme-inducing AEDs, there is an association with lower levels of calcium and vitamin D and raised levels of alkaline phosphatase and parathyroid hormone, although often these may often not be outside normal ranges. The role of measuring newer markers of bone turnover, of osteoclast and osteoblast activity, in this setting, is not yet established. Bone density scans may show reduced density in those at risk but, not surprisingly, do not correlate with biochemical markers. The effect of newer AEDs on bone density may be less but information is limited.

Implications to clinical practice

- Both the physician and patient need to be aware of bone health as a potential issue and be pro-active, where appropriate, about preventing osteopenia.
- Of note is that vitamin D levels are not infrequently suboptimal in the general population, reflecting dietary factors and indoor life-styles. Suboptimal levels may be compounded by the effect of AEDs in epilepsy.
- The potential effect of some AEDs on bone health is one of many considerations in selecting a suitable AED.
- There is debate and conflicting evidence about the efficacy in preventing bone disease of vitamin D and calcium supplementation in epilepsy. The same applies to doses required for clinical benefit. There is, however, evidence of a protective effect in other settings. Therefore we recommend the following.
  - Assess other risk factors in an individual: these include amongst others alcoholism, smoking, immobility, poor diet, GI disease, anorexia, steroid treatment, previous low-impact fractures, thyroid disease, race (older white women most at risk), family history, hypogonadism, and post-menopausal state.
  - Advise patient about life style measures including exercise.
  - Consider bone density scan in those with risk factors. If abnormal refer for management.

- Advise general measures to enhance vitamin D levels including being outdoors if possible and improved diet.
- In patients on enzyme-inducing AEDs or on medications known to affect bone health, and in all those with low or low normal vitamin D and calcium levels, advise supplementation (year round or over the darker months, as appropriate) with vitamin D and calcium or cod liver oil supplements. Make sure the supplement is adequate with optimal vitamin D blood levels achieved in winter. Always check calcium level to avoid supplementation in latent hyperparathyroidism in those with levels around the upper end of the normal range.

Osteoporosis

Osteoporosis is a relatively common age-related progressive, systemic skeletal disorder with low bone mass and micro-architectural deterioration of bone tissue, with a consequent increase in fracture risk. Bone formation exceeds bone resorption until the third decade of life after which there is gradual loss of bone mass (📖 see Box 4b.9). Women are at greater risk with lower peak bone mass and accelerated loss after the menopause.

Diagnosis of osteoporosis is based on a measurement of bone mineral density (BMD), with reference to the number of standard deviations (T-score) from the BMD at peak bone mass. Measurement of BMD can estimate fracture risk:

- Normal: T-score of −1 SD or above.
- Osteopenia: T-score of between −1 and −2.5 SD.
- Osteoporosis: T-score of −2.5 SD or below.
- Established/severe osteoporosis: T-score of −2.5 SD or below with one or more associated fractures (source: 🖰 www.nice.org.uk).

Treatment effective in primary and secondary prevention of osteoporotic fractures is available.

Box 4b.9 Patient information sheet—bone protection in epilepsy

Bone thinning or weakness is common, particularly amongst the elderly, and is often undetected until a fracture occurs. Fractures, which can happen with minor impact, usually affect the wrists, back or hips. Bone thinning can be due to problems with bone structure (osteoporosis) or poor mineralization (osteomalacia). Several medical conditions increase the risk of bone diseases as do drugs such as steroids, excess alcohol/caffeine, and smoking. Sometimes bone disease runs in families. Immobility, lack of exercise, limited sunlight exposure as well as poor diet are also important. Post-menopausal women in general, and particularly women with an early menopause, are at greater risk.

Falls during seizures or from unsteadiness with medication may increase the chances of a fracture. Some of the drugs used to prevent fits can increase the risk of bone diseases, sometimes by reducing important minerals (calcium) and vitamins (vitamin D). People taking these medications need enough of these minerals in their diet and may benefit from supplementation.

There are many simple but important measures that you can take to reduce the risks of fractures such as: taking regular exercise, a good diet, stopping smoking, and reducing alcohol. Your doctor may advise you to take supplements. It is sensible to check calcium level before taking supplements to make sure it is not unexpectedly high from an unrelated cause. There are many different calcium and vitamin D preparations and, initially, a dose of 800IU/day of vitamin D (colecalciferol) is usually recommended. A simple blood test can then ensure that your vitamin D and calcium levels are optimal. If your doctor feels that you are at particular risk, he/she may also arrange a bone density scan. If osteoporosis is detected, there are other treatments that can reduce the risk of fracture.

For more general information about osteoporosis, visit the National Osteoporosis Society (⌁ www.nos.org.uk/)

Vitamin D and mineral calcium
Vitamin D has very important functions; notably it regulates the amount of calcium in the body needed for healthy bones and teeth. Consult ⌁ www.eatwell.gov.uk

Sources of calcium:
- Milk, cheese and other dairy foods.
- Green leafy vegetables—such as broccoli, cabbage and okra, but not spinach.
- Soybean products.
- Nuts.
- Bread and fortified flour.
- Fish where bones are eaten—e.g. sardines and pilchards.

The adult requirement of 700mg a day is easily provided by three portions of dairy foods e.g yoghurt, milk, or cheese.

Sources of Vitamin D:
- Dietary sources: oily fish, liver, cod-liver oil, eggs, fortified foods—e.g. margarine, breakfast cereals, bread and powdered milk.
- Sunlight: most vitamin D is formed under the skin in reaction to sunlight. Caution: take care not to burn. As a fat-soluble vitamin, excess is stored, so daily exposure is not needed to maintain healthy levels. The following are at risk of low vitamin D levels: those with: darker skin; who cover all skin when outside;or rarely get outdoors; and do not consume the foods listed.

Anticoagulants and AEDs
The following AEDs are not thought to have clinically significant interactions with warfarin:
- Clobazam.
- Clonazepam.
- Ethosuximide.
- Gabapentin.
- Lamotrigine.
- Levetiracetam.

- Oxcarbazepine.
- Pregabalin.
- Tiagabine.
- Sodium valproate—but caution required, 📖 see Table 4b.26.
- Vigabatrin.
- Zonisamide.

The following AEDs are thought to interact with warfain (📖 see Table 4b.26 for details). Avoid if possible; close monitoring needed:

- Phenobarbital—reduced anticoagulant effect.
- Primidone—reduced anticoagulant effect.
- Phenytoin—reduced and increased anticoagulant effects noted.
- Carbamazepine—reduced anticoagulant effect.
- Felbamate—isolated case report of increased anticoagulant effect.

Epilepsy and mental health—prescribing AEDs in psychiatric conditions

A detailed account is beyond the scope of this manual. Suffice it to say that there are many interactions between AEDs and drugs used in medical conditions other than epilepsy, and that other medical conditions have direct bearing on metabolism and clearance of AEDs. Furthermore, treatment of conditions that may be associated can alter seizure threshold. Some important conditions are addressed briefly:

Epilepsy, depression, and mental health

Studies of co-morbidity of epilepsy and mental health disorders have methodological limitations. Comorbidity is the co-occurrence of separate conditions at above chance levels, which may be present if one condition causes another, if they share common genetic or environmental risk factors, or if factors associated with one condition lead to the other in a susceptible individual. In adults with epilepsy, anxiety and depression (📖 see Box 4b.10) are the most common psychiatric disorders. Suicide risk is increased with a greater reported risk in temporal lobe epilepsy. Studies also suggest an association between epilepsy and attention deficit hyperactivity disorder (ADHD) with an increased risk of developing epilepsy.

Table 4b.26 Effects of AEDs on warfarin plasma levels

Drug	Effect on warfain plasma levels	Comments
Barbiturates: Phenobarbital	Decrease	Full therapeutic anticoagulation may only be achieved by raising the anticoagulant dosage about 30 to 60%. If the barbiturate is later withdrawn, the anticoagulant dosage should be reduced to avoid the risk of bleeding.
Primidone	Decrease	Primidone is metabolized in the body to phenobarbital and is therefore expected to interact like phenobarbital, although there seem to be no reports of interactions with anticoagulants. Notwithstanding it would be prudent to be alert for reduced anticoagulant effects if primidone is given concurrently.
Benzodiazepines: Diazepam Flurazepam Nitrazepam Chlordiazepoxide	Unlikely to be relevant	An interaction between any oral anticoagulant and a benzodiazepine is unlikely, but there are three unexplained and unconfirmed cases of increased or decreased anticoagulant responses, which were attributed to an interaction.
Carbamazepine	Decrease	The anticoagulant effects of warfarin can be markedly reduced by carbamazepine.
Oxcarbazepine	Unlikely to be relevant	Oxcarbazepine appears not to interact significantly
Felbamate	Increase	An isolated case report describes a marked increase in the effects of warfarin, which were attributed to felbamate.
Valproate	Unlikely to be relevant	Sodium valproate appears not to interact with the oral anticoagulants to a clinically relevant extent. Nevertheless, manufacturers recommend caution with vitamin K-dependent anticoagulants as sodium valproate may displace them from protein binding sites. Transient change has been reported. NB valproate alone can cause altered bleeding time, bruising, heamatoma, and haemorrhage.
Phenytoin	Reduced or increased effect reported	The serum levels of phenytoin are usually unchanged by warfarin and phenindione. However, a single case of phenytoin toxicity has been seen with warfarin. Phenytoin would be expected to reduce the anticoagulant effects of coumarin anticoagulants, and this has been demonstrated for dicoumarol. However, cases of increased effects of warfarin have been reported.

Box 4b.10 Major depression and epilepsy

A number of observational studies link depression with epilepsy. There are many possible explanations for this including shared genetic or environmental susceptibility, effects of treatment and general and specific effects of the epilepsy.

- A history of major depression is associated with an increased risk for *developing* unprovoked seizures, more likely focal. This association holds, though may be reduced in magnitude, after adjustment for alcohol or drug 'abuse' or for therapies for depression.
- There is a positive correlation between seizure frequency and prevalence of depressive symptoms.
- The risk of depression is increased overall in epilepsy in part as a reactive process.
- In addition, the risk of depression is particularly increased in those with temporal lobe epilepsy with involvement of the limbic system, suggesting a shared pathogenic substrate.
- Depression may occur after temporal lobectomy for the treatment of epilepsy.

Antidepressants and epilepsy

- Many antidepressants can reduce seizure threshold and precipitate seizures in those susceptible, with a dose related effect.
- In general, however, wide-spread use of antidepressants has not been associated with a major increase in seizures.
- Where needed and appropriate, antidepressants can and should be prescribed to treat depression in epilepsy.
- Antidepressants with a lower association with seizures and a low interaction rate are preferred. Citalopram, amongst others, is a reasonable choice (📖 see Table 4b.27).
- Antidepressants associated with a higher risk of precipitating seizures should be avoided.

Neuroleptics and epilepsy

- Neuroleptics are associated with a dose-dependent increased risk of seizures.
- Clozapine in particular but also olanzapine, are associated with frequent epileptiform EEG changes, which can be asymptomatic. They are also associated with an increased risk of clinical seizures.
- Where acute treatment is required, haloperidol is considered better than chlorpromazine.
- 📖 See Table 4b.28 for further details.

Electroconvulsive therapy(ECT)

Although associated with an increased risk of unprovoked seizures, electroconvulsive therapy can be used safely where appropriate in epilepsy. However, if an individual with active epilepsy *and* uncontrolled GTCS there seems no indication for ECT, as its efficacy depends on the indication of convulsions.

Tables 4b.27 and 4b.28 refer to antidepressants and antipsychotics when used at therapeutic doses (and not in overdose).

Table 4b.27 Antidepressants in epilepsy. Maudsley guidelines, 2007*

Antidepressant	Safety in epilepsy	Special considerations
Moclobemide	Good choice	Not known to be proconvulsive.
SSRIs	Good choice	Low proconvulsive effect; there is no clear difference in risk between the available SSRIs. Seizure risk is dose related.
Mirtazapine Venlafaxine Reboxetine	Care required	Less data and clinical experience than with SSRIs. Venlafaxine proconvulsive in overdose. Use with care. Mirtazapine may affect EEG.
Duloxetine	Care required	Very limited data and clinical experience. Seizures have been reported rarely.
Amitriptyline Dosulepin (Dothiepin) Clomipramine Buproprion	Avoid	Most are epileptogenic. Ideally should be avoided completely.
Lithium	Care required	Low proconvulsive effect at therapeutic doses. Marked proconvulsive activity in overdose.

*Reproduced with permission from Taylor D, Paton C, and Kerwin R (2007). *The South London and Maudsley NHS Trust & Oxleas NHS Trust 2007 prescribing guidelines*, 9th edn. Taylor and Francis Group, London.

Table 4b.28 Antipsychotics in epilepsy. Maudsley guidelines 2007*

Antipsychotic	Safety in Epilepsy	Special considerations
Trifluroperazine Haloperidol	Good choice	Low proconvulsive effect. Carbamazepine increases the metabolism of some antipsychotics and larger doses of antipsychotic may be required.
Sulpiride	Good choice	Low proconvulsive effect (less clinical experience). No known interactions with AEDs.
Risperidone Olanzapine Quetiapine Amisulpiride	Care required	Limited clinical experience. Use with care. Olanzapine may affect EEG. Myoclinic seizures have been reported. Seizures rarely reported with quetiapine.
Aripiprazole	Care required	Very limited data and clinical experience. Seizures have been reported rarely.
Chlorpromazine Loxapine	Avoid	Most epileptogenic of the older drugs. Ideally best avoided completely.
Clozapine	Avoid	Very epileptogenic. Approximately 4-5% who receive >600mg/day develop seizures. Sodium valproate is the anticonvulsant of choice as it has a lower incidence of leucopaenia than carbamazepine.
Zotepine	Avoid	Has established dose-related proconvulsive effect. Best avoided completely.
Depot antipsychotics	Avoid	None of the depot preparations currently available are thought to be epileptogenic, however: • The kinetics of the depots are complex (seizures may be delayed) • If seizures do occur, the offending drug may not be easily withdrawn Depots should be used with extreme care.

*Reproduced with permission from Taylor D, Paton C, and Kerwin R (2007). *The South London and Maudsley NHS Trust & Oxleas NHS Trust 2007 prescribing guidelines*, 9th edn. Taylor and Francis Group.

Antiepileptic medication and contraception

The effectiveness of contraception depends on the efficacy of the method as well as user-related factors. The efficacy of both combined (COC) and progesterone-only (POP) oral contraceptives can be considerably reduced by interaction with drugs that induce hepatic enzyme activity. NICE (2004) does not recommend the use of the POP for those on enzyme-inducing AEDs. Dose adjustments are advised for those on the COC (☐ see Table 4b.29), but despite this there is still an increased failure rate. This needs to be communicated to women on AEDs who, in considering their options, may find it useful to be aware of failure rates with different methods of contraception, particularly those associated with barrier methods (Box 4b.11).

Box 4b.11 **Failure rates with different methods of contraception as quoted in Guillebaud (2004)***

Method	First year user-failure rate per 100 women
Subcutaneous implant	0–0.1
Depo-Provera®	0–1
Combined pills:	
50mcg oestrogen	0.1–3
<50mcg oestrogen	0.2–3
EVRA® patch	0.6–0.9
Cerazette® POP	0.17–0.9
Old type POP	0.3–4
Levonorgestrel interuterine system (IUS)	0–0.6
Male condom	2–15
Female condom	5–15
Diaphragm	6–20

*Reproduced from Guillebaud J (ed.) (2004). *Contraception: Your questions answered*, 4th edn. Churchill Livingstone, Edinburgh© 2004, with permission from Elsevier.

Failure of oral contraception (OCP) with AEDs

To our knowledge there are no recent data on failure rates of currently used OCPs with enzyme-inducing AEDs. Older data supports an increased failure rate with AEDs, more likely with low dose OCP.

A study by Coulam and Anneggers (1979),[1] identified 82 women with epilepsy on the OCP both with AEDs (total 955 months) and without (total 2278 months). Cases of oral contraceptive failure only occurred in the group also on AEDs. During this period there were 3 contraceptive failures, the expected being 0.12 (relative risk, 25; 95% CI, 5–73).

Another study by Back et al. (1988)[2] evaluated the Committee on Safety of Medicines yellow card reports on oral contraceptive-drug interactions with AEDs for the years 1968–84. A total of 43 pregnancies were reported in women on OCP who concurrently received AEDs (most commonly phenytoin and phenobarbital, reflecting common usage at the time). The largest number of reports related to OCPs containing ethinylestradiol (30mcg) and levonorgestrel (0.15mg).

Women requiring long-term use of an enzyme-inducing drug are encouraged where possible, and if appropriate, to consider a form of contraception that is not affected by hepatic enzyme induction. Where this is not possible, recommendations are listed in Table 4b.29, depending on the method. Where a COC is used, this should include at least 50mcg ethinyestradiol daily, with higher doses often required (unlicensed use). Additional barrier methods should be advised for the first few cycles, and the COC dose adjusted upwards, until the dose is deemed sufficient to suppress ovulation with no mid-cycle bleeding. 'Tricycling' (i.e. taking 3 or 4 packets of monophasic tablets without a break followed by a short tablet-free interval of 4 days) is sometimes recommended on limited evidence. Folic acid supplementation is recommended.

AEDs that induce liver enzymes and REDUCE the efficacy of ethinylestradiol and progestogens:

- Carbamazepine.
- Oxcarbazepine.
- Phenobarbital.
- Phenytoin.
- Primidone.
- Topiramate—dose effect observed with greater decreases in levels with higher doses.

AEDs that DO NOT affect the efficacy of ethinylestradiol and progestogens:

- Gabapentin.
- Levetiracetam.
- Pregabalin.
- Valproate.
- Vigabatrin.
- Zonisamide.

References

1. Coulam CB and Annegers JF (1979). Do anticonvulsants reduce the efficacy of oral contraceptives? *Epilepsia*, **20**, 519–25.

2. Back DJ, Grimmer SF, Orme ML, *et al.* (1988). Evaluation of Committee on Safety of Medicines yellow card reports on oral contraceptive-drug interactions with anticonvulsants and antibiotics. *British Journal of Clinical Pharmacology*, **25**, 527–32.

Table 4b.29 Advice regarding contraceptive use for women using liver enzyme inducing drugs*

Contraceptive method	Advice for women using liver enzyme-inducing drugs
Combined hormonal contraception	
Combined oral contraception (COC)	Use a COC with at least 50mcg ethinylestradiol daily. This can be taken as a 30mcg COC plus a 20mcg COC or as two 30mcg COCs.
	If there is any mid-cycle bleeding increase dose up to 100mcg/day and consider tricycling (NICE 2004).[†] Advise additional contraceptive protection, such as the use of condoms, until the dose is considered appropriate. Information should be given on failure rates with different methods as well as on alternative methods of contraception unaffected by liver enzyme inducers. If additional contraception fails or is not used emergency contraception may be indicated
Combined contraceptive patch	Additional contraceptive protection, such as condoms, is required when taking liver enzyme inducers and for 4 weeks after they are stopped. Use one patch per week as for women not using liver enzyme inducers.
	Information should be given on alternative methods of contraception unaffected by liver enzyme inducers. If additional contraception fails or is not used emergency contraception may be indicated
Progestogen-only contraception	
Progestogen only pills (POPs)	Advise alternative contraceptive methods (NICE 2004)[†]
Progestogen-only implants	Progestogen-only implants are not recommended for use by NICE[†] with enzyme inducing AEDs (2004). Additional contraceptive protection, such as condoms, required when taking liver enzyme inducers and for 4 weeks after they are stopped.
	Information should be given on alternative methods of contraception if liver enzyme inducing drugs are being used long term.
Progestogen-only injectables	Progestogen-only injectables are unaffected by liver enzyme inducers. It is possible to continue with the usual injection interval of 12 weeks with depot medroxyprogesterone acetate and 8 weeks with noristhisterone enanthate. However, NICE (2004)[†] recommends a shorter repeat injection interval of 10 weeks instead of 12 weeks with depot medroxyprogesterone acetate.
Progesterone-only emergency contraception	📖 see Antiepileptic medication and emergency contraception, p.368.
Levonorgestrel-releasing IUS	No additional contraceptive protection required
Non hormonal methods	
Copper-bearing IUD, barrier methods	No additional contraceptive protection required

*Adapted with permission from Faculty of Family Planning and Reproductive Healthcare Clinical Effectiveness Unit Guidance, April (2005). FFPRHC on drug interactions with hormonal contraception. *J Fam Reprod Health Care*, **31**(2), 139–151. [†] NICE: 🕭 www.nice.org.uk

AEDs of unlikely clinical effect on efficacy of ethinylestradiol and progestogens

Ethosuximide: most sources list this as not interacting with the CP and the data sheet does not mention any such interaction. Furthermore ethosuximide, has no effect on CYP450 or UDPGT system and thus has a low potential for such interactions. Some older sources, however, have listed it as of uncertain effect. In the UK Committee on Safety of Medicines adverse reactions register for 1968–84, four pregnancies were identified in women on ethosuximide and an oral contraceptive, but in only one of these was ethosuximide given in monotherapy (other concomitant AEDs being more likely to be implicated). There do not appear to have been any pharmacokinetic/pharmacodynamic studies of the use of ethosuximide with oral contraceptives. According to Stockley no special contraceptive precautions appear to be necessary on concurrent use.[1]

Lamotrigine: despite years of use with advice that it does not affect the efficacy of the OCP, in June 2005, the product licence for lamotrigine (Lamictal® GSK) was changed regarding interaction between lamotrigine and hormonal contraception. It now states that an interaction study showed an effect of lamotrigine on hormonal contraception, and that while the impact of the changes observed is unknown, the possibility of decreased contraceptive efficacy cannot be excluded. It concluded:

'Therefore, women should have a review of their contraception when starting lamotrigine, and the use of alternative non-hormonal methods of contraception should be encouraged. A hormonal contraceptive should only be used as the sole method of contraception if there is no other alternative. If the oral contraceptive pill is chosen as the sole method of contraception, women should be advised to promptly notify their physician if they experience changes in menstrual pattern (e.g. breakthrough bleeding) while taking Lamictal® as this may be an indication of decreased contraceptive efficacy. Women taking Lamictal® should notify their physician if they plan to start or stop use of oral contraceptives or other female hormonal preparations.'

However, the Faculty of Family Planning and Reproductive Health Care Clinical Effectiveness Unit (February 2006) could find no evidence that lamotrigine reduces the effectiveness of hormonal contraceptives (COC, patch and vaginal ring, or POP, implant, injectable or intrauterine releasing system) and claim that there is no good evidence to suggest that non-hormonal methods should be used in favour of hormonal methods when combined with lamotrigine. A reasonable practice is: a) to inform the patient of the above, b) to increase the dose of the pill if there is mid-cycle bleeding, c) to recommend folic acid supplementation.

Caution! There is clear evidence, however, from case series that the OCP reduces lamotrigine levels with a clinically significant effect in some women with the possibility of a) worsening of seizure control when starting an OCP and b) an increase in lamotrigine-associated side effects when the OCP is discontinued.

References

1. Stockley's Drug Interactions. Available at: 🔗 www.medicinescomplete.com

Emergency contraception

Levonorgestrel (a synthetic progestogen) is used as hormonal emergency contraception. Levonorgestrel is available as Levonelle® One Step 1.5mg tablets and Levonelle® 1500 1.5mg tablets. The dose needs to be taken within 72 hours of unprotected intercourse but efficacy is increased by taking the dose as soon as possible. Hormonal emergency contraception is less effective than the insertion of an IUD.

Enzyme-inducing AEDs reduce the effectiveness of hormonal emergency contraception. Where a patient is already taking or has recently taken an enzyme-inducing AED, the dose of levonorgestrel should be increased to a total of 3mg, taken as 1.5mg immediately and 1.5mg 12 hours later (unlicensed dose). If vomiting occurs within 3 hours of the dose, a replacement dose can be given.

Teratogenicity

📖 see Will AEDs affect my baby? pp.450–452.

AEDs and cognitive effects in offspring exposed in utero

- There is concern about the potential of AEDs taken by the mother during pregnancy to cause developmental delay, behavioural problems, and increased educational needs amongst offspring.
- There is evidence in support of this from animal studies with some AEDs studied.
- Adverse effects may not be restricted to the first trimester but may occur throughout pregnancy.
- In general, AED treatment of epilepsy, particularly to prevent GTCS, is recommended during pregnancy and after delivery to minimize the physical risk to the mother, fetus, and infant.
- Comparative data on the safety of different AEDs in pregnancy in terms of physical or 'cognitive' teratogenicity are needed to ensure that the safest medications are prescribed whenever possible.
- This is a difficult area to study in humans because of: a) the long-time scale involved in prospective studies; b) selection bias and incomplete data in retrospective studies; c) the difficulty in assessing very young children with developmental tests carried out too early not being predictive of future intellectual function; and d) the inability to control for many of the potential confounding factors.
- Examples of confounding factors include:
  - Maternal genetic factors as a substrate to the epilepsy or predisposing to adverse drug side effects in the fetus.
  - Maternal IQ.
  - Control of the epilepsy during pregnancy.
  - Polytherapy or comedication with other drugs.
  - Intake of recreational drugs including alcohol and smoking.
  - Socioeconomic factors.
- A Cochrane review in 2004[1] concluded that the majority of studies were of limited quality.
  - *'There was little evidence about which specific drugs carry more risk than others to the development of children exposed in utero. The results between studies are conflicting and while most failed to find a significant detrimental outcome with in utero exposure to monotherapy*

with carbamazepine, phenytoin or phenobarbital, this should be interpreted cautiously. There were very few studies of exposure to sodium valproate. Polytherapy exposure in utero was more commonly associated with poorer outcomes, as was exposure to any AEDs when analysis did not take into account type of AED. The latter may reflect the large proportion of children included in these studies who were in fact exposed to polytherapy.'

- The review concluded 'Based on the best current available evidence it would seem advisable for women to continue medication during pregnancy using monotherapy at the lowest dose required to achieve seizure control. Polytherapy would seem best avoided where possible. More population-based studies adequately powered to examine the effects of *in utero* exposure to specific monotherapies which are used in everyday practice are required.'

- Final conclusions await results of prospective studies such as from the Neurodevelopmental Effects of AEDs (NEAD) study. Despite limitations of data available, current evidence suggests that:
  - The majority of children born to women with epilepsy on AED treatment are within normal limits.
  - AEDs can have an effect on cognitive and behavioural outcomes of offspring of women who take these during pregnancy but there are many other factors that contribute to outcome.
  - Amongst others, reduced verbal IQ and increased incidence of autistic spectrum disorders have been observed in a proportion.
  - The effects observed may range from the offspring being less bright than might have been predicted, but still within normal limits, to severely affected in a small minority.
  - There is an association with subtle physical characteristics/dysmorphic features with some AEDS
  - Reports of affected siblings suggest that there may be a genetic predisposition in some cases.
  - Polytherapy carries a higher risk than monotherapy.
  - The most implicated AED is sodium valproate and the effect seems to be dose related as is the case with major malformations. A proportion of children reported had IQs <70.
  - Some, but not all, studies have shown an effect with phenobarbital, phenytoin, and carbamazepine. While a small effect cannot be excluded with carbamazepine, studies suggest that children born to mothers on monotherapy with carbamazepine have IQs within the normal range.
  - Data on new AEDs is still limited.

References

1. Adab N, Tudur Smith C, Vinten J et al. (2004). Common antiepileptic drugs in pregnancy in women with epilepsy. *Cochrane Database of Systematic Reviews*, **3**, CD004848.

Epilepsy, AEDs, and breastfeeding

Breastfed infants have lower rates of infections and allergies than bottle-fed babies, and breastfeeding is generally recommended where possible. Women with epilepsy often have concerns about AEDs in breast milk.

The following considerations are relevant:
- The baby would have been exposed to the medication in the womb.
- Sudden withdrawal of some medications may give withdrawal symptoms.

The amount of AED that passes into breast milk is often very small although this varies with the medication (📖 see Table 4b.30)

- Drug clearance in the infant is different and accumulation may occur, this being more likely in a premature infant.
- Nocturnal breastfeeding could contribute to sleep deprivation in the mother and increase risk of seizures in those susceptible.
- Physical safety of the infant is a consideration if the mother has uncontrolled epilepsy

Practical advice
- Breastfeeding is generally recommended except in specific situations e.g. if the specific AED is considered high risk (📖 see Table 4b.30) or if the baby is drowsy or not feeding well.
- The choice does not have to be either breast milk or formula feed. In certain situations, a combination of the two may be suitable to reduce drowsiness.
- Sleep deprivation should be avoided. Consider help during the day, to allow the mother to catch up on sleep, and night-time bottle feeding of expressed breast milk or formula feeds.
- If the mother's epilepsy is uncontrolled, breastfeeding at ground level with the mother's back supported, with help present, may reduce risk in the event of a seizure.

Box 4b.12 NICE guidance regarding breastfeeding

'All women with epilepsy should be encouraged to breastfeed, except in very rare circumstances. Breastfeeding for most women taking AEDs is generally safe and should be encouraged. However, each mother needs to be supported in the choice of feeding method that bests suits her and her family.'

AEDSs in breast milk

A number of literature sources categorize medications in terms of risk. The information below is sourced from Dr T Hale's *Medications and Mothers' Milk*:[1]

The amount of drug excreted into breast milk depends on the following factors:
- Concentrations in maternal plasma.
- Molecular weight (MW).
- Protein binding.
- Lipid solubility.

Drugs more likely to transfer into human milk attain high concentrations in maternal plasma, are low in MW, have low protein binding, and high lipid solubility. A popular method of measuring risk is the relative infant dose (RID) calculated by dividing the infant's dose via milk (mg/kg/day) by the mother's dose (mg/kg/day). The RID indicates how much medication the infant is exposed to on a weight-normalized basis. The information in Table 4b.30 applies to term infants. More caution is required in premature infants.

Dr Hale's lactation risk category[1]

L1: safest

Drug which has been taken by a large number of breastfeeding mothers without any observed increase in adverse effects in the infant. Controlled studies in breastfeeding women fail to demonstrate a risk to the infant and the possibility of harm to the breastfeeding infant is remote; or the product is not orally bioavailable in the infant.

L2: safer

Drug which has been studied in a limited number of breastfeeding women without an increase in adverse effects in the infant. And/or, the evidence of a demonstrated risk which is likely to follow use of this medication in a breastfeeding women is remote.

L3: moderately safe

There are no controlled studies in breastfeeding women, however, the risk of untoward effects to a breastfed infant is possible; or, controlled studies show only minimal non threatening adverse effects. Drugs should be given only if the potential benefit justifies the potential risk to the infant. New medications that have absolutely no published data are automatically categorized in this category, regardless of how safe they may be.

L4: possibly hazardous

There is positive evidence of risk to a breastfed infant or to breast milk production, but the benefits from use in breastfeeding mothers may be acceptable despite the risk to the infant (e.g. if the drug is needed in a life-threatening situation or for a serious disease for which safer drugs cannot be used or are ineffective).

L5: contraindicated

Studies in breast-feeding mothers have demonstrated that there is significant and documented risk to the infant based on human experience, or it is a medication that has a high risk of causing significant damage to an infant. The risk of using the drug in breastfeeding women clearly outweighs any possible benefit from breast-feeding. The drug is contraindicated in women who are breastfeeding an infant.

Table 4b.30[1] Relative infant doses (RID) and rating of AEDs during breastfeeding

AED	RID (%)	Rating	Comments
Phenytoin	7.7	L2	One case of methemoglobulinaemia, drowsiness and poor suckling reported
Carbamazepine	4.35	L2	
Phenobarbital	23.9	L3	Sedation and withdrawal symptoms reported
Primidone	Unk	L3	Sedation
Sodium valproate	0.68	L2	Very rare neonate toxicity with thrombocytopaenia, generally considered compatible with breast feeding.
Lamotrigine	22.8	L3	High RID, but no untoward effects reported
Levetiracetam	5.4	L3	
Gabapentin	6.5	L3	
Pregabalin	Unk	Unk	
Zonisamide	*33*	*L5*	
Topiramate	24.4	L3	
Vigabatrin	Unk	L3	
Lorazepam	2.5	L3	
Diazepam	8.1	L3	Reports of lethargy, sedation, poor suckling
Clobazam	Unk	L3	Reports of lethargy, sedation, poor suckling
Clonazepam	Unk	L3	Reports of lethargy, sedation, poor suckling

References
1. Hale T (2006). *Medications and Mothers' Milk*. Hale Publishing.

Vaccination and epilepsy

Reproduced with permission from Epilepsy Research UK Information Leaflet (⁀ www.epilepsyresearch.org.uk/).

I have epilepsy. Does this change what vaccinations I can and can't receive?

- People who have epilepsy can safely be vaccinated with almost all vaccines. Epilepsy itself is not a contra-indication for vaccination. If you regularly have seizures, or are taking any type(s) of antiepileptic drug, you should still be vaccinated absolutely as normal.
- Your children should also be vaccinated as normal. A family history of epilepsy does not affect vaccination in any way.
- You should not receive a vaccine if you have had a confirmed clear allergic reaction to the same vaccine or another vaccine against the same disease.
- If you have an allergy to eggs, then you should not receive influenza or yellow fever vaccines, as these contain egg proteins. If you are allergic to eggs and require these vaccines, your doctor will seek specialist advice about vaccinating you under expert supervision.

My child has epilepsy. Should they receive the normal childhood vaccines?

- Children with epilepsy can safely be vaccinated if their condition is stable. Epilepsy itself is not a contra-indication for vaccination.
- Very young children (under 12 months old) who have epilepsy may have their vaccination postponed while their condition is investigated and stabilized.
- Some vaccines can cause a short rise in body temperature as a side effect. Rarely, this can trigger a seizure (called a febrile seizure). If your child has had a febrile seizure in the past, or if anyone in your family has a history of febrile seizures, then they have a slightly increased risk of having a seizure after their vaccination. However they should still be vaccinated as normal.
- Ask for advice about how to prevent and manage a high body temperature in your child when they receive the vaccine. For example, giving regular paracetamol for the 24 hours after vaccination may be advisable for some children receiving the DTP vaccine.
- Vaccines that may cause a temperature include the DTP vaccine, and the measles, mumps and rubella (MMR) vaccine. The high temperature usually happens within 24 hours with the DTP vaccine, but may take up to a week to develop with the MMR vaccine.

Key reading

1. 'The Green Book', UK Department of Health information on immunisation against infectious disease. 2006 edition. The latest version is available to download from ▣ www.dh.gov.uk/greenbook

2. BMJ Best Treatments website: ⁀ www.besttreatments.co.uk/

3. For the most comprehensive, up-to-date and accurate of information on vaccines, disease and immunization in the UK, visit ⁀ www.immunisation.nhs.uk/

When immunized with diphtheria, tetanus, and whooping cough (DTP) vaccine, children with a family or personal history of seizures had no significant adverse events and their developmental progress was normal.[1]

One study found that 2 to 3 in 10,000 children had a febrile convulsion within two weeks of having their MMR vaccination. These children all recovered fully.[2]

Of interest in this context is the finding in a retrospective study of SCNLA (sodium channel/gene) in 11 of 14 patients with 'alleged vaccine encephalopathy' which clinically resembles severe myoclonic epilepsy of infancy[3].

References

1. Ramsay et al. (1997). CDR Review. 5, R65–7.

2. Barlow WE, Davis RL, Glasser JW, et al. (2001). The risk of seizures after receipt of whole-cell pertussis or measles, mumps, and rubella vaccine. *The New England Journal of Medicine*, **345**, 656–61.

3. Berkovic SF, Harkin L, McMahon JM et al. (2006). De-novo mutations of the sodium channel gene SCN1A in alleged vaccine encephalopathy: a retrospective study. *Lancet Neurol*, **5**(6), 465–6.

AEDs and porphyrias

The *porphyrias* are a group of inherited or acquired disorders of certain enzymes in the haem biosynthetic pathway (also called porphyrin pathway). They are broadly classified as *hepatic* porphyrias or *erythropoietic* porphyrias, based on the site of overproduction and mainly accumulation of the porphyrins (or their chemical precursors). They manifest with either skin problems or with neurological complications (occasionally both).

Most of the older AEDs are strong inducers of hepatic 5-aminolevulinate synthase (Alas1), the rate-limiting enzyme of hepatic porphyrin biosynthesis, and of hepatic cytochromes P450, which account for a significant part of total hepatic heme. Treatment of seizures in patients with acute porphyrias presents a difficult problem, since induction of these enzymes by many AEDs can lead to a porphyric attack. Some newer AEDs do not affect hepatic enzymes and may therefore be safer in cases of acute porphyria although data is limited or anectodal.

The following AEDs are considered definitely (def), probably (prob), or possibly (poss) porphyrinogenic:
- Carbamazepine (def).
- Diazepam (prob).
- Ethosuximide (prob).
- Felbamate (prob).
- Oxcarbazepine (prob).
- Lamotrigine (poss).
- Midazolam (poss).
- Phenobarbital (def).
- Phenytoin (def).
- Primidone (def).
- Sodium valproate (def).
- Tiagabine (poss).
- Topiramate (prob).

The following AEDs are not classified at the time of writing:
- Zonisamide.
- Pregabalin.
- Lacosamide.
- Rufinamide.

AEDs which could be considered for use in acute porphyria and which are listed as 'safe' by some sources include:

- Clobazam.
- Clonazepam—data sheet mentions that 'although Rivotril® has been given uneventfully to patients with porphyria, rarely it may induce convulsions in these patients'.
- Lorazepam.
- Gabapentin—partial epilepsy only.
- Levetiracetam—probably not porphyrinogenic.
- Bromides.

A number of useful web references exist that should be consulted when prescribing in such situations. These include:

- British Porphyria Association: ⌁ www.porphyria.org.uk
- European Porphyria Initiative: ⌁ www.porphyria-europe.com
- American Porphyria Foundation: ⌁ www.porphyriafoundation.com
- Canadian Porphyria Foundation: ⌁ www.cpf-inc.ca
- Drug Database for acute porphyria: ⌁ www.drugs-porphyria.com
- Welsh Medicines Information Specialist Centre: ⌁ www.wmic.wales. nhs.uk/porphyria_info.php

St John's wort and AEDs

- St John's wort, which is sold without prescription, is thought to induce cytochrome P450 3A4 and possibly other enzymes. It can interact with AEDs and other drugs metabolized by these enzymes, which could decrease levels of the AED.

Grapefruit juice and AEDs

- Grapefruit, in the form of juice, segments, and extract is known to interact with a number of medications including some AEDs.
- Furanocoumarins (contained within grapefruit) irreversibly inhibit intestinal CYP P450 3A4 isoenzymes and with very large intake, hepatic 3A4 isoenzymes also. The effect is an increase in blood levels of drugs metabolized via this pathway, the significance of which varies with each drug.
- Other, additional mechanisms of interactions have been postulated.
- The effect can last a number of hours.

Effects on AEDs

- *Diazepam*: increased plasma concentrations. This affects oral administration although is unlikely to be a clinically significant interaction. It is not applicable to parenteral administration. Effects on other routes are not known. Unlikely to be a clinically significant interaction.
- *Midazolam*: increased bioavailability. Only the oral administration has been shown to be affected. Parenteral administration is not affected. The effect on buccal administration is not known.
- *Carbamazepine*: increased bioavailability. Studies have shown that this interaction is likely to be of clinical significance
- *Phenytoin*: although phenytoin is an inducer of CYP3A4, studies have shown that grapefruit juice does not affect the bioavailablity of phenytoin.
- *Other*: the lack of data on other AEDs should not be taken to mean lack of interaction. It may be best to advise against regular use of grapefruit and its juice.

HIV, seizures, and AEDs

HIV and seizures

There is an increased incidence of seizures in those infected with human immunodeficiency virus (HIV) reported in 3–17%. Where seizures occur, they are much more likely in the context of AIDS, opportunistic infections, and low CD4 counts and have been considered a marker for worse outcome.

In adults presenting with a first epileptic seizure, HIV may be the cause, the proportion depending on the cohort studied. Seizures can be the presenting manifestation of HIV-related disease in up to 18% of cases. In the majority, but not in all patients, with HIV and seizures, a cause—other than HIV infection alone—is identified.

Opportunistic CNS infections are commonly reported, including cerebral toxoplasmosis, tuberculosis, and cryptococcal meningitis. JC virus associated progressive multifocal leukoencephalopathy (PML) may also cause seizures. Other causes include primary CNS lymphoma, other neoplasia, stroke, metabolic abnormalities (e.g. hypomagnesaemia, hyponatraemia, hypoglycaemia, and renal impairment), toxic effects of medication including retroviral agents (e.g. zidovudine), antibiotics (e.g. imipenem), and antiviral agents (e.g foscarnet). Factors related to intravenous drug use are also important in certain cohorts and increase predisposition to seizures, chronic epilepsy, and status epilepticus.

The use of AEDs in HIV

In HIV, AEDs may be required for the treatment of acute seizures/status epilepticus as well as long-term prevention of seizures. Other HIV associated disorders such as retroviral induced peripheral neuropathy, post herpetic neuralgia, and mood disorders are other indications. Factors influencing AED choice include:

- Drug–drug interactions with antiretroviral treatment regimens
- Drug–disease interactions.
- Potential drug effects on viral replication.

Drug-drug interactions

It is recommended that potential interactions are considered and that appropriate sources are consulted. A list of drug–drug interactions, along with the website's recommendations can be found on: ⏚ www.tthhiv-clinic.com/interact_tables.html. More detailed information is available on the University of Liverpool website ⏚ www.hiv-druginteractions.org

The use of enzyme-inducing AEDS in those infected with HIV on combination therapy carries the risk of decreasing the efficacy of most treatment regimens, resulting in the emergence of resistant viral strains and treatment failure.

Generally, where patients are on antiretroviral agents, it is preferable to use non-enzyme inducing AEDs, where possible and where cost allows, to manage seizures. The choice of AED is based on seizure type, the urgency of the clinical situation, and concomitant treatment. Benzodiazepines, valproate, and levetiracetam are non-enzyme inducing agents, which are broad spectrum and can also be given intravenously. Tolerance, however, often develops with benzodiazepines. If the patient is loaded with phenytoin or phenobarbital in the acute situation, and if it is considered clinically safe to do so, consideration should be given to an early change over to non-enzyme-inducing AEDs, if possible before enzyme induction occurs. Carbamazepine, oxcarbazepine, phenytoin, phenobarbital, and primidone, are all enzyme inducing. Topiramate also has an enzyme-inducing effect, though weaker than the medications already listed. Lamotrigine does not generally affect combination therapy, but it is not available parenterally and the dose has to be built up gradually to avoid allergic reactions . There are no reported interactions with levetiracetam, which is reasonably broad spectrum. Zonisamide is also broad spectrum and non-enzyme inducing. Clobazam is effective, broad spectrum, and non-enzyme-inducing but habituation can occur in a proportion with loss of effect. Other non-enzyme inducing AEDs used in partial epilepsy include pregabalin and gabapentin.

Protease inhibitors, an important component of combination treatment for HIV, inhibit CYP3A4 and may increase levels of carbamazepine, tiagabine, zonisamide (potentially), topiramate (small increase), and thus enhance toxicity. Ritonavir may also induce glucuronidation and oxidation by CYP2C9 and may decrease plasma concentrations of some AEDs such as phenytoin, valproate, and lamotrigine.

Drug–disease interactions
Drug-relevant physiologic changes in HIV/AIDS include low albumin, increased gammaglobulin levels with an increased risk of hypersensitivity reactions, reduced oral absorption, and decreased integrity of the blood brain barrier.

Potential drug effects on viral replication, viral load, and latency
In vivo studies suggest that some AEDs, can modulate HIV replication. Phenytoin, carbamazepine, and valproate activated HIV replication in latently infected monocytic but not lymphocytic cells at clinically relevant dosages, but the clinical relevance of these observations is unknown. A potential role for valproate in reducing latent infections, as a histone deacetylase (HDAC) inhibitor, by inducing expression of HIV from resting CD4 T cells, remains unproven. There are also reports of a putative neuroprotective effect with valproate as well as reports of an association with cognitive decline in advanced HIV. It is used currently for seizures in HIV with combination treatment with the advise that viral load is monitored.

General principles for prescribing AEDs in renal disease

Patients requiring antiepileptic medication with co-existing renal disease must be carefully assessed before the prescription of any drug in order to determine the risks and benefits. Renal reserve is low in comparison to the liver, and indeed renal impairment has consequences on liver function and vice versa.

Renal function is usually expressed in terms of glomerular filtration rate (GFR), the rate at which plasma is filtered at the glomeruli. The clearance of creatinine, owing to its characteristics of secretion by the kidneys and low reabsorption, is used as a measure of GFR.

The calculation most commonly performed is the Cockcroft–Gault (Box 4b.13):

Box 4b.13 Cockcroft–Gault calculation

Creatinine clearance (mL/min) = [F·(140-A)·W] / Sc

where:
F = 1.23 (male)
F = 1.04 (female)
A = age (years)
W = weight (kg)
Sc = serum creatinine (micromol/L)

The Cockcroft–Gault equation is, however, subject to many limitations and should be interpreted with caution especially in patients who are elderly, pregnant, with high/low levels of muscle mass, amputees, and those with rapidly fluctuating renal function.

Definitions of renal function based on this equation are described as follows:

- Mild renal impairment: 20–50mL/min.
- Moderate renal impairment: 10–20mL/min.
- Severe renal impairment: <10mL/min.

Whilst the BNF provides some guidance on doses in renal impairment, information provided by the summary of product characteristics (SPC) for a drug, or the use of specialist handbooks such as the *Renal Drug Handbook* or the American *Drug dosing in renal failure* is often more informative.[1,2]

A number of factors, both patient and drug, must be taken into consideration prior to the prescription of AEDs in the renally impaired adult. These include:

Patient factors:
- Degree of renal impairment.
- Applicability of Cockcroft–Gault equation.
- Concomitant medication.

Drug factors:
- Is the drug renally cleared?
- Is the drug nephrotoxic?
- Is it likely to interact with, have a synergistic effect with concomitant drugs?

- Can plasma levels of the drug be monitored and are they useful?
- Are there alternatives?

Patients who are undergoing renal replacement therapies pose a further challenge.

The clearance of AEDs via haemodialysis will depend on a number of factors:
- Water solubility.
- Protein binding.
- Volume of distribution.
- Dialysate conditions—including type of filter and flow rates.

Molecular size is also a factor to consider with drugs in general, however, all AEDs are all molecularly small enough to pass through filters and thus this does not need to be considered here.

AEDs with high water solubility, low protein binding, and low volumes of distribution are more readily dialyzable (□ see Table 4b.31). Where drugs are dialysed, some references and or their SPC provide recommendations for supplemental dosing in order to maintain adequate plasma concentrations post dialysis.

References
1. Bunn R and Ashley C (eds.) (1999). *The Renal Drug Handbook.* Radcliffe Medical Press, Oxford.

2. Aronof GR, Berns JS, Brier ME et al. (1999). *Drug prescribing in renal failure: dosing guidelines for adults,* 4th edn. American College of Physicans, Philadelphia.

General principles for prescribing AEDs in liver disease

Patients requiring antiepileptic medication with co-existing liver disease must be carefully assessed before the prescription of any drug in order to determine the risks and benefits. Liver disease affects both pharmacodynamic and pharmacokinetic parameters of medication use, increasing the risk of adverse effects.

The term 'liver disease' itself is rather broad and unhelpful when considering the prescription of medications and thus further categorization of the type of liver disease is required. Whilst it is not possible to describe the levels of liver impairment as accurately as in renal impairment, liver disease could be sub categorized as follows:
- Mild hepatitis without cirrhosis.
- Cholestasis.
- Compensated liver sclerosis.
- Decompensated liver sclerosis.
- Acute liver failure.

The first 2 categories are unlikely to pose a significant problem when prescribing AEDs. The intrinsic liver function is essentially normal and is unlikely to be acutely affected by the prescription of hepatically metabolized AEDs.

Patients within category 3 may well have reasonably preserved liver function at this stage, however, have the potential to deteriorate rapidly. Hepatically active drug choice in this case may therefore be considered more carefully. Patients falling in to category 4 and 5 include patients where the prescription of hepatically active AEDs should be avoided in the majority of occasions.

The management of status epilepticus should not vary particularly in these patients once the risks and benefits have been considered.

The prescription of simple AED regimens is of even greater significance in patients with liver disease, as the consequences of drug interactions are likely to be more severe.

AEDs associated with drug-induced hepatotoxicity should be avoided in patients with liver disease, as the effects are more severe in these patients subsequent to reduced hepatic reserve.

Table 4b.31 A table to indicate likely dose changes of AEDs in patients with renal impairment and/or on dialysis

AED	Dose change in renal impairment	Dialysed
Clobazam	No change	No
Clonazepam	No change	No
Ethosuximide	No change	Yes
Felbamate	Unknown	Unknown
Fosphenytoin	↓ dose; see SPC/Renal Drug Handbook[1]	No
Gabapentin	↓ dose; see SPC/Renal Drug Handbook[1]	Yes
Lamotrigine	Use low dose initially	No
Levetiracetam	↓ dose; see SPC/Renal Drug Handbook[1]	Yes
Oxcarbazepine	↓ dose; see SPC	Unknown
Phenobarbital	↓ dose; see SPC/Renal Drug Handbook[1]	Yes
Phenytoin	No change	No
Primidone	↓ dose; see SPC	Some degree of dialysis
Tiagabine	No change	No
Topiramate	↓ dose; see SPC/Renal Drug Handbook[1]	Yes
Sodium valproate	No change	No
Zonisamide	Likely to require dose ↓	Some degree of dialysis

↓ decreased. 1. Bunn R and Ashley C (eds.) (1999). *The Renal Drug Handbook*. Radcliffe Medical Press, Oxford.

Follow-up of patients with epilepsy

This is closely linked with general principles of management. It is only too easy to follow-up patients in clinic to no purpose and it is helpful to keep certain aims in mind. These include:

Aims

To diagnose and monitor the condition causing the epilepsy

To prevent seizures

An important goal is that of seizure freedom since seizures carry a physical risk, with increased morbidity and mortality, seizure freedom is associated with a better quality of life. There are exceptions, as in the following examples:

- If seizures are very mild without significant risk of injury, i.e. without associated falls, significant impairment of function, or post-ictal symptoms, and if the patient does not care to drive, the patient may prefer living with seizures to further drug manipulation.
- If the patient has intractable epilepsy with multiple seizure types and previous many unsuccessful medical and surgical attempts at controlling seizures, then the chances of seizure freedom with additional intervention are very small indeed. The goals may be then modified depending on the individual case. For example, goals may be:
  - To prevent convulsive seizures especially if prolonged.
  - To abort prolonged seizures or clusters of seizures with rescue medication.
  - To prevent injury—e.g. by preventing seizures associated with falls or by supervision when ambulant or the wearing of head protection.
  - To prevent frequent emergency hospital attendance or admission.
  - To prevent seizures on important days or outings.
  - To achieve stability with a predictable pattern of seizures.
  - To minimize medication side effects.

To prevent complications of treatment

There are potential side effects with all treatments as discussed in other sections. These can be short, medium, or long term. They can, amongst others, affect the individual's quality of life, educational attainment, and cognition. There are also effects on the unborn child. Awareness of potential side effects and their proactive management helps to minimize their impact.

To maintain a record of the epilepsy and its treatment for current and future reference

We cannot over-emphasize how important this is. Documentation is essential in a long-term condition and is unfortunately largely deficient. Keeping accurate records of seizure frequency, responses to treatment, side effects, doses used and escalation rates, reasons for withdrawal, as well as the rationale behind therapeutic decisions can inform future treatment. Relying on physicians' or patients' recall is insufficient. Copying letters to patients can help in this regard as well as reinforcing decisions made and advice given.

To provide support and continuity

This is best achieved by a multidisciplinary service. Although occasionally a new 'fresh' assessment is helpful by another physician, in general continuity of care is advised and is favoured by both patients and physicians given the nature of management of a long-term condition such as epilepsy.

To prevent, identify, and treat associated co-morbidity

What to record at clinic visits?

The following information is needed to aid treatment decisions and for future reference. We advise that this information is included in clinic letters and copied to patients and carers:

Summary:

Epilepsy diagnosis, classification, seizure types, date of onset, aetiology, summary of previous investigation results, and treatments given, status episodes, major/complications and allergies.

Seizures:

Seizure type, frequency, and pattern: 1-year planners are best for easy reference (□ see example of seizure chart in Management of epilepsy, p.245). Some patients may wish to supplement this with a more detailed diary.

Recent seizure-triggers: this information is essential to guide management.

Medication/treatment:

- *Regular AED treatment*: with information on preparation, dose schedule, last change in doses, adherence to treatment (on history and if appropriate blood levels), response to recent change etc.
- *As required treatment*: with information on doses, how often this is used and in what circumstance.
- *Treatment for other conditions*: this should include any recent change.
- *Contraception.*
- *Supplements, herbal, and other self-administered medication.*
- *Side effects*: in polytherapy, these, if possible, should include which drug is considered most likely to cause the side effect reported.
- *VNS*: the device needs to be checked and adjusted as appropriate.

Adherence to treatment

In general, nonadherence to treatment does not receive the attention it deserves. It is so easy to prescribe medication and so difficult to make the effort to take it on a regular basis. The association of nonadherence with seizures for many patients, in time, may provide an incentive to take the medication, but this is not always the case. Whenever, there is a break-through seizure, and before decisions are made about treatment, it is essential to ask the specific question of whether that seizure was precipitated by forgetting doses. Occasional general discussions can be helped by the following (gentle) probing: *many people find it difficult to take their tablets regularly, and occasionally forget; does this happen to you? how often? do you forget altogether or just delay the dose? what do you make it easier to remember? do you sometimes run out altogether? how long have you gone without the tablets? what happened? etc.* It is our impression that most of us do not enquire regularly, sensitively or expertly regarding adherence.

A recent retrospective study (Fraught et al. 2008)[1], based on Medicaid claims data amongst 33,658 adults with a diagnosis of epilepsy in Florida, Iowa, and New Jersey, USA, looked at the relationship between nonadherence to AEDs and mortality as well as serious clinical events (emergency department visits, hospitalizations, motor vehicle accident, injuries) over more than 9 years. Adherence was assessed using 'medication possession ratio (MPR)' on a quarterly basis with MPR > or = 0.80 considered adherent and <0.80 nonadherent. There were 388,564 AED-treated quarteres, 26% of which were nonadherent. Nonadherence was associated with an over threefold increased risk of mortality compared to adherence (hazard ratio = 3.32, 95% CI = 3.11–3.54) Nonadherence was also associated with a significantly higher incidence of serious clinical events.

Relevant life-style issues

These are diverse and include potential seizure triggers, driving, education, supervision, potential physical risk, employment, rehabilitation and social integration. In women of reproductive age they also include relation of seizures to monthly cycle, contraception, plans for pregnancy and care of young children.

Other comorbid conditions

Management plan

These needs to be very clearly stated to include the following:

- Rationale for changes in drug therapy; doses recommended with changes guided by clinical response; suggested interim maximum doses; contact number if any concerns between appointments; situations where a newly introduced medication is withdrawn promptly etc
- If appropriate, investigations and consideration of surgery for epilepsy
- A record of information/advice given to patient or carers in clinic or of referrals to other services/members of team
- Options for future treatment
- Long-term goals/plan

An example of a seizure chart can be seen in 📖 Management of epilepsy, p.245.

References

1. Fraught E, Duh MS, Weiner JR et al. (2008). Nonadherence to antiepileptic drugs and increased mortality: findings from the RANSOM Study. *Neurol* **11**, 1572–8.

'Would you like to take part in a drug trial?'

When a new promising drug for the treatment of epilepsy is identified, it is first tested on animals to establish if there are toxic effects. The efficacy of the drug to treat epilepsy is also tested on animal models of epilepsy.

If the drug is still promising and no toxic effects are observed, it is then tested on human volunteers and patients with epilepsy.

Assessing the value of new compounds for the treatment of epilepsy is difficult because the main symptoms of the disease (epileptic seizures) have the following characteristics:

- Seizures are intermittent events.
- During most of the time, patients do not have seizures.
- When seizures occur, they are relatively brief events that can be missed.
- The frequency of seizures for each patient is variable, often erratic.
- Other signs which are easier to observe, such as the incidence of interictal epileptiform discharges, do not clearly correlate with the frequency of seizures in a given patient.

Such difficulties have led to the creation of rather sophisticated experimental designs ('drug trials') to test the efficacy and safety of new drugs for the treatment of epilepsy.

In the context of epilepsy, the general objectives of drug trials on human subjects are:

- To estimate the safety profile of the new drug.
- To establish the doses at which the new drug can be considered safe.
- To evaluate the efficacy of the new drug to treat epilepsy.
- To identify the epilepsy syndromes for which the new drug is effective.
- To meet ethical concerns: not to deny effective treatment to patients while the possibly ineffective new drug is being tested on them. Generally, patients will be treated with already approved (presumed effective) AEDs while the new drug is being tested.

📖 See Box 4b.14 for frequently used terminology used in drug trials.

Evaluation of safety

Generally the safety profile of the new drug is evaluated by identifying adverse events—either actively or from a checklist—and by identifying changes in physical examination and other tests before and after starting treatment with the new drug.

Box 4b.14 Frequently used terminology in drug trials

- *Randomized (controlled) trial:* patients are randomized to new drug or control.
- *Open label:* patient and dispensing physician know if the patient is taking the new drug or the control.
- *Single blind:* the patient does not know if he/she is taking the new drug or the control, but the dispensing physician does know.
- *Double blind:* neither the patient nor the dispensing physician knows if the patient is taking the new drug or the control.
- *Add-on trial:* the new drug is tried while patients are still taking their habitual approved AEDs.
- *Monotherapy trial:* patients take the new drug and no other AEDs.
- *Parallel group design:* patients are randomized to new drug or control for a single period.
- *Cross-over:* patients are initially randomized to new drug or control, stay on either for a period, and then switch over.
- *Carry-over effects:* long-term effects of effective treatment that can persist after crossing-over.
- *Washout period:* the period where the patient does not take either the new drug or placebo before crossing over for the second treatment period. Washout periods are necessary because of the possibility that the drug administered first can affect the outcome variable for some time after administration ceases due to carry-over effects.
- *Attenuated active controlled trial or pseudo-placebo trial:* the test drug is compared with a low dose of an approved antiepileptic drug.

Evaluation of efficacy

This is difficult because of the spontaneous fluctuations in seizure frequency and severity. It might be difficult to identify true changes in seizure frequency or severity in the context of natural erratic fluctuations. In addition, patients tend to volunteer to take part in testing new, possibly effective, drugs while they are having more frequent and severe seizures, during a period that can naturally be followed by a length of time with fewer or less severe seizures (regression to the mean effect). This might suggest that the new drug is effective when in reality it is not. To paliate this effect, patients must be stratified according to pre-treatment seizure frequency.

To overcome such difficulties, patients can be randomized to taking either the new drug at a presumed effective dose or a control (tablets that look identical to those with the new drug but do not contain it at a presumed effective dose).

The control can contain:
- No drug at all—placebo.
- A standard AED at a standard dose—the so called reference drug.
- A standard AED at low, ineffective dose—low-dose reference drug or pseudo-placebo.
- The new drug at low, presumably ineffective dose—low-dose test drug.

Recording seizure characteristics during a period before starting the new treatment (baseline period, typically lasting for 8–12 weeks) can help in taking into account the spontaneous fluctuations in seizure frequency and characteristics. Nevertheless, an additional difficulty in establising efficacy of new AEDs is that patients' beliefs about the efficacy of their treatment can apparently influence seizure frequency via psychosomatic mechanisms, at least for some time. Thus if the patient thinks that he or she is getting an effective treatment, seizure frequency might temporarily decrease, suggesting that the drug is effective when it might not be (the so-called placebo effect).

To cancel the placebo effect, patients are randomized to new drug or control and results are compared (randomized or controlled trial). Since patients do not know whether they are on the new drug or the control (they are blind to the condition) it is assumed that the placebo effect is similar in both populations and cancels out when both populations are compared. Since the attitude of the dispensing physician may somehow suggest to the patient whether he/she is receiving new drug or control, many drug trial designs demand that the prescribing/dispensing physician is also blind to the condition (double blind).

Meeting ethical concerns

Approaching ethical concerns in drug trial design is complicated because meeting one ethical concern can lead to not meeting another.

Two general ethical concerns must be taken into consideration in designing a drug trial:
- **Safety**: because seizures are serious by events—potentially lethal— patients must be protected randomized to treatment with approved AEDs in case the new drug is not effective or if the patient happens to be randomized to the control group.
- **Patient benefit**: if the drug is effective, patients should benefit. Patients should have a period where they try the new drug, and if it is effective, they are given the option to remain on it.

To meet the first ethical concern before efficacy of the new drug is demonstrated, the new drug is tried while patients are still taking their habitual approved AEDs (add-on trials). This has the drawback that if the new drug is less effective than the approved drugs, an effective drug could be discarded as ineffective. Such a drug can still be useful, for instance because it could have fewer interactions, fewer side effects or be more effective in specific syndromes.

Testing the new drug in the absence of other AEDs (monotherapy trials) is ethically justified in specific circumstances, for instance, during pre-surgical assessment, when AEDs can be withdrawn in order to record seizures within an acceptable period of time. It could be claimed that testing the new drug during this period could abolish seizures if effective, defeating the initial purpose. Nevertheless, if the new drug is so effective, the patient might then continue on it and avoid surgery! Controlled monotherapy trials can also be ethically acceptable when immediate treatment is not deemed necessary by physician and patient.

To meet the second ethical concern, patients can be initially randomized to the new drug or control, stay on either condition for a period, and then switch over condition (cross-over design). Patients that appear to respond during either period can be asked to remain on the new drug after the trial. The drawback is that if the patient appears to be responsive to the first period, he/she might not be willing to cross-over. In an effort to protect responders, a response-dependent trial design has been proposed where only non-responders are crossed over.

In an effort to meet ethical concerns while maximizing the chance of detecting efficacy, the *response-dependent (enriched) design* can be used. In this design, only responders to an open-label test period will be randomized to a double-blind test. The purpose is to estimate whether the new drug is sufficiently efficacious compared to placebo to warrant further development as an AED.

General candidates suitable to take part in drug trials:
- Outpatients or inpatients with incomplete control of seizures. Incomplete control is defined as suffering seizures despite maximum tolerable serum concentrations of standard AEDs.
- Previously untreated patients can be recruited in some phases if severe drug interactions are observed in earlier phases.
- Good drug compliance is usually a prerequisite.
- Often women of childbearing potential are excluded, or are included if carefully using reliable contraception methods (provided that animal testing has not shown evidence of teratogenicity).
- Concomitant antiepileptic therapy consisting of a single drug is preferred, but two may be acceptable.

Sample size
The sample size varies depending on the estimated difference between the effects of the new drug and the control. Whereas initial trials often included <50 patients, it is not uncommon for modern multicentre trials to include hundreds of patients.

Cross-over design requires fewer patients than parallel group design (they have more power). However, the analysis of cross-over trials is more complicated and needs to rule out the long term effects of effective treatment (carry-over effects). To minimize carry-over effects, there must be a period where the patient does not take the new drug or placebo before crossing over (washout period).

Outcome measures
In many trials for focal epilepsy, the primary outcome measures for efficacy are percentage change in seizure frequency from baseline, or the proportion of responders (the percentage of patients with 50% or more seizure reduction). Other measures include seizure-free rates, the percentage of seizure–free days, the response ratio (the ratio of the difference between treatment and baseline seizure rates to the sum of treatment and baseline seizure rates).

Advantages and disadvantages of add-on trials

Advantages
- Unequivocal interpretation if efficacy is shown.
- Mimics clinical practice.
- Universally accepted by regulatory agencies.

Disadvantages
- Might not detect efficacy if new drug less effective than standard drugs.
- Pharmacokinetic and phamacodynamic interactions may be difficult to control.
- Provides no evidence for activity of test drug in monotherapy use.
- Overestimates toxicity of new drug.

In adults, accomplishing the drug trial objectives detailed above often involves a series of separate drug trials to test for safety and efficacy according to the following phases:

Early phase I:
Objectives: the primary objective is to characterize the pharmacokinetic behaviour of the drug (half-life, absorption, protein binding, excretion, metabolism) with single dose or multiple dose studies. The secondary objective is to evaluate the safety of the new drug by determining the maximum tolerated dose during a period of at least 4 weeks.

Procedure: single and multiple dose administration

Subjects: healthy adult volunteers. Women of childbearing potential, smokers, drug or alcohol abusers should be excluded.

Evaluation parameters: physical and neurological examination, ECG, EEG, blood and urine samples, neuropsychological tests.

Late phase I:
Objectives: preliminary evaluation of the safety and efficacy of the new drug, definition of the dose ranges within which the new drug can be safely tested, and determination of pharmacokinetics in chronically co-medicated patients.

Procedure: new drug is added to the usual antiepileptic medication as an open label, initially as a single dose, followed by a stepwise increase to maximum tolerated dose.

Subjects: patients with epilepsy whose seizures are not completely controlled. Good drug compliance is required. Patients with expanding cerebral tumours or progressive neurological disorders, patients with cardiac, renal, or hepatic disorders, women of childbearing potential should be excluded.

Evaluation parameters: change in seizure frequency, adverse reactions, serum levels of new and standard medicaton, other laboratory tests, evaluation of interactions.

Early phase II:
Objectives: the primary objective is to evaluate the efficacy of the new drug through controlled, randomized trials. The secondary objective is to

establish the effective dose range and to further evaluate the drug safety profile.

Procedure: the new drug is added to the usual antiepileptic medication in a randomized double blind fashion (cross-over or parallel designs). Monotherapy trials might be performed if pronounced drug interactions were identified in late phase I trials.

Subjects: patients with epilepsy whose seizures are not completely controlled. Patients with cardiac, renal, or hepatic disorders patients with expanding cerebral tumours or progressive neurological disorders should be excluded. If animal data do not show evidence of teratogenicity, women of childbearing potential can be included if carefully using reliable contraception methods.

Evaluation parameters: changes in seizure frequency of the different seizure types, seizure-free intervals, seizure duration, seizure patterns, functional capacity, percentage of responders, adverse reactions as monitored by a checklist, serum levels of test drug and co-medication, other laboratory tests.

Late phase II:

Objectives: the objectives are to evaluate the efficacy and toxicity of the new drug in monotherapy and the persistence of its antiepileptic effects in the long term.

Procedure: new drug is added to concomitant antiepileptic medication in a randomized double-blind fashion for a long period. This can be followed by a response-related gradual withdrawal of previous medication. Previously untreated patients can be randomized to new drug or placebo/reference drug.

Subjects: patients with epilepsy whose seizures are not completely controlled with good drug compliance. Patients with cardiac, renal, or hepatic disorders and patients with expanding cerebral tumours or progressive neurological disorders should be excluded. If animal data do not show evidence of teratogenicity, women of childbearing potential can be included if carefully using reliable contraception methods. Previously untreated patients can be recruited if severe drug interactions are observed in early phase II trials.

Evaluation parameters: changes in seizure frequency, seizure-free intervals, seizure duration, seizure patterns, or functional capacity, percentage of responders, adverse reactions as monitored by a checklist, serum levels of test drug and co-medication, other laboratory tests.

Phase III:

Objectives: to better define the efficacy and toxicity profiles of the new drug in in larger patient groups and for longer periods. This permits the evaluation of potential tolerance, efficacy in specific epilepsy syndromes and as monotherapy.

Procedure: various randomized designs as add-on or monotherapy.

Subjects: patients with epilepsy whose seizures are not completely controlled with good drug compliance. Patients with cardiac, renal, or hepatic disorders and patients with expanding cerebral tumours or progressive neurological disorders should be excluded. If animal data do not show evidence of teratogenicity, women of childbearing potential can be included if carefully using reliable contraception methods. Previously untreated patients can be recruited if strong proof of efficacy has been obtained in earlier phases.

Evaluation parameters: changes in seizure frequency, seizure-free intervals, seizure duration, seizure patterns, functional capacity, percentage of responders, adverse reactions as monitored by a checklist, serum levels of test drug and co-medication, other laboratory tests.

Phase IV:

Objectives: to evaluate post-marketing performance of the new drug with focus on safety profile and on the role of the new drug among the established drugs.

Procedure: new drug administered alone and in open label in a large population for prolonged periods.

Subjects: patients with epilepsy whose seizures are not completely controlled with good drug compliance. Patients with cardiac, renal, or hepatic disorders should be included. Patients with expanding cerebral tumours or progressive neurological disorders should be excluded. If animal data do not show evidence of teratogenicity, women of childbearing potential can be included if carefully using reliable contraception methods and after careful consideration of the risk/benefit ratio. Previously untreated patients can be recruited in accordance with the approved indication.

Evaluation parameters: changes in seizure frequency, seizure-free intervals, seizure duration, seizure patterns, or functional capacity, percentage of responders, adverse reactions as monitored by a checklist and number of drop-outs, serum levels of test drug and co-medication, other laboratory tests.

Trials in children

- The use of new AEDs in children traditionally has been delayed until sufficient knowledge has been attained from adult trials. Nevertheless, since children are not small adults, AEDs need not be effective in adults to be effective in children.
- Generally, if animal studies and preliminary observations in humans suggest that the new compound might be active in paediatric syndromes, children can be included in phase II trials and above.
- Guidelines on trials in children have been published by the Commission on Antiepileptic Drugs of the International League Against Epilepsy.[1]

References

1. International League Against Epilepsy: First Commission on Antiepileptic Drugs (1973). Principles for clinical testing of antiepileptic drugs. *Epilepsia*, **14**, 451–8.

Key reading

1. Commission on Antiepileptic Drugs of the International League Against Epilepsy (1994). Guidelines for Antiepileptic Drug trials in Children. *Epilepsia*, **35**, 94–100.

2. Schmidt D (ed.) (1998). *Drug Trials in Epilepsy: A physician's guide.* Martin Dunitz, London.

Management of status epilepticus

Definitions

Status epilepticus has been defined as a seizure lasting >30min or as recurrent seizures over the same time course without recovery in between. Although the time scale had been reduced from 60min, the definition is wanting at an operational level. The time course is still too long, as most self-limiting seizures terminate much earlier, usually within a few minutes, and a shorter time is appropriate for starting timely treatment of convulsive seizures.

Status epilepticus is also said to occur when a seizure persists for a sufficient length of time or is repeated frequently enough to produce a fixed or enduring epileptic condition. This is conceptually a useful definition but offers little practical guidance.

The same applies to the ILAE current, rather cumbersome, if accurate definition:

'A seizure which shows no clinical signs of arresting after a duration encompassing the great majority of seizures of that type in most patients or recurrent seizures without resumption of baseline central nervous system function interictally.'

Background

- Status epilepticus may be classified as convulsive and non-convulsive.
- Status epilepticus is more common in children and in the elderly with a minimum overall incidence of 10–20/100,000 of the general population. Approximately half the cases are convulsive. Of the non-convulsive cases, the large majority are partial with only a small minority being absence status.
- Status epilepticus is associated with an overall case fatality of about 13%, with a wide range depending on the underlying condition. The mortality is lowest in children and highest in the elderly and is determined to a large extent by the underlying disease causing status. A common cause of status epilepticus in children is prolonged febrile seizures. In a population based study of convulsive status epilepticus in childhood, case fatality was 3%.
- In those presenting with a first episode of status epilepticus, long-term mortality is significantly increased, this being related to the aetiology of the status. Long-term mortality is comparable to the normal population in those with idiopathic/cryptogenic status.
- Status may occur de novo or in the context of a previous diagnosis of epilepsy.
- Status can be recurrent and this is more likely in remote symptomatic cases.
- Prolonged status epilepticus is associated with the early development of resistance to drugs. One possible mechanism observed in animal models is the internalization of $GABA_A$ receptors from synaptic membranes, where they are accessible to drug effects, to endosomes.
- Refractory status epilepticus, mainly if convulsive, is associated with secondary neuronal injury with a risk of cognitive decline and secondary epilepsy, the latter estimated at between 25–40%.

- Early and prompt treatment is indicated with clearly defined protocols, adapted to the setting in which treatment is administered.
- Recognition of non-epileptic or pseudo-status is important to avoid iatrogenic complications.

Non-convulsive status epilepticus (NCSE)

The category is very broad with diverse seizure manifestations, duration, severity, classification, and prognosis (☐ see Non-convulsive status epilepticus pp.199–204). Indeed it is said there are as many forms of status as there are seizure types. The term non-convulsive differentiates it from tonic–clonic generalized status epilepticus and should not be taken to mean lack of any motor activity.

The definition in italics below is favoured by Shorvon[1] who stated that NCSE can be 'viewed as a form of cerebral response which is dependent largely on the level of cerebral development of the individual (age and cerebral integrity/development/maturity), epilepsy syndrome and the anatomical location of the epileptic activity.'

'Non-convulsive status epilepticus is a term used to denote a range of conditions in which electrographic seizure activity is prolonged and results in non-convulsive clinical symptoms.'

The implication is for a change from baseline a) of function and b) of EEG, a change which is of reasonable duration but which may remit. In the more severe epilepsy syndromes, particularly in childhood, there is overlap between NCSE and epileptic encephalopathy, a more enduring state.

Classification of NCSE is problematic and will no doubt evolve.

NCSE may be:
- Absence—typical or atypical.
- Myoclonic.
- Tonic.
- Simple or complex partial.

NCSE occurs in known epilepsy syndromes at any age, with many presenting in infancy or childhood. It can also occur de novo in adulthood, often secondary to an acute neurological insult or drug withdrawal. Thus, NCSE may occur in diverse aetiologies and syndromes. Examples of NCSE include:
- West syndrome.
- Ohtahara syndrome.
- Dravet's syndrome or severe myoclonic epilepsy in infancy.
- Myoclonic astatic epilepsy.
- Panayiotopoulos syndrome or early onset benign childhood occipital epilepsy.
- Ring chromosome 20—atypical absence or complex partial status.
- Angelman syndrome.
- ESES—electrical status epilepticus in slow-wave sleep.
- Landau–Kleffner syndrome.
- Lennox–Gastaut syndrome—usually atypical absence or tonic status.
- IGE—absence status or myoclonic status.
- Progressive myoclonic epilepsies—myoclonic status.
- Mitochondrial cytopathies—often partial status.
- De novo absence status of late onset.

- Aura continua.
- Post-ictal post GTCS—complex partial status.
- Epilepsia partialis continua.
- Simple partial status including focal motor status.
- Complex partial status—limbic or non-limbic.
- Post-anoxic myoclonic status epilepticus in coma.

Management of NCSE involves:

- Recognition and confirmation of the diagnosis.
- Establishing and treating the underlying aetiology.
- Treating the NCSE as appropriate with an urgency dictated by the clinical situation.

Recognition and confirmation of the diagnosis

An index of suspicion is required. There is a:

- Change in function, which may fluctuate, such as persistent aura, focal movement, or, commonly, clouding of consciousness.
- An association with electrographic change.

Emergency EEG is required to confirm the suspected clinical diagnosis. Generally EEG shows either absence or complex partial status. EEG changes, however, are varied, can be difficult to interpret and require expertise. Sometimes it is only after serial EEGs are recorded with evolution over time that the diagnosis is confirmed. Clear epileptiform discharges, slow background, fluctuations in EEG, rhythmicity of epileptiform discharges, change from previous EEG recordings, and clear electrographic seizures all favour NCSE, as does a clinical and EEG response to benzodiazepines. Some EEG patterns appear epileptiform, such as PLEDS or periodic lateralized epileptiform discharges, but these reflect underlying structural brain pathology, and suppressing them is not necessarily helpful. Other features in the EEG and clinical change would need to be also present for the diagnosis of NCSE to be made and treatment recommended. In some cases sleep EEG is also required.

Establishing and treating the underlying aetiology

A detailed account here is outside the scope of this section. Briefly, assessment requires a detailed general and neurological history including of previous seizures, development, neurological history/insult infection and use of medication/recreational drugs. Investigations, in addition to urgent EEG, may include imaging, biochemical, toxicological, metabolic, autoimmune and infection screens, lumbar puncture and others investigations as indicated.

Treating NCSE as appropriate with an urgency dictated by the clinical situation

This differs so much depending on the type of NCSE. Sometimes NCSE is a medical emergency, treated along similar lines to convulsive status epilepticus, but this is by no means always the case. It is important in this situation to tailor the treatment to the individual case and not 'to crack a nut with a sledgehammer' to avoid unnecessary iatrogenic complications. On the other hand, NCSE can be associated with neurological and cognitive impairment, risk of injury, and, importantly, may progress to convulsive status epilepticus. In such cases, early treatment is advisable. Where appropriate, medications that minimize need for ventilation are used, while recognizing that this may be required in some cases. High dependency care is required whenever the patient is obtunded and emergency medication administered. It is self-evident that treatment is less aggressive in the ambulant patient. Medications that may be appropriate for use in NCSE are also discussed in relation to convulsive status epilepticus addressed below. Some illustrative examples are provided next:

- *Epilepsia partialis continua*: this can be a chronic condition, akin to a movement disorder, sometimes persisting for years, with focal myoclonic irregular twitching of a group of muscles which may have a cortical or sub-cortical basis. The affected individual is usually alert and impairment of function relates to the muscle groups involved and may be very minor. It may be associated with secondarily generalized convulsions. Control of the latter is more easily achieved. Suppression of the former may be partly possible with medication. But it is important to be clear of the goals of therapy, and potential side effects, where functional deficit is minimal.
- *Myoclonic status epilepticus in coma*: this describes myoclonic jerking with epileptiform EEG discharges in acute cerebral damage, usually anoxic. It indicates a poor prognosis and is associated with a significantly increased mortality. Treatment is appropriate, if there are clear features of NCSE, to suppress symptoms and prevent GTCS. However, sometimes the changes noted reflect the brain injury and intervention may be of limited benefit.
- *Absence or myoclonic status in IGE:* this usually responds to benzodiazepines, the route selected depending on the clinical situation. It is not thought to result in any long-term sequelae.
- *Complex partial status*: e.g. complicating acute brain lesions: These should be treated vigorously as seizures associated with the brain lesion may worsen outcome.

Convulsive status epilepticus

This is generalized tonic–clonic status which may evolve to continuing electrical status without motor activity. It is a medical emergency which requires aggressive and prompt treatment.

Management of convulsive seizures/status epilepticus in adults

- Treatment of convulsive epileptic seizures should generally start after 5–10min if there is no evidence of the seizure subsiding, this being considered potential status epilepticus. This is based on the observation that most seizures last <5min. The exception is where habitual seizures are known to cease spontaneously shortly after.
- In those with known epilepsy, where the information is available, treatment is according to individually drawn protocols based on habitual seizure duration and pattern.
- Prompt treatment of the prodromal phase of increasingly frequent or serial seizures can prevent evolution into status.
- Treatment of potential status epilepticus may begin in the community using easily administered medications not requiring special expertise or intravenous access, following training and individually adapted guidelines.

Pre-hospital treatment of serial/prolonged seizures

- This can be provided by emergency services with expertise and supportive facilities and can follow hospital status guidelines adapted to local needs
- Effective pre-hospital treatment can also be provided by trained carers, according to a previously agreed individualized protocol based on usual seizure type, pattern, and duration in the individual case. Doses are also adjusted based on previous response with the aim of recommending an effective dose while minimizing sedation or risk of respiratory depression. Emergency services can be called upon to support carers when this is first used, if appropriate, and at any time there is concern.
- Benzodiazepines (Box 4b.15) are the mainstay of treatment in the community.
- It is advisable not to delay treatment and not to undertreat, as early adequate treatment is more likely to be effective.

Box 4b.15 Benzodiazepines, options, and methods of administration

Clobazam can be given orally at 10–20mg for clusters of, usually minor, seizures, with recovery in between, if the patient is safely able to swallow and if the delayed duration time of action is compatible with the desired effect.

Diazepam is sometimes given orally in similar situations as clobazam, where indicated it is given intravenously (10mg at 2–5mg/min, repeated if required after 5min up to 20mg total) or rectally at 5–30mg. *Diazepam must not be given intramuscularly*

Lorazepam is given intravenously usually in hospital (📖 see p.401).

Midazolam use in epilepsy is outside licence. It can be given intravenously (5mg with a maximum rate of 4mg per min); rectally 5–10mg; intramuscularly 5–10mg, although absorption by the intramuscular route can be erratic and delayed respiratory compromise can occur; and by the buccal or nasal route **usually at 5–10mg** (2.5–5mg starting dose if <50kg, elderly or considered potentially sensitive to benzodiazepines; the standard buccal midazolam dose for an adult patient is 10mg, a repeat dose may be given after 10min).

Experience with the buccal route for midazolam is increasing and it is much preferred by carers over the less practical rectal diazepam route. The concentrated intravenous preparation of 10mg in 2mL can be used or the specially prepared buccal preparation (Epistatus® 10mg/mL), if available. For both this indication, and the latter preparation, are outside licence.

Hospital management

Management of status epilepticus involves:
- General measures *and*
- Specific drug treatment.

These should proceed in tandem, the former dictated by the patient's condition and the latter along a predefined time scale to ensure prompt effective treatment. Pharmaco-resistance and neuronal injury are more likely the more prolonged the seizure.

There are a number of published protocols for the treatment of status epilepticus which can be adapted for local use. These include the Scottish Intercollegiate Guideline Network,[2] NICE (🕮 also see Tables 4b.32 and 4b.33),[3] European Federation of Neurological Science,[4] and Italian League Against Epilepsy.[5] Also see Cochrane review of drug trials in status epilepticus.[6]

General measures:

General medical measures:
- Administer oxygen and secure airway.
- Monitor ECG, BP, oximetry, temperature.
- Establish intravenous access in large veins. Take blood for electrolytes, glucose, calcium, magnesium, FBC, liver function tests, AED levels, creatine kinase, alcohol and toxicology screen, as well as cultures as appropriate. Urea and electrolytes, blood glucose, calcium and phenytoin, where appropriate, should be obtained urgently.
- Check BM stick for glucose and immediately correct any hypoglycaemia.
- If poor nutrition/ alcohol abuse is suspected, give thiamine intravenously.
- Check blood gases.
- Provide supportive treatment, including ionotropic agents, as necessary.

Seizure-related measures:
- Investigate the cause of status and treat accordingly.
- Reinstate any recently withdrawn AEDs.
- Continue existing AEDs.
- Start maintenance therapy promptly.

Caution:
- 25% of 'refractory status epilepticus' referred to specialist units reportedly have pseudo-status.
- EEG is extremely useful in diagnosis and management of status and pseudo -status.
- Iatrogenic complications of inappropriate treatment in pseudo-status are significant.

Specific hospital drug treatment of convulsive seizures/status epilepticus in adults:

Important! This should be carried out promptly with careful monitoring and resuscitation facilities as per the steps in Box 4b.16. Patients in convulsive status are at high risk. Close observation is required throughout including the post-ictal state.

Box 4b.16 Treatment of convulsive status epilepticus

- **Step 1:** first-line agent: benzodiazepine.
- **Step 2a:** second-line agent.
- **Step 2b:** (in selected cases only) another second-line agent.
- **Step 3:** anaesthesia and ventilation.
- **Step 4:** maintenance treatment (this must not be forgotten—📖 see p.406)

There are a number of drug options for each of these steps as discussed next. Placebo-controlled double-blind trials are limited and, for many, the use of these drugs is based on experience and therapeutic success in clinical practice. Practice differs in different countries, partly on the basis of local experience but also on the availability of medications. The Veterans Affairs Status Epilepticus Cooperative Study Group randomized trial, summarized in Box 4b.17, was a landmark study in which four treatment regimens were compared as first-line treatment. This study supports the use of lorazepam, a benzodiazepine, as first-line treatment (step 1). If unsuccessful this is followed by step 2a, where a second-line agent is used. Where this fails, rather than give another second-line agent, general anaesthesia is usually recommended as it is considered that only a small proportion of cases given another second-line agent respond. However, data are limited; there may be a role for step 2b in selected cases with convulsions of shorter duration in an otherwise stable patient. *If there are severe systemic disturbances at any stage, proceed directly to anaesthesia.*

Box 4b.17 Veterans Affairs Status Epilepticus Cooperative Study Group randomized trial[6]

This landmark study compared four intravenous treatments for generalized convulsive status epilepticus (percentages below are for patients with over status and verified diagnosis):

Agent	Success rate*
Lorazepam (0.1mg/kg)	64.9 %
Phenobarbital (15mg/kg)	58.2 %
Diazepam (0.15mg/kg), followed by phenytoin (18mg/kg):	55.8 %
Phenytoin (18mg per kg)	43.6 %

*cessation of all motor and electroencephalographic seizure activity within 20min after the beginning of the drug infusion with no return during the next 40min.

P was 0.02 for the overall comparison among the four groups; lorazepam was significantly superior to phenytoin alone (P = 0.002). There was no difference among the treatments with respect to recurrence during the 12-hour study period, the incidence of adverse reactions, or the outcome at 30 days.

The authors concluded: 'As initial intravenous treatment for overt generalized convulsive status epilepticus, lorazepam is more effective than phenytoin. Although lorazepam is no more efficacious than phenobarbital or diazepam plus phenytoin, it is easier to use.'

Step 1: Benzodiazepine
Although lorazepam's onset of action is a little delayed compared to diazepam, its use is associated with a lower recurrence rate and it has a longer duration of action. Its rate of administration is less critical as it is less lipid-soluble and therefore crosses the blood–brain barrier less quickly than diazepam which has to be administered slowly. A disadvantage of lorazepam is that tolerance develops more quickly with repeated use. If diazepam is used in status epilepticus, then, to avoid recurrence, phenytoin, if not already prescribed, is given in a loading dose. Some countries use alternative benzodiazepines, such as clonazepam, effectively.

- *Lorazepam*: lorazepam is administered intravenously up to 0.1mg/kg (some recommend a maximum of 8mg). If used early, an initial dose of 4mg is usually given at 2mg/min, and repeated if seizures continue after 10min. Small veins should be avoided and the patient monitored for hypotension, respiratory depression, and cardiac arrhythmias. Median onset of action is reported as 3min (1–15min) and CSF concentrations are said to peak within 7min of injection.
- If seizures continue 10min after lorazepam intravenously, a second-line agent is indicated.

Step 2a/b: agents used as second line
Overview: the main second-line agents are *phenytoin/fosphenytoin*, *phenobarbital*, and possibly *valproate*. Phenytoin is given after a benzodiazepine in many protocols, including in the UK. An advantage is that phenytoin is less sedating but hypotension, arrhythmias, and severe local reactions are potential serious disadvantages. Local irritation is minimized with the use of the pro-drug fosphenytoin, but the extra cost has limited its use. Phenobarbital is effective but more sedating, with potential for respiratory depression. Valproate is less sedating and usually well tolerated but experience in its use in status is less widespread. Cumulative experience from many studies including >400 adults and children suggest that valproate is effective and reasonably well tolerated, but data are limited from randomized controlled trials regarding its use as a second-line agent. It should be avoided if mitochondrial disease is suspected. It is reasonable to use any of the above-mentioned as second-line after benzodiazepines depending on local experience, local guidelines, and requirements for individual patients.

There are other options briefly mentioned below. Of interest is emerging experience in the use of levetiracetam in status epilepticus, which like valproate appears well tolerated and non-sedating. This, however, is outside licence and its role in this setting is still to be defined.

- Phenytoin or fosphenytoin:
  - If the patient is not likely to be already on phenytoin, load with phenytoin/or fosphenytoin.
  - This is contraindicated in those with severe hypotension or second-degree heart block and in those with known allergy to it.
  - Monitor BP and ECG for hypotension and arrhythmia.
  - Phenytoin dose is 15–18mg/kg. In obesity, use adjusted body weight with a suggested maximum of 1500mg. The recommended rate of administration is 25–50mg/min(maximum) to be administered into *a large vein*. Do not mix with any other medication in the same intravenous line.

- Fosphenytoin (Pro-Epanutin®) is a phenytoin pro-drug which is less alkaline with less adverse effects on peripheral veins. It is also associated with a risk of severe cardiovascular reactions (📖 see Committee of Safety of Medicines warning ⌐ www. mhra.gov.uk/Publications/Safetyguidance/Convert problems in pharmacovigilance/CONOO 746). It is prescribed in 'phenytoin sodium equivalent (PE) units'. Although it can be administered more quickly than phenytoin, its speed of action is similar as its effect depends on its conversion to phenytoin. The usual dose is 15–18mg PE per kg. It is given at a rate of between 100–150mg PE per min and should not be administered faster. Unlike phenytoin, fosphenytoin can be given intramuscularly.
- With a history of recent phenytoin withdrawal, phenytoin is loaded. Otherwise, in those already loaded with phenytoin or if phenytoin is contraindicated, use alternative second-line agent. In those on phenytoin, obtain urgent phenytoin levels within the hour. Make up deficit as follows: dose of phenytoin in mg/kg = $0.7 \times$ (blood level required in mg/L—actual blood level measured in mg/L).
- If the patient has not responded to 18mg/kg of phenytoin by the end of the infusion or within 10min of ending the equivalent fosphenytoin infusion go to next step. Some protocols suggest an additional 5mg/kg of phenytoin (or PE of fosphenytoin).
- Phenobarbital (phenobarbitone):
  - This was shown to be effective in Veterans Affairs Status Epilepticus Cooperative Study as a first-line agent.[6] In the patient not already loaded with phenobarbital, load with phenobarbital 10–15mg per kg. Some suggest a maximum of 1g, at a rate not exceeding 100mg per min. Some protocols suggest a total of up to 20mg per kg. NICE suggests 10–15mg/kg at a rate of 100mg/min. Mean elapsed time for cessation of seizures is 5min from onset of infusion. Administer with BP, ECG, and respiratory monitoring. Sedation, hypotension and respiratory depression may occur and respiratory support may be required. Respiratory arrest has been reported when given with benzodiazepines
- Sodium valproate:
  - Valproate was not included as first- or second-agent in the Veterans Affairs Status Epilepticus Cooperative Study Group[7] and it is therefore difficult to make comments on comparative efficacy between it and the other agents tested. In a randomized pilot study from India[8], it was compared with phenytoin alone as a first-line agent in 68 patients with convulsive status epilepticus. Seizures were aborted in 66% in the valproate group compared to 42% in the phenytoin group. In the same study, VPA was effective in 79% and PHT in 25% as a second line in refractory patients. As mentioned already, despite limited trial data, there is reasonable reported experience in the use of valporate intravenously in status epilepticus. Hypotension, dizziness, and thrombocytopenia may occur in a minority with a low incidence of haemodynamic effects. It may thus be preferred in those with cardiopulmonary compromise or in certain syndromes such as some progressive myoclonic epilepsies, (but not mitochondrial disease) but it has

also been used in a wide range of status aetiologies. Advantages include lack of enzyme-inducing effect and less sedation. Caution and dose adjustment is needed if valproate is added in someone on lamotrigine therapy as it prolongs the latter's half-life significantly. In those with possible underlying metabolic abnormalities or mitochondrial disease, who may be at increased risk of liver failure, other second-line agents should be used.

- Sodium valproate intravenously is given as a bolus of 15mg/kg in adults (some recommend 30mg/kg bolus or ~ up to 2500mg), followed by continuous or repeated infusion of 1mg/kg/hour up to a maximum of 2500mg/day. Optimal doses are still to be determined.
- More than one preparation is available. In the UK, intravenous Epilim® is available as 400mg vial to which 4mL of water for injection is added to provide 100mg/mL concentration. Episenta® is available as a 300mg vial to which 3mL of water for injection should be added again providing 100mg/mL concentration.
- Some other possible agents:
  - Levetiracetam intravenously: levetiracetam is available as an intravenous preparation, with equivalent bioavailability to the oral preparation, but it is not licensed for use in status epilepticus. Nevertheless its successful use for this indication has been reported. It appears to be generally well tolerated without excessive sedation and with early efficacy. The lack of drug interactions is an additional advantage. Doses used successfully have varied and optimum doses are yet to be determined. A bolus dose is usually given followed by maintenance treatment.
  - Clomethiazole intravenously: can be used on high dependency units as a short term measure. It can accumulate precipitously and cause cardiorespiratory collapse. It should not be a mainstay of treatment and should not be given on medical wards. It is available as 8mg per mL (0.8%) solution. A loading dose of 32mg/min by intravenous infusion (4 mL/min) is given until seizures are controlled (up to total dose of 320–800mg (40–100mL)), followed by continuous infusion titrated according to response usually 4–8mg per min (0.5–1.0mL per min).
  - Paraldehyde intramuscularly or rectally: if plastic syringes are used, and as paraldehyde softens plastic, it must be given within 10min of being drawn up. *If diluted for rectal administration,* olive/sunflower oil is recommended rather than arachis oil to avoid risk of peanut allergies. Paraldehyde used to be widely used despite its drawbacks because of reportedly lower respiratory suppression and may still be useful in selected situations.
    —rectal dose: 10–20mL at 50% solution (mixed with equal volume of sunflower or olive oil).
    —intramuscular: usually 5–10mL: no more than 5mL at any one site. Paraldehyde can cause necrosis.
  - Lidocaine: this has been used in status and is sometimes listed but is not generally recommended. There is no comparative trial data, it requires expertise in its use and there is a risk of hypotension, bradyarrhythmias and hallucinations.

Step 3: general anaesthesia

If there are severe systemic disturbances at any stage (e.g., hypotension, respiratory compromise, acidosis, etc.) *or* if seizures continue despite a second line agent, proceed directly to anaesthesia with *propofol* or *thiopental* and ventilate with EEG monitoring until clinical and EEG seizures cease. Give pressor therapy as appropriate. *Midazolam* may also be used in conjunction. Some advise aiming for depth of anaesthesia sufficient to achieve EEG burst suppression. It is possible, however, for seizure activity to continue despite this pattern. Thus, suppressing seizure activity should be the primary aim. Keep the patient ventilated for a period without any electrical or clinical seizure activity. This period should be a minimum of 12 hours, but a longer minimum period of 24–48 hours is preferable if the status was difficult to control and of longer duration. Note that EEG monitoring in this situation is essential. It is possible for motor activity to cease and for electrical status to continue and this occurs in a significant proportion of cases with prolonged status. Some advocate antiepileptic medications with reported efficacy in status with a neuroprotective effect in animal models, such as oral topiramate, although it must be stated that there is no evidence for neuroprotection in this setting in humans. Isoflurane has also been used. Anaesthetists are very familiar with the use of these medications and the following initial doses are only included as a general guide to other physicians:

- *Propofol*: initially 1–2mg/kg bolus, then 2–10mg/kg/hour titrated to effect.
- *Thiopental*: 3–5mg/kg bolus, then 3–5mg/kg/hour titrated to effect.
- *Midazolam*: 0.1–0.2mg/kg bolus, then 0.05–0.5mg/kg/hour titrated to effect.

NICE guidelines 2004

📖 See Tables 4b.32 and 4b.33, reproduced with permission from NICE.[3]
Caution: background (long-term) AED medication must be reviewed and continued throughout.

Table 4b.32 Treating convulsive status epilepticus in adults[3]

General measures

1st stage (0–10min)   Early status
- Secure airway and resuscitate
- Administer oxygen
- Assess cardiorespiratory function Establish
  intravenous access

2nd stage (0–30min)
- Institute regular monitoring
- Consider the possibility of non-epileptic status
- Emergency AED therapy
- Emergency investigations
- Administer glucose (50mL of 50% solution) and/or intravenous thiamine
  (250mg) as high potency intravenous Pabrinex if any suggestion of alcohol
  abuse or impaired nutrition
- Treat acidosis if severe

3rd stage (0–60min)   Established status
- Establish aetiology
- Alert anaesthetist and ITU
- Identify and treat medical complications
- Pressor therapy when appropriate

4th stage (30–90min)   Refractory status
- Transfer to intensive care
- Establish intensive care and EEG monitoring
- Initiate intracranial pressure monitoring where
  appropriate
- Initiate long-term, maintenance AED therapy

Emergency investigations

Blood should be taken for blood gases, glucose, renal and liver function, calcium
and magnesium, FBC (including platelets), blood clotting, AED drug levels;
5mL of serum and 50mL of urine samples should be saved for future analysis,
including toxicology, especially if the cause of the status epilepticus is uncertain.
Chest radiograph to evaluate possible risk of aspiration. Other investigations
depend on the clinical circumstances and may include brain imaging, lumbar
puncture.

Monitoring

Regular neurological observations and measurements of pulse, BP, temperature.
ECG, biochemistry, blood gases, clotting, blood count, drug levels. Patients
require the full range of ITU facilities and care should be shared between
anaesthetist and neurologist. EEG monitoring is necessary for refractory status.
Consider the possibility of non-epileptic status. In refractory status epilepticus,
the primary end-point is suppression of epileptic activity on the EEG, with a
secondary end-point of burst-suppression pattern (i.e. short intervals of up to
1sec between bursts of background rhythm).

Table 4b.33 Emergency AED therapy for convulsive status epilepticus[3]

Premonitory stage (pre-hospital)	Diazepam 10–20mg given rectally, repeated once 15min later if status continues to threaten
	or midazolam 10mg given buccally
	If seizures continue, treat as below
Early status	Lorazepam (intravenously) 0.1mg/kg (usually a 4mg bolus, repeated once after 10–20min; rate not critical)
	Give usual AED medication if already on treatment
	For sustained control or if seizures continue, treat as below.
Established status	Phenytoin infusion at a dose of 15–18mg/kg at a rate of 50mg/min or fosphenytoin infusion at a dose of 15–20mg PE/kg at a rate of 50–100mg PE/min
	and/or phenobarbital bolus of 10–5mg/kg at a rate of 100mg/min
Refractory status*	General anaesthesia, with one of:
	• Propofol: 1–2mg/kg bolus, then 2–10mg/kg/hour, titrated to effect
	• Midazolam: 0.1–0.2mg/kg bolus, then 0.05–0.5mg/kg/hour, titrated to effect.
	• Thiopental: 3–5mg/kg bolus, then 3–5mg/kg/hour, titrated to effect; after 2–3 days infusion rate needs reduction as fat stores are saturated
	Anaesthetic continued for 12–24 hours after the last clinical or electrographic seizure, then dose tapered

*In this scheme, the refractory stage (general anaesthesia) is reached 60/90min after the initial therapy.

This scheme is suitable for usual clinical hospital settings. In some situations, general anaesthesia should be initiated earlier and, occasionally, should be delayed.

Experience with long-term administration (hours or days) of the newer anaesthetic drugs is very limited. The modern anaesthetics have, however, important pharmacokinetic advantages over the more traditional barbiturates.

Long-term AED therapy long-term, maintenance, and AED therapy must be given in parallel with emergency treatment. The choice of drug depends on previous therapy, the type of epilepsy, and the clinical setting. Any pre-existing AED therapy should be continued at full dose, and any recent reductions reversed.

If phenytoin or phenobarbital has been used in emergency treatment, maintenance doses can be continued orally or intravenously guided by serum level monitoring. Other maintenance AEDs can be started also, with oral loading doses. Care needs to be taken with nasogastric feeds, which can interfere with the absorption of some AEDs. Once the patient has been free of seizures for 12–24 hours and provided that there are adequate plasma levels of concomitant AEDs, then the anaesthetic should be slowly tapered.

Treatment of status epilepticus in children

A published guideline exists for the treatment of status epilepticus that was produced by the status epilepticus working party of the British Paediatric Neurology Association, based on a systematic review of evidence[9] and subsequently published by NICE (2004). The guideline was primarily designed for a child presenting in status epilepticus to the A&E department or the hospital paediatric ward. For the purpose of this guideline it is stated that the approach to the child who presents with a tonic–clonic convulsion lasting >5min should be the same as a child in 'established' status—to stop the seizure and to prevent the development of status epilepticus. What it does not address is where to start within the guideline dependent on prehospital treatment—the most common cause of admission to ITU in a recent epidemiological study was overdose of benzodiazepines (i.e. more than two doses given). More than two doses of benzodiazepines should therefore not be given in total. The role of buccal midazolam in out of hospital treatment is increasing, more socially acceptable than rectal administration; equal efficacy has been shown in trials to date. There would appear to be little place for rectal or buccal treatment where intravenous access has been secured.

Treatment of NCSE in children

Often the most difficult aspect to the mangement of non-convulsive status (NCS) is recognition; defined as continuous epileptiform activity on EEG without convulsive clinical movement (Fig. 4b.5). It is defined as a change in EEG with associated change in behaviour from baseline. It is most commonly seen in children in those with an underlying difficult refractory epilepsy (e.g. Lennox–Gastaut syndrome)—often when baseline measures are not secure. Whether the brain is at risk from NCS to the same degree as to convulsive status remains unclear. Prognosis appears dependent on underlying aetiology rather than the duration or continuation of NCS. In the context of a subacute situation oral benzodiazepines are the treatment of choice. Acute abrupt changes of behaviour with unresponsiveness and cognitive regression may require a course of high dose steroids (prednisolone 2mg/kg/day for 6 weeks followed by a 6-week wean) (NICE 2004). It is important to consider that certain AEDs may provoke NCS e.g. carbamazepine.

References

1. Shorvon S (2007). What is non-convulsive status epilepticus and what are its subtypes. *The First London Colloquium on Status Epilepticus 2007 abstract.*

2 Scottish Intercollegiate Guideline Network (2003). *Diagnosis and management of epilepsy in adults. A National Clinical Guideline.* Available at: 🖳 www.sign.ac.uk/pdf/sign70.pdf

3. NICE. The epilepsies: the diagnosis and management of the epilepsies in adults and children in primary and secondary care. Available at: 🖳 www.NICE.org.uk/cg020.

4. Meierkord H, Boon P, Engelsen B, *et al.* (2006). EFNS guideline on the management of status epilepticus. *European Journal of Neurology,* **13**, 445–50.

5. Minicucci F, Muscas G, Perucca E *et al.* (2006). Treatment of status epilepticus in adults: guidelines of the Italian League Against Epilepsy. *Epilepsia,* **47**(Suppl. 5), 9–15.

6. Prasad *et al.* (2007). Anticonvulsant therapy for status epilepticus. *Cochrane Database of Systematic Reviews* **4**.

7. Treiman DM, Meyers PD, Walton NY, *et al.* (1998). Veterans Affairs Status Epilepticus Cooperative Study Group randomized trial. *New England Journal of Medicine,* **17**, 339(12), 792–8.

8. Misra UK, Kalita J, Patel R. *et al.* (2006). Sodium valproate vs phenytoin in status epilepticus: a pilot study. *Neurology,* **67**, 340–2.

9 Appleton R, Choonara I, Martland T, *et al.* (2000). The treatment of convulsive status epilepticus in children. The Status Epilepticus Working Party, Members of the Status Epilepticus Working Party. *Archives of Disease in Childhood,* **83**, 415–9.

Surgical treatment of epilepsy

Who can be operated on and when to suggest surgery?

Epilepsy is one of the most common neurological disorders, with a prevalence of 1/200 and an incidence of 46/100,000 per year. Approximately 300,000 people in the UK have epilepsy. About 20–30 % of patients are not satisfactorily controlled by medical treatment and are potential candidates for surgery.

Before surgery can be performed for the treatment of epilepsy, detailed preoperative assessment has to be carried out in order to confirm the nature of the attacks, and to establish if there is a single source for the patient's seizures and where it is.

The general admission criteria for patients to enter a programme for preoperative assessment of epilepsy are the following:

- *Reliable diagnosis of intractable epilepsy*: there should be no doubt that attacks are epileptic, the possibility of attacks being non-epileptic seizures should be ruled out, the patient must have been on appropriate medication at the correct doses for at least 2 years without adequate seizure control, and the patient must have been compliant with medication.
- *Seizures should be disabling*: seizures should pose an obstacle to the patient's lifestyle, capabilities, and aspirations, because of the nature, timing, and/or frequency of seizures.
- *Patient has resources to cope with assessment:* patients should be able to tolerate the procedures, have realistic expectations about the results, and be able to accept failure of surgery.
- *Absence of general contraindications to neurosurgery.*

For specific admission criteria, 📖 see Box 4c.1.

Surgical assessment

Overview of surgical strategies

- **Lesionectomy, focal or lobar resection:** to remove, destroy, or deactivate a discrete, functionally and structurally abnormal brain region ('epileptogenic zone') causing partial seizures. Seizures must be partial, with or without secondary generalization.
- **Multiple subpial transection:** multiple cortical sections that divide the cortex into small cortical islands to abolish seizure spread without compromising function.
- **Hemispherectomy and hemispherotomy:** to remove or isolate a grossly dysfunctional hemisphere that generates seizures.
- **Callosotomy:** section of the corpus callosum to prevent interhemispheric spread of seizures that cause injury due to falling.
- **Vagus nerve stimulation:** intermittent electrical stimulus of left vagus nerve in the neck by a generator implanted below the clavicle. Mode of action unknown.
- **Brain stimulation:** electrical stimulation applied either directly to the cortical focus or to deeper subcortical structures (deep brain stimulation, DBS) such as the thalamus. Electrical stimulation of the thalamus can relieve epilepsy, particularly frontal lobe epilepsy and epilepsy associated with learning difficulties. Perhaps effective in other syndromes. Still under evaluation.

Purpose of presurgical assessment

- To confirm that the patient suffers from epileptic seizures.
- To decide if the severity of epilepsy warrants surgery.
- To identify the source of the patient's seizures.
- To decide the type of surgical procedure: resection of a lesion (lesionectomy), wider resection, multiple subpial transection, callosotomy, hemispherectomy, hemispherotomy.
- To identify the risks of surgery: particularly the function of the area which the surgeon plans to resect.
- To identify contraindications for surgery.

> ### Box 4c.1 Admission criteria for surgical assessment programme*
>
> *General criteria for admission:*
> - Reliable diagnosis of intractable epilepsy:
>   - Attacks are epileptic, no pseudoseizures (or pseudoseizures distinguishable from epileptic seizures and the latter being the major cause of morbidity—the conditions frequently co-exist).
>   - Failure of appropriate medication.
>   - Patient is compliant
> - Seizures of such a frequency and nature that they are disabling, having regard to the patient's lifestyle.
> - No other contraindication of surgery, for example a coagulation defect.

Criteria for investigation for resective surgery:
- Partial (focal) seizures, whether or not secondarily generalized
- Does not fulfil criteria for hemispherectomy and hemispherotomy as detailed in the next section.
- Full scale IQ generally not <70: a low IQ used to be regarded as a contraindication as it suggested a widespread brain dysfunction. This criterion is less rigidly applied nowadays, as it is recognized that focal lesions may cause severe epilepsy and affect IQ.
- Age generally not >55: again this is less frequently applied nowadays as outcome seems only slightly less favourable in the over 55s.
- Patient has emotional resources to cope with the procedures, and possible inoperability.

Note:
- A single inter-ictal EEG focus is not a requirement.
- Psychiatric or behavioural disorder is not an automatic exclusion criterion.
- If patient does not satisfy the criteria for resective surgery, apply selection criteria for hemispherectomy or callosotomy as detailed next.

Criteria for hemispherectomy and hemispherotomy:
- Long standing unilateral hemispheric damage evidenced by hemiplegia, and brain imaging. Pre-existing hemiplagia in most.
- Partial seizures, whether or not secondarily generalized, arising from the diseased hemisphere.

Criteria for callosotomy:
- Generalized seizures, particularly atonic or tonic seizures, causing injury, in the context of partial or symptomatic generalized epilepsy.
- This may be a preferred solution in patients with unilateral hemisphere disease, not severe enough for hemispherectomy.
- Associated partial seizures, if any, are not amenable to resective surgery.

Criteria for VNS:
- Ineligibility for all the above, or a <50% probability even of palliation.
- Arguably, all possible callosotomy candidates.

Reproduced from Binnie CD and Polkey CE (1992). Surgery for Epilepsy, *Recent Advances in Clinical Neurology*, **7**, 55–93, with permission from Elsevier.

Contraindications to surgery for epilepsy
- Severe depression: some procedures (temporal lobectomy) can induce or worsen depression.
- Chronic psychosis: although post-ictal or ictal psychosis is not a contraindication.
- General contraindications for neurosurgery.

Methods used in surgical assessment
- Medical history, including review of old notes.
- Seizure description.
- Neuropsychiatric assessment.
- Neuroimaging: mainly CT, MRI, PET, SPECT.
- Neuropsychology.
- Inter-ictal scalp EEG: awake and sleep.
- Ictal scalp EEG: video telemetry.
- Amytal® test.
- Video telemetry with intracranial EEG: ictal and inter-ictal.
- Functional mapping:
  - Non-invasive, e.g. fMRI.
  - Invasive via intracranial electrodes.
  - During surgery under local anaesthetic.
- Intraoperative electrocorticography (ECoG)

Underlying philosophy of surgical assessment for resective surgery
- Resective surgery is unlikely to succeed unless resected tissue is both functionally and structurally abnormal.
- Evidence from the methods listed in the previous section should converge onto a single region.
- If evidence is not convergent, an explanatory hypothesis must be proposed and tested, or resective surgery abandoned.

Medical history
Apart to the general issues regarding history taking in epilepsy (📖 see Role of history, pp.158–160), special emphasis should be placed on the description, frequency, and severity of seizures, with the purpose of identifying both the source of the patient's seizures and the impact of seizures in the patient's life.

The following features should be carefully recorded:
- Documentation and descriptions of all seizure types.
- Descriptions of specific attacks:
  - *Last attack witnessed:* better remembered.
  - *First seizure:* the first seizure may differ from the rest as in febrile convulsions. In addition, the first seizure can provide an indication on impact to patient's life and patient's reaction to it.
  - *Worst seizure:* indicates the scale of the clinical problem, risk to life, circumstances of occurrence.
- Frequency of attacks for each seizure type:
  - Average frequency per week.
  - Highest frequency per week.
  - Longest attack-free period.
  - Number of seizure-free days per month.

In addition, the patient's educational and working history should be carefully documented to estimate the handicap associated with epilepsy, which could in part be reversed by surgery.

Seizure semiology

- The area responsible for seizures can be lateralized to a hemisphere by studying the clinical features of seizures alone in around 78% of patients.
- Although history taking is a cornerstone in epileptology, seizure semiology is most accurately studied by observing videos of seizures. Often video recording from each seizure must be seen several times before a complete description can be made.
- The main lateralizing and localizing signs are:
  - Dystonic posturing suggests contralateral onset.
  - Unilateral automatisms suggests ipsilateral onset.
  - Ictal speech suggests onset in the non-dominant hemisphere.
  - Forced head version (slow, gradual, sustained and extreme rotation of the head) suggests onset contralateral to the side towards which the head rotates (patient looks away from focus).
  - Unilateral clonic movements suggest contralateral onset.
  - Preserved consciousness with automatisms (very rare) suggests right hemisphere onset.
  - Blinking suggests occipital seizures.
  - Unilateral blinking suggests ipsilateral onset.
  - Vomiting suggest right temporal seizures.
  - Retching suggest an insular onset.
  - Post-ictal dysphasia suggests onset in the dominant hemisphere.
  - Todd's paralysis (post-ictal unilateral paralysis or weakness) suggests contralateral onset.
  - Post-ictal nose wiping suggests ipsilateral temporal onset.

Auras (simple partial seizures)

- Déjà vu (feeling that what is happening has already happened) suggests medial temporal onset.
- Epigastric rising sensation suggests medial temporal onset.
- Hearing sounds or melodies suggests lateral temporal onset.
- Unilateral tingling suggests contralateral onset close to somatosensory area.
- Elementary visual symptoms (flashing lights, circles, colours) suggest occipital onset.
- Unilateral elementary visual symptoms suggest contralateral occipital onset.
- Complex visual hallucinations suggests occipital, parieto-occipital or frontal onset.
- Thought disorder (e.g. thought implanted on someone's head) suggest frontal onset.

Neuropsychiatric assessment

- Neuropsychiatric assessment is essential before surgery because there is high psychiatric co-morbidity in patients with epilepsy. Treatable conditions should be identified and treated before surgery.
- Psychiatric morbidity is not as such a contraindication to surgery, particularly if symptoms are related to seizures (peri-ictal), which may be relieved by surgery.

Neuroimaging

- Neuroimaging has become paramount in the surgical assessment of patients with epilepsy.
- MRI is the main imaging modality.
- MRI should include coronal (perpendicular to the long axis of the temporal horn/hippocampus) and T1- and T2-weighted images (preferably with a volumetric T1W acquisition with partitions of 1mm or less). FLAIR images are also helpful, particularly to look for subtle grey matter and subcortical white matter high signal associated with focal cortical dysplasia and the high signal seen in hippocampal sclerosis.
- CT is occasionally useful as an adjunct to MRI to show calcified lesions (tumours such as oligodendroglioms, phakomatoses such as tuberous sclerosis) and in an emergency. CT is also useful after surgery (to show surgical complications or electrode positions).
- 85% of patients with intractable epilepsy show a structural abnormality on neuroimaging. However, the absence of a structural abnormality on neuroimaging does not rule out surgery, as the source of seizures may be identified with intracranial electrodes (📖 see Intracranial EEG recordings, pp.423–431).

Quantification of MR images (hippocampal volume, hippocampal T2 measurements): may be helpful but are time consuming to perform in every patient.

Positron emission tomography (PET): fluoro-deoxyglucose (FDG) is the most commonly used PET tracer. The vast majority of PET studies are inter-ictal, since it is unlikely that patients have seizures during the period of PET acquisition. Between 60–90% of patients with temporal lobe epilepsy, show unilateral temporal hypometabolism on the side of seizure onset (Fig. 4c.1). Hypometabolism tends to be more widespread than the structural lesion, often involving most of the affected temporal lobe. In frontal lobe epilepsy, hypometabolism is reported to be lower, in the region of 60% or less of patients.

Single proton emission tomography (SPECT): the most commonly used tracer is 99mTc-HMPAO (99mTc-hexamethylpropylamine oxime). SPECT studies can be inter-ictal, ictal, or post-ictal. Since the tracer fixes in the brain shortly after intravenous injection, the technique has relatively high temporal resolution and can image seizures if injected shortly after seizure onset. This can be achieved in combination with video telemetry. Ictal SPECT shows appropriately lateralized hypermetabolism in 97% of temporal lobe seizures and in 92% of extratemporal seizures, the interpretation being dependant on timing of injection in relation to seizure onset.

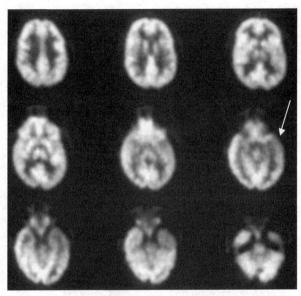

Fig. 4c.1 ^{18}FDG-PET showing right temporal hypometabolism in a patient with right mesial temporal sclerosis (the right hemisphere is on the right side of the page). Note: hypometabolism involves most of the affected temporal lobe, affecting cortex beyond the hippocampus.

Neuropsychology

- Neuropsychological assessment may demonstrate a lateralized functional deficit associated with epileptogenesis.
- A discrepancy >15 points between the verbal and performance (non-verbal) IQ suggests a lateralized dysfunction and hence unilateral pathology. A depressed verbal IQ suggests pathology in the dominant hemisphere for language (usually the left). A depressed non-verbal IQ would suggest pathology in the non-dominant hemisphere (usually the right).
- Differences between verbal and non-verbal memory scores have similar implications.
- The lateralizing value of verbal and non-verbal IQ differences is particularly high in right-handed patients because approximately 96% of right handed patients have language on the left hemisphere. The lateralizing value of IQ difference is much lower in left- or mixed-handed patients, because only 70% have language on the left hemisphere. These figures apply to patients with late brain damage; for those with early damage, the figures fall to approximately 80% and 30% respectively.
- Preoperative IQ and memory have prognostic value: the patients with higher IQs tend to show higher postoperative deficits—possibly because they had more to lose.

Inter-ictal scalp EEG

- Awake and sleep EEGs typically last for 30–90min and usually contain only inter-ictal EEG, since it is unlikely that seizures will occur during the period of recording.
- Abnormalities can manifest as epileptiform discharges, slowing of the background activity (more slowing on the abnormal region) or asymmetry in alpha or beta activities (less activity on the abnormal side).
- Hyperventilation can activate discharges.
- Patients assessed for surgery are only very rarely photosensitive.
- Sleep is useful because it can enhance epileptiform discharges or demonstrate new foci.
- The incidence of bilateral independent epileptiform discharges in temporal lobe epilepsy is around 40% and their presence should not preclude surgery. Discharges are usually more prominent in the epileptogenic side, particularly during sleep.

Ictal scalp EEG

Analysis of the EEG during a seizure (ictal EEG) may be of value in determining the side and site (i.e. laterality and localization) of the seizure focus.

- Since seizures are not usually seen during standard EEG recordings, video telemetry is often necessary to obtain recordings during seizures.
- EEG changes associated with seizures can be ictal or post-ictal. Ictal changes can consist of flattening of the EEG (electrodecremental event), low amplitude fast activity (10–50Hz), rhythmic sharp waves or spikes, or slowing in the delta or theta ranges.
- EEG changes can be absent during simple partial seizures, and less commonly during frontal seizures.

- The initial ictal changes can be unilateral or bilateral. If unilateral and focal, they have localizing and lateralizing value (Fig. 4c.2). If the first scalp EEG changes are bilateral, they should not preclude surgery. This is because seizures may still have a focal origin, although EEG changes may be seen on the scalp only after bilateral propagation has occurred. Intracranial recordings may be necessary to show a focal onset.

As it is important to establish if there is a single site of onset, several seizures should be recorded during video telemetry (preferably five or more). In order to increase the chance of recording several seizures, activation procedures such as one-night sleep deprivation can be carried out, or AED medication may have to be reduced or withdrawn. Reductions in AED medication should be carried out slowly (over 2–3 days or longer) to reduce the risk of triggering status epilepticus or withdrawal seizures which may show an anomalous onset or rapid generalization, making difficult to localize seizure onset. Under these circumstances, drug reductions do not generally change the clinical and electroencephalographic characteristics of patients' seizures.

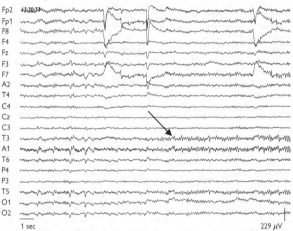

Fig. 4c.2 Focal seizure onset observed on scalp EEG recordings. Note a diffuse flattening of the EEG (electrodecremental event) followed by onset of fast activity showing largest amplitude at the left mid-temporal (A1) and Sylvian (T3) regions (arrow).

The Amytal® test—carotid amobarbital test, Wada test

In some patients with suspected temporal lobe epilepsy, an amytal test may be performed to identify the side of speech dominance, and to determine if speech or memory deficits may result from surgery. To carry out this test, sodium amobarbital (around 75–100mg) is injected through a catheter placed into one internal carotid artery. This induces selective anaesthesia of the injected hemisphere for around 4min. During this period, speech is assessed and material is presented to be memorized. Recall is tested 10min after the effects of anaesthesia wear off. With this method, speech and memory performance of the non-anaesthetized hemisphere are estimated. Once one hemisphere is tested, the cannula is moved to the other internal carotid artery to test speech and memory abilities present in the remaining hemisphere.

Patient's performance when one hemisphere is anaesthetized estimates the function present in the non-anaesthetized hemisphere, and what deficits may result from surgery on the side of injection.

The scalp EEG can be recorded during the Amytal® test in order to confirm that the effects of the injection are unilateral, on the appropriate side, and outlast the period of psychological testing.

Some authors have questioned the value of the Amytal® test to predict postoperative deficits. There is presently an interesting debate about whether modern functional MRI techniques can replace the Amytal® test. At present, functional MRI appears to be reliable enough to lateralize speech, but not memory.

In patients with generalized epileptiform discharges with suspected secondary bilateral synchrony (discharges arising from one hemisphere and rapidly generalizing), the Amytal® test can be used to establish which is the hemisphere that drives the discharges. When the driving hemisphere is anaesthetized, discharges disappear bilaterally. On the other hand, when the driven hemisphere is anaesthetized, discharges disappear only on the injected side. Since secondary bilateral synchrony is generally studied in children with behavioural problems who have generalized spikes mainly during sleep, the amytal test to study this phenomenon is best performed under general anaesthesia. Extensive adjustments with the levels of anaesthesia might be necessary to induce a regular rate of generalized discharges. If generalized discharges still fail to occur, methohexital (a rapid acting barbiturate) can be administered intravenously at progressively higher doses (up to 70–75mg) until electrocerebral silence is observed on the EEG. Under such conditions, 'primary epileptogenic foci' show more resistance to synaptic blockade. The hemisphere showing epileptiform activity that disappeared latest and/or reappeared earliest after injection is considered as the driving hemisphere. These pharmacological tests are sometimes carried out as part of presurgical assessment in patients with Landau–Kleffner syndrome where multiple subpial transection of the perisylvian cortex is contemplated to treat acquired aphasia.

Intracranial EEG recordings

In patients where seizure semiology, neuroimaging findings, neuropsychological testing, scalp inter-ictal and ictal EEG abnormalities converge to suggest a single region as the source of seizures, surgery can be undertaken. If evidence is not convergent, an explanatory hypothesis must be proposed and tested, or resective surgery abandoned. Often, such an explanatory hypothesis can be tested by implanting electrodes close to the candidate site(s) for seizure onset. Compared to scalp electrodes, intracranial electrodes allow recording of much larger EEG signals from a much smaller region of brain with fewer muscle artifacts.

Once the patient recovers from electrode implantation, standard video telemetry is carried out with the intracranial electrodes to record the EEG until sufficient numbers of seizures are recorded. This is often referred to as chronic or subacute intracranial recordings (as opposed to the acute recordings obtained during intraoperative ECoG, 📖 see below).

It has been claimed that recent advances in MRI technology will eventually abolish the need for chronic intracranial recordings. While improved imaging, particularly MRI, has undoubtedly been a major advance in epilepsy surgery, our experience in recent years is that intracranial recordings continue to be indicated in a proportion of patients. As with any diagnostic test, improvements in MRI sensitivity will necessarily be associated with increments in the number of true and false positive detections. In some patients multiple lesions are detected, raising the question of whether there is a single focal seizure onset and, if so, which lesion generates seizures. In other patients, mild non-specific unclear abnormalities can be seen, raising doubt of whether they are indeed epileptogenic.

Several types of intracranial electrodes are available:

Foramen ovale electrodes

These are multicontact electrode bundles that can be inserted through the foramen ovale under fluoroscopic control and under general anaesthesia. The deepest contacts lay close to medial temporal structures. Removal does not require general anaesthesia. Because no craniotomy or burr holes are required for their implantation, they are often considered less invasive than subdural and depth electrodes. However, the use of these electrodes has declined as they are rather disagreeable, often irritating the trigeminal nerve while implanted. 📖 See Fig. 4c.3.

Subdural electrodes

These come as groups of electrodes arranged in either mats (grids) or strips (📖 Figs. 4c.4, 4c.5, and 4c.6). For simplicity, each electrode within a mat or strip is called a contact. Mats are arrays of contacts. Strips are single rows of contacts. Contacts are embedded in Silastic® or Teflon® sheets. Each contact typically has 5mm diameter and contact centres are located 1cm apart. Mats need to be introduced through a craniotomy, and can be placed under the dura over the cerebral convexity, or carefully inserted between brain and dura (at some risk of venous bleeding). Mats are suitable for functional mapping with electrical stimulation or with evoked responses to sensory stimulation. Strips come in single rows, typically of 4 or 8 contacts, and several can be inserted through a burr hole. If inserted through a burr hole anterior to the ear, an 8 contact strip can be slipped under the temporal lobe and provide excellent recording from the parahippocampal gyrus. Used in this way, they serve similar purpose to foramen ovale electrodes. General anaesthesia is required for insertion and removal. Strips can be combined with mats to cover the cerebral convexity and, if inserted parasagittally, the medial aspect of the cerebral hemispheres.

Depth (intracerebral) electrodes

These are multicontact electrode bundles that can be inserted stereotactically through the brain under neuroimaging control. They provide excellent recordings form deep brain regions (hippocampus, amygdala, cingulum) with some simultaneous EEG sampling from more superficial regions. 📖 See Figs. 4c.7 and 4c.8.

Epidural peg electrodes

A stainless steel disc mounted in a mushroom-shaped Silastic® support. They can be fixed on a burr hole with the top of the mushroom outside the skull. They are useful in addition to other intracranial electrodes when it is found during recording that an additional area needs exploring.

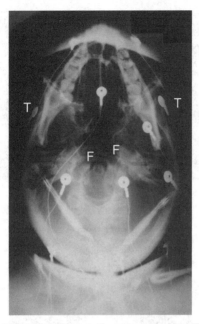

Fig. 4c.3 Skull X-radiograph of implanted foramen ovale electrodes (F) and scalp electrodes. T = anterior temporal scalp electrodes. (Reproduced from Fernandez Torre, JL; Alarcón, G.; Binnie, CD, et al. (1999). Comparison of sphenoidal, foramen ovale and anterior temporal placements for detecting interictal epileptiform discharges in presurgical assessment for temporal lobe epilepsy. *Clinical Neurophysiology* **110**, 895–904,© 1999, with permission from Elsevier.)

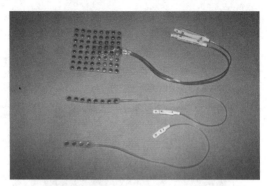

Fig. 4c.4 Subdural strips and mat (grid) electrodes.

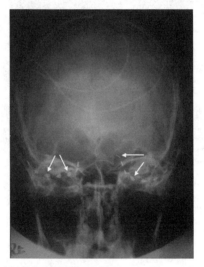

Fig. 4c.5 Implanted bilateral subtemporal strips.

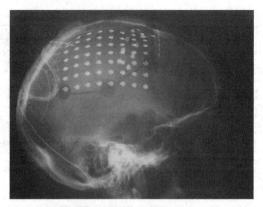

Fig. 4c.6 Implanted lateral and medial mats.

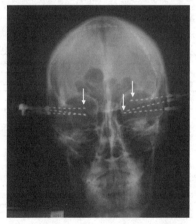

Fig. 4c.7 Bilateral temporal intracerebral (depth) electrodes (arrows point to the tip of the bundles, i.e. the deepest contacts).

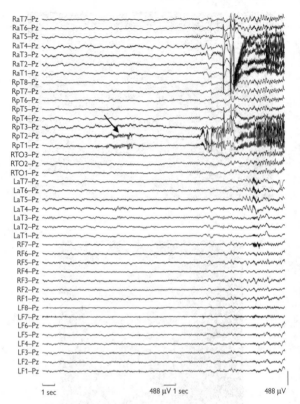

Fig. 4c.8 Seizure onset (arrow) recorded with depth electrodes at electrodes 1 and 2 (deepest) of the right posterior temporal electrode bundle (RpT1 and RpT2). Right anterior temporal (RaT), right posterior temporal (RpT), right temporo-occipital (RTO), left anterior temporal (LaT), right frontal (RF), left frontal (LF), mid parietal scalp electrode (Pz).

Indications for implantation of intracranial electrodes

The following three resective procedures can be performed without the need to employ intracranial electrodes:

- *Lesionectomy:* patients with a discrete, cerebral, non-atrophic lesion demonstrated by neuroimaging at a non-functionally eloquent site, with location concordant with seizure semiology, topography of inter-ictal discharges, topography of ictal onset on scalp EEG, distribution of background abnormalities in the inter-ictal EEG, and neuropsychological findings.
- *Temporal lobectomy:* patients with a consistent, single, temporal site of seizure onset on scalp EEG telemetry, with EEG changes preceding clinical semiology, concordant with seizure semiology, distribution of background abnormalities in the inter-ictal scalp EEG, neuroimaging, and neuropsychological findings.
- *Hemispherectomy:* 📖 see Surgical techniques, p.435.

Patients not fulfilling these criteria can have studies with intracranial electrodes. These are patients where a hypothesis is available to explain findings to date, particularly any non-convergence of evidence from different tests, and this hypothesis is testable with intracranial electrode implantation. The choice and placement of intracranial electrodes depends on the working hypothesis with regard to the site of seizure onset. As intracerebral (depth) electrodes are perceived to be more invasive than subdural recordings, the latter are generally preferred if possible. When temporal lobe seizures are suspected, but laterality is uncertain, recordings with bilateral 8-contact subtemporal strips inserted through fronto-temporal burr holes can be carried out. If this procedure yields inconclusive results, a second intracranial recording can be performed with bilateral temporal intracerebral electrodes. When seizures are thought to arise from the frontal lobes, but laterality is uncertain, bilateral intracerebral electrodes can be used. When the seizures are thought to arise from the cerebral convexity, from peri-central regions or from the supplementary motor area, mats or strips can be used, usually implanted unilaterally.

Resective surgery can be excluded if:

- The EEG shows predominantly generalized inter-ictal EEG discharges in the absence of a discrete lesion on neuroimaging.
- Independent sites of electrographic seizure onset are demonstrated in more than one lobe.
- Generalized discharges are seen at or immediately preceding clinical seizure onset
- A site of seizure onset is identified, which could not be resected without unacceptable complications, and is unsuitable for multiple subpial transection.
- Bilateral or multilobar seizure onset is seen with intracranial recordings and no clear alternative hypothesis exists for further studies with intracranial recordings.

Complications of intracranial electrodes

The main complications are infection and cerebral haemorrhage. The likelihood of complications from intracranial recordings is roughly proportional to the number of electrodes implanted. We have found <2% risk of permanent neurological deficits. Transitory deficits and complications are more common (almost 5%). Transmission of Creutzfeldt–Jakob disease has been reported but can be avoided by disposing of used electrodes. Chronic implantation of mats can be associated with leakage of cerebrospinal fluid that can be managed by keeping the head high and changing the head bandage regularly. Mat recordings appear to have a 0.85% risk of infection, which can be reduced with prophylactic antibiotics, minimizing duration of implantation and passing the cables through the scalp at a point far from the craniotomy. Frank meningitis or encephalitis is rare. Depth electrodes have a very low risk of infection, a 1.9% risk of haemorrhage with transitory deficits, and a 0.8% risk of haemorrhage with permanent deficits.

Interpretation of intracranial recordings

Epileptiform discharges recorded inter-ictally with intracranial electrodes are larger, sharper, and occur more frequently than those seen on the scalp. Each patient usually exhibits several patterns of epileptiform discharges occurring independently at different sites, often including the hemisphere opposite to seizure onset. For this reason, inter-ictal activity recorded with intracranial electrodes should be interpreted cautiously. Ictal changes consist of flattening of the on-going EEG (electrodecremental event), low amplitude fast activity (10–50Hz), rhythmic sharp waves or spikes, or slowing in the delta or theta ranges. Fast activity appears to be the pattern with the highest localizing value. Generalized electrodecremental events (diffuse flattening of the EEG) are common at seizure onset but should not discourage surgery, since they do not seem to be associated with worse outcome. Any other form of changes occurring diffusely at seizure onset would suggest that the seizure is generalized or, more commonly, electrodes are not placed at the site of seizure origin.

Functional mapping

If the proposed resection is close to an area relevant for vital functions (motor, sensory, or speech areas), the risk of major postoperative functional deficits can be reduced by accurate identification of such functional areas with the purpose of avoiding their resection. The role of functional MRI for this purpose is still undetermined. At present, functional mapping can be reliably obtained in patients with intracranial electrodes. Sensory areas can be plotted from sensory evoked potentials recorded with mat electrodes. Alternatively, functional regions can be identified by electrical stimulation in the conscious patient. Mapping can be obtained intraoperatively or during chronic recordings in telemetry. Constant current electrical stimulation of progressive intensity and duration is used (up to 6-sec trains of electrical pulses, up to 10mA, 1ms bipolar pulses at 50Hz). Pairs of adjacent electrodes are used consecutively to deliver current. Stimulation of the somatosensory area induces tingling, numbness, or other paraesthesiae in the corresponding cutaneous region. Stimulation of the motor strip is associated with focal twitches of the corresponding muscle group(s). Stimulation of the speech area induces speech arrest.

Electrical stimulation that induces the patient's habitual auras or seizures can be used to aid the identification of areas responsible for spontaneous seizures.

Intraoperative (acute) ECoG

Once a patient has been found suitable for resective surgery or for multiple subpial transection, and the general location of the procedure has been decided, it is possible to further define the surgical procedure at the time of surgery. This can be achieved with intraoperative EEG recordings obtained with electrodes in contact with the cortex in the operating theatre (intraoperative ECoG). 📖 See Fig. 4c.9.

Electrocorticographic recordings are obtained covering most of the area around the proposed resection or transection. If epileptiform discharges are not seen, they can be induced by reducing the levels of anaesthesia, or by progressive injection of thiopental (25mg every 20sec, up to 250mg in adults). Post-resection or post-transection recordings should be carried out to confirm the abolition of discharges following the procedure. If discharges remain, the procedure should be extended if safely possible. Electrocorticographic evaluation is largely restricted to inter-ictal activity.

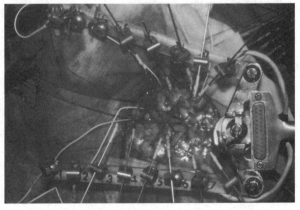

Fig. 4c.9 Electrocorticographic recordings.

Phased evaluation

Surgical assessment requires a multidisciplinary team and the interpretation of multiple tests. 📖 See Box 4c.2. and Fig. 4c.10

Box 4c.2 Phases of investigation for possible surgical treatment*

- *Phase Ia*: baseline outpatient investigations routinely performed on referral.
  - Clinical assessment.
  - High resolution MRI with FLAIR.
  - Routine and sleep EEG
- *Phase Ib:* further non-invasive investigations.
  - Scalp telemetry.
  - Neuropsychology.
  - Volumetric MRI.
  - FDG-PET.
  - Flumazenil PET.
  - Ictal SPECT.
- *Phase IIa:* minor invasive procedures.
  - Telemetry with subdural strips.
  - Telemetry with foramen ovale electrodes.
  - Carotid amylobarbital test (Wada test).
- *Phase IIb:* major invasive procedures.
  - Telemetry with subdural mats or depth (intracerebral) electrodes.

*Reprinted from Binnie C, Cooper R, Mauguière F, et al. (eds.) (2003). *Clinical Neurophysiology*, vol 2. Elsevier Science B.V., Amsterdam© 2003, with permission from Elsevier.

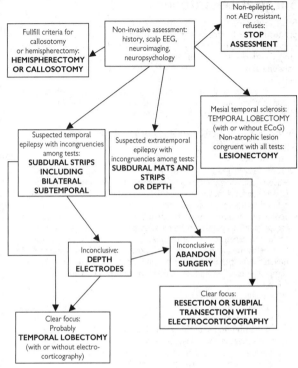

Fig. 4c.10 Flow chart of presurgical assessment at King's College Hospital, London.

Surgical techniques

Because seizures necessarily arise from tissue that is functional, surgical procedures for the treatment of epilepsy can affect cortex that is relevant to normal function (memory, speech, motor and sensory functions, mood, etc.). Therefore the aim of surgery should be to obtain a compromise between achieving seizure control and avoiding unacceptable functional deficits.

Generally, in focal resections, the greater the resection the better seizure control but the higher the likelihood of inducing functional deficits (speech problems, motor deficits, poor memory).

Summary of available surgical procedures to treat epilepsy and their indications

Local resection

To remove the area from where focal seizures arise. Several approaches are used depending on the location of the area generating seizures:

- *Lesionectomy:* removal of a well-defined non-atrophic lesion clearly related to the source of seizures.
- *Temporal lobectomy:* this is the most common local resection because temporal lobe epilepsy is the most common type of epilepsy amenable to surgical treatment. After lesionectomy, it is also the procedure that yields the highest rate of good postsurgical seizure control. Only unilateral temporal lobectomies can be carried out, because bilateral temporal resections induce permanent amnesia. Two approaches are adopted:
  - *Standard resection ('en bloc'):* removal of the hippocampus, half of the amydala and most of the anterior temporal neocortex. Measured from the temporal pole, the resection can extend as far as 6cm on the non-dominant hemisphere for speech. On the dominant hemisphere, it should not extend further than 4cm, and should spare the posterior half of the superior temporal gyrus, in order to minimize postoperative speech deficits.
  - *'Tailored resection'* whose limits are defined according to pre- and intraoperative intracranial EEG recordings.
- *Selective amygdalohippocampectomy:* removal of the amygdala, hippocampus and parahippocampal gyrus. For patients with seizures arising in these structures, it may induce less memory deficits than temporal lobectomy and, consequently, some centres offer this operation in patients with memory lateralized to the side where surgery is proposed (i.e. in patients who show low memory scores on the amytal test when injecting the side of the proposed surgery).
- *Extratemporal resections (sublobar, lobar, or multilobar):* no anatomically standardized procedures are available. Resections are tailored according to MRI and EEG findings (often requiring invasive intracranial recordings and intraoperative electrocorticography).

Radiosurgery ('gamma knife')

Destruction of epileptogenic tissue by radiation concentrated on imaging defined targets. Its safety and efficacy is not clearly established. Good results have been claimed on mesial temporal sclerosis, cavernous hemangiomata, and hypothalamic hamartomas. Stereotactic seed implantations optimized by intracranial EEG recordings have also been used.

Hemispherectomy or hemispherotomy

Removal or isolation of most of the diseased hemisphere. This is indicated when seizures arise from a large region of one hemisphere that is grossly damaged and dysfunctional. It is essentially restricted to patients with long-standing unilateral hemispheric disease, preferably since early childhood, with severe hemiparesis, and partial seizures arising only from the damaged hemisphere. On the whole, there should be no evidence of structural contralateral damage. The EEG often shows bilateral dysfunction, often with most epileptiform discharges on the healthy side—the diseased side being perhaps so damaged that the amplitude of discharges is small.

Hemispherectomy consists of the removal of one cerebral hemisphere, sparing the basal ganglia. Hemispherectomy is a major neurosurgical procedure often requiring blood transfusion and a stay in the intensive care unit. Postoperative complications may include hydrocephalus, subdural haematoma, and superficial cerebral haemosiderosis with consequent hydrocephalus. Hemosiderosis may occur many years after surgery and consists of a dementing illness with blood products deposited on the brain surface. It is thought to result from repeated minor injury to the remaining brain occupying a cavity much larger than required. Various modifications to the operation have been employed to reduce this risk, such as Adams' modification (leaving an extradural rather than a subdural space), culminating in the hemispherotomy in which the hemisphere cortex remains in situ but is completely disconnected from the opposite hemisphere and deep nuclei. Hemispherotomy has become more common than hemispherectomy, as it include less blood loss, which is an obvious advantage, particularly in children, and it requires less operating time.

Functional procedures

- *Callosotomy:* section of the corpus callosum. It prevents interhemispheric spread of seizures, decreasing the risk of falling and associated injury. Sectioning is often restricted to the anterior two-thirds of the corpus callosum to prevent disconnection syndrome (□ see Complications of Callosotomy, p.442). This can result in impaired speech function and some subtle alteration in the ability to integrate sensory input managed by the two hemispheres. It is a palliative procedure that prevents generalization of seizures. It is indicated in patients with seizures associated with sudden fall and frequent injuries (the so called 'drop attacks', which can be tonic or atonic seizures). Most of these patients have symptomatic generalized epilepsy. The EEG usually shows bilaterally synchronous epileptiform discharges. If focal abnormalities are seen resection should be considered.

- *Multiple subpial transection:* multiple parallel transections of the cortex are carried out perpendicular to the cortical surface at <5mm spacing. The purpose is to divide the cortex into small islands to prevent seizure spread without affecting function, since section of horizontal fibres produces no deficit. This blocks propagation of seizures and discharges across the cortex without compromising cortical function which is organized in a columnar fashion (📖 see Surround inhibition, p.20). Sections should be carried out perpendicular to the surface and transversely across each gyrus under the pia to avoid severing blood supply. It blocks local epileptogenesis but it is considered less effective in controlling seizures than resective surgery. It is indicated in patients with seizures arising from areas where resection would cause an unacceptable functional deficit (motor, sensory, and speech areas). Results are less satisfactory than resection of the relevant cortex in terms of seizure outcome but the technique is associated with a low risk of major neurological deficit. Subtle deficits, especially of a sensory nature are common however. It has also been used to treat acquired aphasia in patients with Landau–Kleffner syndrome.

- *Vagus nerve stimulation:* intermittent stimulation of the left vagus nerve in the neck. Its mechanism of action is unclear. It is a palliative procedure only, to be considered if resective surgery has been excluded as an option. In essence, it is associated with close to 50% seizure reduction in 50% of patients, and some improvement in seizure severity. Effects may take weeks or months to appear. It is associated with few side effects, including voice distortion when the stimulator is on. It is contraindicated in the presence of dysphagia.
- *Deep brain stimulation with electrical currents:* this is still experimental. Several sites have been or are being tested: midthalamic nuclei, subthalamic nuclei, centromedial nuclei, substantia nigra, mesial temporal structures, lesions. Optimal stimulation sites and protocols are yet to be determined. This may be considered if resective surgery has been excluded.

Summary of general surgical strategy

- Focal seizures arising unilaterally from a localized resectable area: focal/lobar resection.
- Frequent seizures with unilateral onset associated with unilateral widespread cortical damage and hemiplegia: hemispherectomy or hemispherotomy.
- Focal seizures arising from motor, sensory or speech areas (non-resectable areas): multiple subpial transaction.
- Drop attacks (atonic or tonic seizures) associated with sudden falls inducing multiple injuries: callosotomy or vagus nerve stimulation.
- If none of these is applicable, or other strategies have failed: vagus nerve stimulation or cerebral stimulation with electrical currents.
- Lesional radiosurgery is an experimental alternative to focal resection at present.

Outcome from surgery

When evaluating the outcome of surgery for the treatment of epilepsy, seizure control is commonly emphasized. Nevertheless, the degree of seizure control should be balanced against the risks of the neurological and neuropsychiatric deficits after surgery. Ultimately, the success or failure of surgery must be determined by its overall effects on daily activities and the patient's sense of well being.

Outcome with respect to seizure control

As in the case of medical treatment, assessment of the efficacy of surgery is complicated by the fact that the frequency and severity of seizures can spontaneously fluctuate widely.

After surgery, seizure control should be assessed periodically, initially every 6 months and later once a year, depending on the patient's response to treatment. A number of patients will have a relatively long seizure-free period after surgery, but seizures can reappear years later. Several variables related to seizure control should be assessed: seizure frequency, seizure severity and duration, ictal incontinence, presence of an aura that provides an opportunity to avoid injury or embarrassment.

There is often concern on the reliability of accounts based on patient's reports. Some patients might be unwilling to admit to themselves or to their physicians that seizures are still occurring. Other patients may be psychosocially dependant on their seizures, causing patients to report seizures when they are seizure free or to develop psychogenic seizures. Relatives and other witnesses should be involved, and a detailed account should be obtained on whether the nature of the seizures has changed since surgery. Sometimes, postoperative video monitoring might be necessary to establish the nature of the attacks.

A number of scales have been proposed to quantify the benefits of post-surgical seizure control. Perhaps the most widely used is that shown in Box 4c.3, proposed by Engel.[1] This scale has the advantage of combining seizure control with a degree of impact on quality of life.

It is generally agreed that the best seizure control is obtained after lesionectomies and temporal resections, which usually include the hippocampus and part of the amygdala. Nearly 70% of patients become seizure free after temporal lobectomy or amygdalohippocampectomy, a result only matched by lesionectomy and hemispherectomy. After callosotomy few patients become seizure free but many improve, as would be expected from a palliative procedure. A summary of outcome expected for different procedures is shown in Table 4c.1.[1]

It is important to note that 'seizure-free' applies only to the period for which the patient has been followed up. A recent large study suggested that of patients who had enjoyed 1 year seizure free following temporal lobe surgery, 36% would suffer at least one more seizure in the next decade.

Box 4c.3 Classifications of postoperative outcome[1]

Class I: free of disabling seizures (excludes early postoperative seizures during the first few weeks).
- A. Completely seizure-free since surgery.
- B. Non-disabling simple partial seizures only since surgery.
- C. Some disabling seizures after surgery, but free of disabling seizures for at least 2 years.
- D. Generalized convulsion with AED withdrawal only.

Class II: rare disabling seizures ('almost seizure-free').
- A. Initially free of disabling seizures but has rare seizures now.
- B. Rare disabling seizures since surgery.
- C. More than rare disabling seizures after surgery, but rare seizures for at least 2 years.
- D. Nocturnal seizures only.

Class III: worthwhile improvement.
- A. Worthwhile seizure reduction.
- B. Prolonged seizure-free intervals amounting to greater than half the follow-up period, but not less than 2 years.

Class IV: no worthwhile improvement (determination of "worthwhile improvement" will require quantitative analysis of additional data such as percent of seizure reduction, cognitive function, and quality of life)
- A. Significant seizure reduction.
- B. No appreciable change.
- C. Seizures worse.

Table 4c.1 Outcome expected for different procedures

Procedure	Seizure free	Improved	Not improved	Number of patients
Temporal lobectomy	67.9%	24%	8.1%	3579
Amygdalohippocampectomy	68.8%	22.3%	9%	413
Lesionectomy	66.6%	21.5%	11.9%	293
Extratemporal resections	45.1%	35.2%	19.8%	805
Multilobar resections	45.2%	35.5%	19.3%	166
Hemispherectomy	67.4%	21.1%	11.6%	190
Callosotomy	7.6%	60.9%	31.4%	563

*Data from Engel Jr J, vanNess P, Rasmussen T, *et al.* (1993). Outcome with respect to seizures. In *Surgical Treatment of the Epilepsies*, 2nd edn. Engel Jr J (ed.), Raven Press, Ltd. New York.

Complications from surgery

Complications of electrode implantation have been described in 📖 Complications of intracranial electrodes, p.430.

Epilepsy surgery may involve the removal or sectioning of tissue which is functional. Thus, it might be associated with neurological, psychiatric, and neuropsychological deficits, in addition to the general complications of neurosurgery under general anaesthesia.

A distinction must be made between complications and expected deficits. For instance, hemiplegia is a deficit that occurs after hemispherectomy as a trade off for improving seizure control. It can hardly be considered a complication of surgery. Complications can occur in a proportion of patients, and measures should be taken to minimize the risk of these occurring. For instance, speech deficits can occur after temporal lobectomy, which can be minimized by adjusting the extent of the resection on the dominant side.

The general complications of major neurosurgical procedures include: infection, haematoma, vascular compromise, brain oedema, hydrocephalus, brain injury, and death. Epilepsy can result from any brain surgery and it is probable that some cases of late failure of epilepsy surgery relate to this issue.

The specific complications of different procedures are summarized here:

Complications of temporal lobectomy: transient hemiparesis (4%), permanent hemiparesis (2%), mild superior visual field defects usually undetected by patients (50%), severe visual field defects such as quadrantanopsia or hemianopia (2–4%), mortality (0% in recent series), infection (<0.5%), epidural hematoma (<0.5%), transient 3rd cranial nerve palsy (<0.1%), transitory naming problems (>20%), persistent dysphasia (1–3%), global memory deficits (1%), transitory psychosis or depression (2–20%, more likely after right temporal lobectomy). Visual defects are due to disruption of optic radiation fibres in the roof of the temporal horn of the lateral ventricle. Such disruption can be due to direct sectioning when entering the ventricle to expose the hippocampus or to vascular injury during resection of medial temporal structures.

Complications of selective amygdalohippocampectomy: it has been claimed that selective amygdalohippocampectomy induces less memory deficits than temporal lobectomy, particularly verbal deficits in dominant hemisphere surgery. Data is not consistent on this point however, and some recent data has actually shown the converse. This aspect remains controversial. Most series show a very similar outcome and complication profile to temporal lobectomy.

Complications of frontal resections: dysphasia due to resection or infarction of Broca's area is the most common complication. Broca's area tends to occupy the posterior 2.5cm of the inferior frontal gyrus in the dominant hemisphere. Nevertheless, due to the variable location of Broca's area, functional mapping might be necessary. Transitory aphasia is frequently elicited when resections are carried to within 1.5cm of areas detected by functional mapping.

Complications of central (peri-Rolandic) resections: resection of the motor cortex is associated with transitory or permanent paralysis of the corresponding muscle group. Face and lower limb paralysis are often transitory or partially recover. Resections of the hand area invariably generates a permanent highly disabling deficit of fine motor control and should be avoided if the hand is functional preoperatively. Resections involving the somatosensory cortex are associated with sensory deficits of tactile and joint position discrimination. Functional mapping is mandatory if a central resection is contemplated. Rarely, resections involving the supplementary motor cortex may result in paucity of volitional movements and mutism for 6 weeks to 3 months.

Complications of parietal resections: large parietal resections in the non-dominant hemisphere have a low risk of hemiparesis (0.5%). Very occasionally patients show a degree of contralateral neglect. In the dominant hemisphere, speech mapping might be necessary. Resections involving the parietal operculum may be associated with contralateral inferior visual field defects and more rarely hemianopia.

Complications of occipital resections: the main complication is contralateral homonymous hemianopia. Thus, if vision is intact preoperatively, calcarine cortex and optic radiations should be spared if possible. Resections above or below the calcarine fissure can induce contralateral inferior or superior quadrantanopia.

Complications of hemispherectomy: candidates for hemispherectomy are usually already hemiplegic. The procedure induces little further motor deficit provided that prehensile hand, fine finger movement, and foot tapping are absent preoperatively. In some circumstances, a hemianopia may be an inevitable but acceptable complication. The original anatomical (complete) hemsipherectomy involved removal of most of the cerebral hemisphere with the exception of the basal ganglia, hypothalamus, and diencephalon. This procedure removes large amounts of brain tissue and leaves large dead space in the operated hemicranium. Postoperatively, patients are vulnerable to minor head trauma, repeated haemorrhages, obstructive hydrocephalus, and subdural haematoma. They can suffer superficial cerebral haemosiderosis characterized by insidious neurological deterioration (somnolence, tremor, ataxia, headache) and increased intracranial pressure. Because this severe complication was common (20–35%), the procedure has been repeatedly modified. Subtotal or functional hemispherectomy combines a large central and temporal resection with deafferentation of frontal, occipital, and parasagittal cortices, which are left in situ with intact blood supply. This procedure has fewer complications.

Complications of callosotomy: this procedure, used to treat drop attacks, shows a number of direct surgical complications such as frontal brain swelling and infarction, left hemiplegia, hydrocephalus, and meningitis. Many of these complications are relatively common (10%) and may arise from retraction of the hemispheres in order to expose the corpus callosum. They can be minimized by staged callosal divisions and by restricting section to the anterior two-thirds of the corpus callosum, although it has been claimed that this may compromise seizure control. In addition, there are complications directly derived from severing the corpus callosum:

- *Acute disconnection syndrome*: usually transitory (days to weeks) and characterized by decreased speech or mutism, left apraxia or hemiparesis (leg more than arm), left hemineglect, increased focal motor seizures, and occasionally urgency and incontinence.
- *Posterior (sensory) disconnection syndrome*: posterior section of the corpus callosum isolates the language dominant hemisphere from contralateral sensory information. These patients cannot name objects exclusively presented to the non-dominant hemisphere, such as those placed in the non-dominant hand or tachistoscopically presented to the non-dominant visual hemifield. In normal life, this syndrome is not clinically disabling due to bihemispheric sensory input.
- *Split brain syndrome*: complete disconnection of both hemispheres may be disabling in 3–5% of patients who suffer disordered speech initiation, unresponsiveness of the non-dominant hand to verbal commands that may act antagonistically to the other hand, inability to pursue multiple strategies simultaneously, forgetfulness, inattention. In most cases it is transitory (months).

Withdrawal of AEDs after surgery

There is still no agreement as to when to withdraw AED medication in patients who remain seizure-free after surgery. In those with polytherapy, medication is simplified. Risk factors for seizure recurrence after withdrawal have not been determined. Patients, including those who are driving, are often reluctant to stop medication. Pragmatically, it is often considered that at least 2 years of seizure freedom should elapse before gradual medication withdrawal is contemplated and discussed with the patient. There is a risk of occurrence of convulsive seizures. In seizure-free children, medication withdrawal should be tried before adolescence, when patients are not driving and recurrence of seizures is less likely to cause embarrassment or injury.

Employment

- Rehabilitation of the individual after epilepsy surgery is important.
- Controlled studies have shown that the chances of obtaining employment and the quality of employment improve after surgery.

References

1. Engel Jr J, vanNess P, Rasmussen T, *et al.* (1993). Outcome with respect to seizures. In *Surgical Treatment of the Epilepsies*, 2nd edn. Engel Jr J (ed.), Raven Press, Ltd. New York.

Surgical treatment of epilepsy in children

There is no minimum age at which a child may come to surgery. The range of surgical candidates in childhood epilepsy is wide, wider than may be seen within the adult population. The general principle remains the same: the primary aim to alleviate seizures by removal of functionally silent responsible cortex. This may involve a focal resection, multilobar resection or even hemispherectomy in selected cases. However there is no benefit to waiting should there be evidence a child may be a surgical candidate. Evidence suggests that early cessation of seizures is more likely to optimize developmental outcome.

Early onset epilepsy that fails to respond to AED medication is uniformly associated with poor neurodevelopmental outcome.

Differences between adult and paediatric population coming to surgery

- Semiology of seizures often unclear, e.g. automatisms often immature in the very young.
- Ictal EEG recording may be bilateral in the presence of unilateral pathology.
- Imaging may change over the first few years of life—developmental lesions may 'emerge' whereas others may 'disappear' as myelination becomes complete.
- Likely significant degree of learning difficulties in children coming to surgery; no evidence this ultimately influences seizure outcome.
- High rate of behaviour disorder as classified by DSM IV criteria.
- Greater proportion of hemispherectomy/multilobar resection as opposed to temporal or focal extratemporal resection.

Selection of surgical candidates—who should be assessed?

- Children with focal epilepsy resistant to an appropriate trial of AED medication—adult criteria of at least 2 years inappropriate in the very young.
- Seizures arise from functionally silent area of the brain.
- Children with epilepsy associated with congenital hemiplegia, and structurally abnormal contralateral hemisphere.
- Children with persistent drop attacks failing to respond to medication.

All children presenting in the first 2 years of life with a localized or lateralized brain lesion should be referred for assessment since it is likely they will fail AED medication.

What is the likely underlying pathology?

Developmental malformations are by far the most common pathology for which surgery is performed—usually with lobar, multilobar operations, or hemispherectomy. Benign tumours then take up a significant proportion, followed by various other pathologies such as hippocampal sclerosis, ischaemic insults, and Rasmussen's encephalitis.

Pathologies in surgery for epilepsy in children

- Developmental malformations:
  - Focal cortical dysplasia.
  - Hemimegalencephaly.
- Benign tumours:
  - Dysembryoplastic neuro epithelial tumours.
  - Gangliogliomas.
- Hippocampal sclerosis.
- Rasmussen's encephalitis.

Presurgical evaluation—what does it entail?

The aims of the presurgical evaluation, as in adults, are to determine whether seizures arise from one area, and whether that area can be removed without detriment in function to the individual. Investigations are aimed to be as non-invasive as possible, although in a selected number of children invasive EEG recording will be required to delineate the seizure focus in relation to areas of eloquent cortex.

Differences in children to adults include:

- Initial review with regard to localization of seizure onset/abnormal area of brain:
  - Clinical review.
  - Inter-ictal EEG recording.
  - Optimized MRI including volumetric sequences.
- Subsequent investigation:
  - Video EEG to document seizures for localization of onset.
  - Functional imaging such as ictal/inter-ictal SPECT or FDG PET.
- Further evaluation to determine localization of function:
  - Full neuropsychology/neurodevelopmental assessment.
  - Functional MRI for language and/or motor function.

The range of children coming to assessment is wide. Many have significant learning difficulties and/or behavioural problems. Surgery will always be guided toward seizure relief. Gains in cognitive ability or improvement in behaviour profile, although they do occur, can never be guaranteed. It is important that the aims of surgery are explained and discussed. A full neuropsychiatric evaluation, where appropriate, is therefore recommended as part of any surgery programme.

When all the required information has been gathered, a full discussion is undertaken within a multidisciplinary meeting and a decision made about whether surgery can be offered with an assessment of likely benefit and risk.

What is the likely outcome of surgery?

The outcome with regard to seizure relief in children is directly related to the underlying pathology, and the extent of resection that has been achieved (📖 see Box 4c.4). Functional outcome relates to the likelihood of there being useful function in the tissue removed, which is unlikely in the majority. Children with congenital hemiplegia with no fine finger movement on the affected side and epilepsy onset under 5 years are unlikely to see deterioration in function following hemispherectomy; visual field defect (hemianopia) is inevitable if not already present. The functional outcome from focal resection will be related to the area to be resected, and full presurgical evaluation will allow for prediction or estimation of risk of deficit. Overall the premise is that the early cessation of seizures will lead to improved developmental outcome. This has been difficult to prove. However, it is likely that IQ is preserved allowing a developmental trajectory which may not have occurred should seizures have continued. Studies of children undergoing temporal lobe resection have suggested that children show a greater rate in recovery from any inflicted memory deficit than adults.

Box 4c.4 Rates of seizure freedom following surgery in children

- Hemispherectomy:
  - Malformations   37–58%
  - Vascular/acquired   67–88%
- Temporal resection   60–78%

Women's issues

Many aspects included in this chapter are discussed in more detail in other chapters. An overview is presented here, focussing on questions frequently asked by patients.

Epilepsy, contraception, and pregnancy

- It is essential that all women with epilepsy who are of childbearing age receive advice on epilepsy and pregnancy. Emphasize the advantages of a planned pregnancy. Start in the teenage years and reinforce all information regularly as pregnancy may be unplanned. Give specific preconception advice if a woman is planning a pregnancy.
- Give broad advice about commonly asked questions. Then tailor advice to the individual depending on their clinical state and drug regimen.
- Remember you are treating the woman first and foremost—not potential pregnancies

Will my tablets affect the pill?

The combined oral contraceptive pill can be used as an effective method of contraception for women taking valproate, gabapentin, levetiracetam, tiagabine, pregabalin, and zonisamide. More detailed information may be found in section ▢ Antiepileptic medication and contraception, pp.364–368, and in sections addressing individual drugs in Chapter 4b.

Effectiveness of the combined oral contraceptive pill is reduced by enzyme-inducing drugs e.g. carbamazepine, oxcarbazepine, phenytoin, primidone, and phenobarbital.

- Ideally offer other forms of contraception e.g. intra-uterine device (IUD) or depo-progesterone (though note warning from the Committee on Safety of Medicines on 10 Nov 2004 regarding loss of bone mineral density).[1]
- If using the combined oral contraceptive pill, prescribe a combination of pills with 50mcg oestrogen content, while recommending additional barrier methods of contraception for the time being. If there is breakthrough bleeding, increase the dose of oestrogen initially to 75mcg, then 100mcg if needed.
- Some recommend tricycling the pill (taking three packs consecutively without a break) and advise a shorter, 4 day, break between cycles of pill-taking.

Women on enzyme-inducing anti-epileptic medication taking the combined oral contraceptive pill (even at higher dose) are at increased risk of contraceptive failure and unexpected pregnancy.

Levels of lamotrigine can be reduced by the contraceptive pill. Thus, introduction of the contraceptive pill can in certain cases cause loss of seizure control and require increased doses of lamotrigine.

What other contraceptives can I use?

- The progesterone-only oral contraceptive and progesterone implants are not recommended because progesterone metabolism is increased by enzyme-inducing AEDs.
- The Depo-Provera® injection has been found to be effective. Some recommend it every 10 weeks for patients taking enzyme-inducing AEDs (see CSM Advice[1]). Medroxyprogesterone acetate (Depo-Provera®) is used with caution due to the potential risk of reduction in bone mineral denisty.
- IUD is a very effective form of contraception and is not affected by any AEDs. The Mirena® coil is probably the best option. This is only to be used as a last resort in women who have not had children due to risk of pelvic inflammatory disease and ectopic pregnancy.
- Contraceptive patches (Evra®) and the vaginal ring which releases oestrogen progesterone are not indicated if a woman is taking enzyme-inducing drugs.

Emergency contraception can be used as normal except for those on enzyme-inducing drugs who should take a higher dose: 1.5mg levonorgestrel followed by 1.5mg 12 hours later. This use of levonorgestrel is unlicensed; a copper-containing IUD is a possible alternative.

Will my fertility be affected?

There is some evidence that women with epilepsy have a slightly lower fertility rate than the normal population.

This is thought to be related to multiple factors including:

- Women with epilepsy being anxious about having children due to the potential effects of their AEDs on the unborn child.
- Difficulties with forming and maintaining relationships.
- The effect of AEDs on fertility and sexual function.
- Reproductive endocrine disorders—more common among patients with epilepsy than the general population.

Will AEDs affect my baby?

The association between AEDs and fetal malformations has been evident for many years but it is only relatively recently that large-scale prospective registers have been set up. It is hoped that these registers will allow for management decisions in this context to be based on more robust data than has hitherto been available. Women with epilepsy taking AEDs have an increased risk of having a child with minor or major malformations (Tables 4d.1 and 4d.2). There is also an association with an adverse effect on cognition and behaviour with certain drugs particularly in polytherapy (📖 see pp.368–369).

- The background risk of a major malformation in the general population is approximately 1–2%. This is increased to between 4–9% if there is prenatal exposure to AEDs.
- The malformation rate can increase up to 15% on polytherapy.
- The recently published Belfast Pregnancy Register identified a dose-related response associated with lamotrigine and valproate.[2,3]

Women need to be aware of the risk and may consider changing AED therapy preconception. This is a significant decision which should be made with the guidance of a neurologist. Any drug change could potentially destabilize someone's epilepsy. Difficulties in making decisions relate to the limited information available on many AEDs in this regard and the sometimes conflicting aims of avoiding structural on cognitive teratogenicity, while maintaining seizure control and, thus, safety of the mother and fetus. We recommend seeking up-to-date information regarding specific AEDs and combinations, some of which should be avoided where possible. We also recommend using the lowest doses to control seizures and, empirically, splitting doses into 3 per day to minimize peak levels. Use of long acting preparations is also advised. Below is a brief overview regarding three commonly used AEDs. 📖 See Table 4d.1 and 4d.2 for malformation rates published by the UK and Pregnancy Registers. Please note that more up-to-date data has been presented at meetings but have yet to be published.

Carbamazepine

Carbamazepine has a relatively good profile in pregnancy (Table 4d.1) and is a good choice in pregnancy, if appropriate for the syndrome.

Sodium valproate

Sodium valproate, an excellent treatment for those with idiopathic generalized epilepsy, is unfortunately associated with a higher malformation rate, of 6.2 % (4.6–8.2) (Table 4d.1) and a greater risk of developmental delay in offspring although the latter observation is mainly in retrospective studies and further investigation is required. The general consensus is to avoid valproate in women of child-bearing age if there is a potentially safer alternative. The risk should be discussed with the patient. Particular caution is needed if there is a history of a previously affected pregnancy. If deemed necessary despite this risk, doses below 1000 mg/day using long acting preparations in divided doses are advised.

Lamotrigine

Lamotrigine has a relatively good profile in pregnancy, in relation to teratogenicity (Table 4d.1) at doses <400mg daily but there is a distinct rise in malformation rate with doses >400 mg once a day according to the UK epilepsy and pregnancy register. Lamotrigine levels drop in pregnancy and this can be clinically significant.

> **There remains limited data regarding most new generation drugs therefore these should be used with caution in women of childbearing age.**

Certain malformations are far more devastating than others for example a cardiac abnormality or neural tube defects carry more implications than a facial cleft or hypospadias.

For up-to-date information about pregnancy contact the UK Epilepsy and Pregnancy Register.[4]

Table 4d.1 The MCM rate by monotherapy drugs exposure[2]

Drug	Number of informative outcomes*	Number of MCMs	MCM rate (9.5% CI)	OR (95% CI)
Carbamazepine	900	20	2.2% (1.4–3.4)	1.0
Valproate	715	44	6.2% (4.6–8.2)	2.78 (1.62–4.76)
Lamotrigine	647	21	3.2% (2.1–4.9)	1.44 (0.77–2.67)
Phenytoin	82	3	3.7% (1.3–10.2)	1.64 (0.48–5.62)
Gabapentin	31	1	3.2% (0.6–16.2)	1.33 (0.17–10.20)
Topiramate	28	2	7.1% (2.0–22.6)	2.75 (0.62–12.20)
Levetiracetam*	22	0	0.0% (0.0–14.9)	–

CI, confidence interval; MCM, major congenital malformation; OR, odds ratio. *Pregnancy losses with no MCM excluded.

*More than 100 pregnancies on monotherapy with levetiracetam have been presented by the UK pregnancy register with no malformations so far.

Table 4d.2 Types of MCMs by AED[2]

Drug	Number of case	NTD	Facial cleft	Cardiac	Hypo-spadias/ GUT	GIT	Skeletal	Other
CBZ	900	2 0.2%	4 0.4%	6 0.7%	2 0.2%	2 0.2%	3 0.3%	1 0.1%
VPA	715	7 1.0%	11 1.5%	5 0.7%	9 1.3%	2 0.2%	8 1.1%	2 0.3%
LTG	647	1 0.2%	1 0.2%	4 0.6%	6 0.9%	3 0.5%	2 0.3%	4 0.6%
PHT	82	0 0.0%	1 1.2%	1 1.2%	0 0.0%	1 1.2%	0 0.0%	0 0.0%

CBZ, carbamazepine; GUT, genitourinary tract; GIT, gastrointestinal tract defects; LTG, lamotrigine; NTD, neural tube defect; PHT, phenytoin; VPA, valproate.

Folic acid

- In the general population, folic acid supplementation has been shown to reduce the incidence of neural tube defects (NTDs). This also applies in women who have previously had an affected child (secondary prevention).
- Women in general are advised to take preconception folic acid (400mcg).
- Evidence regarding effect and specific dose in pregnancy in epilepsy is lacking. In the UK, NICE recommend that a 5mg dose should be taken preconception by women with epilepsy, and for the first trimester of pregnancy.[5]
- There is no strong evidence that folic acid exacerbates seizures.
- It has been reported that folic acid supplementation reduces spontaneous abortion in women with epilepsy on AEDs.

Effect of pregnancy on seizure control

As a general rule, women with well controlled epilepsy tend to continue with good control whereas those with more severe epilepsy can experience an exacerbation of their seizures.

A recent observational study (EURAP)[6,7] showed:
- 63.6% had unaltered seizure control.
- 15.9% had improved seizure control.
- 17.3% had worsened seizure control.
- Some authors have suggested that poor seizure control can occur as the pregnancy progresses as a result of non-adherence to treatment or change in AED serum levels.
- EURAP involved 300 collaborators from over 300 countries. The study reported 58.3% of women were seizure-free throughout pregnancy. Occurrence of any seizures was associated with localization-related epilepsy and polytherapy and for tonic–clonic seizures, with oxcarbazepine monotherapy.

Vitamin K

- Vitamin K_1 is recommended for women on enzyme-inducing drugs from 36 weeks to reduce the risk of neonatal cerebral haemorrhage.
- 10mg is given once daily. This is usually prescribed by the obstetrician.

Labour

The vast majority of women will have an uncomplicated labour and delivery.
- Approximately 2–5% of women are at increased risk of seizures during or 24 hours after labour.
- EURAP reported 3.5% of women experienced seizures during delivery; the only factor significantly associated with risk of seizures during delivery was the occurrence of seizures earlier in pregnancy.
- Delivery should occur in a medical unit.

Will my child have epilepsy?

In practice the risk of the mother's offspring developing epilepsy to a large extent depends on the classification of their epilepsy. If this is unknown, and there is no family history suggestive mendelian inheritance, one can quote a <10 % chance depending on the syndrome (see p.427).

Catamenial seizures and the menopause

Female hormones and epilepsy

The observation that hormones affect seizure frequency has been recognized for many years.

Catamenial epilepsy

- True catamenial epilepsy is defined as at least 75% or more of the total number of seizures occurring within the 4 days before and after 6 days the onset of menstruation. Where this possibility is raised, a seizure/menstruation diary should be kept to confirm it.
- Often women report a strong relationship between seizures and menstruation but this is often not confirmed if a diary is kept.

Treatment

- Clobazam, 10mg once or twice per day for a few days each month, depending on case.
- Acetaozolamide perimenstrually may be useful if clobazam fails.

Menopause

- The effect of the menopause on a woman's epilepsy is unclear. Further studies are required but currently the major risk appears to be an increased risk of bone demineralization, particularly affecting women taking enzyme-inducing AEDs. (📖 see Bone health and AEDs, pp.356–358).
- There is no current contraindication for the use of combined hormone replacement therapy in epilepsy, but there may be other general contraindications. Efficacy of oral preparations is reduced in those on enzyme-inducing drugs.

Chapter 5

Seizures in special circumstances/syndromes

Seizures in the intensive care unit (ICU)

In comatose patients, the following questions regarding seizures often arise:

- Is non-convulsive status epilepticus the cause of the patient's coma?
- If the comatose patient suffers odd movements, are they seizures?
- Is status epilepticus under control?

Diagnosis of seizures can be complicated because many causes of coma can also cause seizures and, conversely, non-convulsive status epilepticus can manifest as unresponsiveness (see Non-convulsive status epilepticus, pp.199–203.)

Four general rules are useful in this scenario:

- If the patient is not sedated and lies unresponsive and immobile for long periods (minutes or hours), he/she is unlikely to be suffering non-convulsive status epilepticus.
- If the comatose patient (other than neonate) suffers sporadic, subtle, small or jerky movements or blinks, they are unlikely of be due to seizures unless there are also clear manifestations of seizures (convulsions, tonic movements, automatisms, eye deviation, confusion, clear myoclonic jerks).
- Conversely, repetitive and continuous regular movements such as continuous repetitive blinking or focal jerking can be a manifestation of status epilepticus.
- An urgent EEG is of paramount importance to establish the diagnosis of status epilepticus, but is less useful in establishing the ictal nature of subtle sporadic movements.

EEG diagnosis of status epilepticus is always an emergency and requires skilled recording and immediate interpretation at the bedside. If status epilepticus is diagnosed, discussion with the ICU team will help in planning intravenous therapy under continuous or intermittent EEG control to guide therapeutic management.

In the ICU, status epilepticus can occur in the context of two different situations:

- Patients with a history of epilepsy, or as the first manifestation of epilepsy—status epilepticus de novo.
- Patients who develop seizures in the context of a major medical or surgical acute emergency—encephalitis, meningitis, post-traumatic coma, post-neurosurgery, metabolic coma, post-anoxic coma, etc. In this context, seizures may prove slow to respond to AEDs and may also require concomitant treatment of the underlying condition.

Regardless of the underlying aetiology, the EEG in comatose patients typically shows slow or flattened background activity, sometimes with periods of flattening alternating with periods of fast activity every few seconds—an EEG pattern called burst-suppression.

Occasionally, epileptiform discharges are also seen. In acute disorders—encephalitis, cardiac arrest, metabolic disturbance, etc.—three distinct patterns of epileptiform discharges can be observed:

- Irregular slowing of background activity with superimposed epileptiform discharges or burst suppression patterns. This is commonly seen in the ICU in the absence of epilepsy or status epilepticus, and should not be misinterpreted as status epilepticus.

- Repetitive discharges in patients with status epilepticus.
- Bursts of repetitive epileptiform discharges or continuous discharges in patients without any clinical evidence of status epilepticus (electrographic status epilepticus). This might be due to the presence of non-convulsive status epilepticus masked by sedation.

Seizures in post-anoxic coma are often myoclonic and sometimes stimulus sensitive, usually associated with generalized discharges in the context of a low amplitude or flattened EEG background.

In general, it is essential to treat status epilepticus urgently regardless of whether it occurs in the context of a seizure disorder or an acute illness, in order to avoid brain damage or death. Response to treatment and outcome are worse the longer the delay in treatment. Outcome is influenced to a range degree by underlying pathology.

Epilepsy and learning disability

A learning disability (LD) involves a significant deficit in cognition, communication, self-care, and social interaction. The criteria may vary, but generally those with an IQ of 70 or below are categorized in the UK as having a diagnosis of LD.

- About 30% of patients with severe-to-moderate mental disabilities also have epilepsy.
- Approximately 50% of those with severe LD (IQ <50) develop epilepsy.

Diagnosis in this group of patients can be fraught with difficulties:

- *Communication:* those with a physical and/or intellectual impairment may have difficulties communicating effectively which will have an impact on the following:
  - Obtaining a clear medical history.
  - Obtaining a clear description of events and their frequency.
  - Monitoring treatment and adverse side effects.
- *Risk of neuroleptic or drug induced seizures:* this is uncommon, but a full history of past and recent medication, particularly those prescribed by psychiatrist colleagues, is essential
- *Concurrent illness:* often these patients may have multiple health needs and there is a large potential differential diagnosis.
- *Difficulties with performing investigations:* depending on the degree of LD one must balance the risk–benefit ratio of performing diagnostic tests, and whether anesthesia or sedation for this purpose is justified (Table 5.1).
- *Limited information:* if there are frequent changes in carers.
- *Stereotypic behaviour:* may be mistaken for epilepsy.

Although often easily recognizable, epilepsy may take unusual forms and pose diagnostic difficulties in the mentally disabled, particularly when widespread cerebral damage is present. Multiple seizure types may be present, and non-epileptic events may resemble seizures. Some seizure types are more frequent in patients with learning difficulties. These include atonic and tonic seizures, atypical absence seizures, and myclonus. Stereotypies are common and can be mistaken for seizures. In addition, nonspecific inter-ictal EEG abnormalities are frequent in the mentally disabled, even in the absence of epilepsy, often showing diffuse slowing, multifocal background abnormalities, multifocal sharp waves and frank spikes, and even generalized or widespread sharp waves. It is therefore important that an abnormal inter-ictal EEG should not be misinterpreted as evidence that behavioural disturbances are of epileptic nature.

Table 5.1 Investigation difficulties in LD

Investigation	Difficulties/risks
Neuroimaging	Often those with significant LD cannot tolerate CT or MRI scans, e.g. some patients may require sedation or general anesthetic which may pose a risk. The benefit must be balanced against the risk to the patient
EEG	Some patients may not tolerate an EEG and pull electrodes off. A specially made electrode cap may be useful.
Blood tests	Some patients will not tolerate blood tests. Saliva and hair testing is useful for monitoring AED but are generally not widely or easily available.

Differential diagnosis

The following can be misdiagnosed as seizures in this population (☐ also see Box 5.1):

- Repetitive stereotyped motor behaviours.
- Episodes of self-gratification.
- Apnoea.
- Hyperpnoea.
- Psychogenic non-epileptic attacks.
- Cardiac disorders.

Box 5.1 Practical tips for taking a history

- Ensure that, where possible, a family member can attend the appointment to provide a past medical history.
- Ensure the 'key' worker or carer is at the appointment, as they are most likely to have seen recent events.
- Request an 'event' diary from day services and carers/relatives—i.e. day centre or respite centre.
- Where possible ensure the person does not have to wait too long for the consultation—these patients can get very agitated in an unfamiliar environment.
- Ensure all members of the multidisciplinary team, especially community LD nurses, are aware of consultation and copied into all clinic letters.
- Ensure where possible that the person with LD is included in the consultation—it is all too easy to talk only to the carer and relatives and not the patient.
- Consider that carer education and participation on a long-term basis is a necessary and essential component of management.

Seizures

- Often multiple seizure types. Those with LD can experience a vast range of seizure types.
- Duration of seizures may be longer than usually seen in those without learning difficulties, and protocols for rescue medication may be needed.
- Often high risk of seizure related injuries—particularly those who experience atonic or tonic clonic seizures.

AEDs and potential adverse side effects

- Once the diagnosis is secure, management principles should not differ from the general epilepsy population.
- Drugs should be introduced or withdrawn slowly. People with cerebral damage are more susceptible to drug side effects even when drug levels suggest this is not the case.
- Ensure the preparation is appropriate i.e. elixir, chewable, or sprinkle preparations. Some patients are not able to tolerate tablets.
- Assessment of adverse side effects can be difficult to monitor due to communication difficulties. As a general rule any behavioural change may indicate difficulties in tolerating a drug e.g. dizziness may manifest as irritability or reluctance to mobilize.
- Educate carers (this should include day centre/respite care staff) about risk and possible presentation of adverse side effects.
- If blood serum monitoring is not possible consider saliva testing or hair testing (these tests are only available at specialist centres)
- Provide a clear treatment plan, which is copied to all those involved in the person's care. This is essential
- If patient is drug resistant, it is likely numerous drug combinations have been tried in the past. Change AEDs with caution (Box 5.2).
- Often AEDs are blamed for behavioural problems which may pre-date initiation of drug treatment. Ensure you are certain that the drug is causing difficulties before changing an AED if the person is well controlled.
- Make management decisions in consultation and agreement of those involved.

Box 5.2 Changing AEDs

Beware that any drug change could destabilize a person's epilepsy. If there is a long history of drug resistance be cautious—sometimes a person who appears to be very poorly controlled is actually at their optimum control when compared to past seizure control. Consider asking 'If you look at Jim's seizures from birth until now… is this the best control, worst, or has he remained the same?' Ask about previous convulsive seizures and their duration, falls, or admission to hospital.

Conversely, appropriate investigations and optimal seizure control have in some cases been overlooked, because it is sometimes accepted that those with learning difficulties experience seizures, where in actual fact there is potential for improved control with AED adjustment/change.

Some syndromes commonly associated with epilepsy and LD

Angelman syndrome (happy-puppet syndrome)

A syndrome named after a British paediatrician, Dr. Harry Angelman, who first described the syndrome in 1965. The alternative term 'happy-puppet syndrome' refers to the puppet-like and happy appearance of those affected.

Characteristics
- Microcephaly.
- LD.
- Flat occiput.
- Ataxia.
- Jerky limb movements 'puppet-like movements'.
- Hyperactive behaviour.
- Characteristic smiley faces.
- Inappropriate laughter.
- Light hair and eye colour.
- Wide mouth and protruding tongue.
- Hypotonia.
- Tuning fork test.

Seizures
- Seizures occur in approximately 80–90% of children.
- Seizures usually begin within the first 3 years of life.
- Drug resistant epilepsy develops in around 50% of children.
- Seizure frequency and severity often reduce with age.

The following seizure types are seen:
- Atypical absence.
- Myoclonic including episodes of myoclonic status: hypotonia, drowsiness, and mild clonic jerking—rare after age 6 years.
- Tonic.
- Unilateral clonic.
- Complex partial with eye deviation and vomiting.

EEG

Diffuse, bi-frontally dominant usually high amplitude 1–3Hz, notched triphasic or polyphasic slow waves and sharp waves often seen in stage 3 and 4 sleep.

Treatment
- Use of valproate or ethosuximide is often successful in combination with a benzodiazepine.
- *In some cases carbamazepine can make myoclonus and absence seizures worse.*
- Genetic counselling should be offered to parents which may help predict in future offspring.

Prognosis
- Poor.
- LD and premature death.
- Most people will live into adulthood.
- Late deterioration with Parkinsonian rigidity is described.

Aicardi syndrome

A syndrome affecting females, characterized by a triad of:
- Retinal lacunae and small eyes—microphthalmia.
- Absence of the corpus callosum.
- Infantile spasms.

Seizures
- In the majority of patients, seizures occur within 3 months.
- Focal seizures may precede the first infantile spasms.
- Infantile spasms are usually asymmetrical.

EEG
Often asymmetric diffuse abnormalities, asynchronus with burst/ suppression and/or atypical hypsarrhythmia

Treatment
- Steroid treatment.
- Long-term AED therapy.
- Patients often resistant to AED and multiple combinations are tried.

Prognosis
- High mortality rate.
- Those that survive are usually affected by severe LD.

Rett's syndrome

An X-linked syndrome that is caused by sporadic mutations in the gene *MECP2* located on the X chromosome. It affects largely females.

Characteristics
- LD, screaming, inconsolable crying, avoidance of eye contact, lack of social/emotional reciprocity.
- Acquired microcephaly.
- Progressive language impairment—expressive and receptive.
- Gait apraxia.
- Loss of purposeful hand movements.
- Impairments of growth—i.e. scoliosis.
- Spasticity, tremor.
- Bruxism.
- Brainstem dysfunction and apnoea.
- Cardiac arrhythmias.
- Social withdrawal.
- Progressive physical and mental deterioration.
- The spectrum of clinical features associated with this mutation is wider than originally thought.

Usually normal development until 6 months. Categorized by 4 stages:
- Early developmental stagnation.
- Rapid regression.
- Usually over years to decades, plateau of symptoms.
- Late motor deterioration—usually wheelchair dependency

Seizures

Seizures are common, affecting up to 80% of patients, and usually devolving between the ages of 3–10 years. Common seizure types:

- Complex partial seizures.
- Atypical absences.
- Generalized tonic–clonic.
- Atonic.
- Myoclonic.

EEG

- Usually normal until approximately 2 years.
- There is diffuse slowing of the background, particularly over fronto-central regions, and focal, multifocal, or generalized epileptiform discharges.
- EEG abnormalities often deteriorate in parallel with clinical deterioration.

Treatment

- No specific treatment exists for Rett's syndrome.
- Seizure control may improve with age.
- AEDs may be required and some patients are drug resistant.

Prognosis

- Poor. Usually severe LD.
- Premature death although cases cited into middle age.

Fragile X-syndrome

Most common form of inherited LD after downs syndrome. It is a genetic disorder caused by mutation of the *FMR1* gene on the X chromosome.

Characteristics

- Hyperkinetic behaviour.
- Hypotonia.
- Large testicles—macro-orchadism—in males.
- LD.
- Autistic features.
- Dysmorphic facial features—i.e. long face, prominent forehead, large ears, and broad nose.
- Delayed language and speech.
- Affects both boys and girls although girls are less severely affected than boys.

Seizures

Occur in approximately 25–40% of boys and 5–8% of girls. Common seizures include:

- Focal motor seizures.
- Complex partial seizures.
- Secondarily generalized tonic–clonic seizures.
- Atypical absences.
- Akinetic seizures.

EEG
- Background can be normal or slow.
- Rolandic or midtemporal monophasic or diphasic spikes often increase dramatically in NREM sleep.
- Sometimes resembles benign epilepsy of childhood with centrotemporal spikes.

Treatment
- There is no treatment for fragile X except supportive treatment.
- Seizures are usually well controlled on monotherapy or first-line treatments such as sodium valproate or carbamazepine. Usually control improves with age.
- Genetic counselling to parents.

Further information
Photos of affected individuals can be seen at:
 www.fragilex.org/FragileXCommunityPictures/index.html

Down syndrome (trisomy 21)
Trisomy 21 is the most common chromosomal disorder causing a LD affecting 1 in 1000 births.

Characteristics
- LD.
- Characteristic dysmorphic facial features—i.e. flattened occiput, brachycephaly, flat nasal bridge, low set ears, and sparse hair growth.
- Small for gestational age.
- Slow growth.
- Hypotonia.
- Joint hypermobility.

Seizures
- The occurrence of seizures increases with age.
- Only 2% of children with Down syndrome experience seizures.
- The risk of seizures increases to around 25% after the age of 50 years.

Seizures commonly seen:
- Infantile spasms—in children.
- Tonic–clonic seizures.
- Myoclonic.
- Simple partial.
- Complex partial.
- Secondarily generalized tonic–clonic.
- Startle seizures.
- Reflex seizure.

EEG
- Usually normal.
- Hypsarrhythmia can be seen in those children with infantile spasms.
- Generalized spike-and-wave has been seen in those with generalized seizures and focal discharges in those with partial seizures.
- No specific EEG abnormalities exist.

Treatment
- Usually good response to treatment.
- Treatment should be chosen dependant on seizure type.
- Broad spectrum treatment is advised.

Prognosis
- Other than in those where Alzheimer's develops, there is generally a good response to drug treatment, but this depends on presentation, and epilepsy may be difficult to treat in those with early dementia.
- Usually live well into adulthood. Early dementia is common.
- Associated cardiac defect may be present.

Ring chromosome 20, ring-shaped chromosome 20, or r(20) syndrome
Ring chromosome 20 is a rare human chromosome abnormality where the two arms of chromosome 20 fuse to form a ring chromosome. This abnormality is associated with epileptic seizures, learning difficulties, and behavioural disorders. Behavioural problems vary widely from relatively minor concentration and attention difficulties to profound behavioural problems. Unlike other chromosomal syndromes with and without epilepsy, abnormal facial (dysmorphic) features are often absent.

The seizure types seen in patients with r(20) are:
- Complex partial seizures.
- Subtle nocturnal seizures.
- Nocturnal frontal lobe seizures.
- Non-convulsive status epilepticus.

The interictal EEG is usually abnormal, showing a variety of findings:
- Bursts of sharp theta waves.
- Runs of high voltage, frontally dominant slow waves and spikes-and-wave.
- Continuous spike and wave discharges during sleep similar to that seen in Lennox–Gastaut and Landau–Kleffner syndromes, which can delay the diagnosis of r(20) syndrome.

Neurocutaneous syndromes
Tuberous sclerosis, Sturge–Weber syndrome, and other neurocutaneous syndromes are described later in this chapter (📖 see Neurocutaneous syndromes, pp.470–477). They can be associated with epilepsy with or without LDs.

Social and economic aspects
The impact of having a family member with a LD is far reaching. Currently in the UK all children and adults with a LD should have access to assessment by a LD team. This multi-disciplinary team usually includes:
- Paediatric LD consultant or adult psychiatrist.
- Community nurses.
- Physiotherapy.
- Speech therapy.
- Psychologist.
- Social worker/case manager.
- Occupational therapy.

Team roles
- Usually initial assessments by two or more members of the team recommend the appropriate services.
- Funding for these services is co-ordinated by the social worker or case manager.
- Health needs are provided by the community health team.
- Daycare—i.e. respite, day centre placements—are provided by local social services.
- Social services also fund basic self-care needs—i.e. assistance with washing and dressing and practical care in the form of shopping.
- In many areas these teams have amalgamated, ensuring a more seamless service.
- Parents/carers may encounter difficulties obtaining services which can become very frustrating.

Rectal diazepam and buccal midazolam

Ensure carers have appropriate training if a client requires rectal diazepam or buccal midazolam. The JEC have developed an excellent rectal diazepam and buccal midazolam care plan.[1] The NSE provides training and buccal midazolam on general epilepsy care and rectal diazepam training.[2] Community nurses and ESN can also provide this training.

Day care services may need training to ensure that those who experience multiple and prolonged seizures are not sent home or to the local A&E department after every seizure, which can be very disruptive for the person and their family/carers. Provision of an individualized management plan can be very useful.

Social care

- Carers for adults with LDs in many cases are the elderly parents. Close monitoring is essential to ensure they can still cope with the physical and emotional demands.
- Support by the local LD team is essential with regular assessment to ensure all self care and health needs are met.
- Respite care should be provided.
- Ensure appropriate benefits are being claimed—i.e. Carers allowance, Disability Living Allowance, Free travel pass, etc.
- For those with a mild disability consider referral to supported employment scheme i.e. Shaw Trust or College course e.g. life skills courses.
- If the home setting is not appropriate, the following can be considered:
  - Warden-controlled accommodation varies from large accommodation sites containing numerous self-contained flats to small units within a house taking only 2–3 persons.
  - Specialist residential homes for those with severe epilepsy (☐ see Residential care and special centres of epilepsy, pp.548–550).

Special equipment

- Various seizure alarms including bed wetting and movement alarms exist—see Epilepsy Action and NSE websites.[2,3]
- Also the NHS will provide funding for protective head wear (helmets). Contact local occupational therapy departments for manufactures.

Contacts

- British Institute for Learning Disability: ⌂ www.bild.org.uk
- Foundation for People with Learning Disabilities:
  ⌂ www.learningdisabilities.org.uk
- Mencap: ⌂ www.mencap.org
- NSE LD booklet: ⌂ www.epilepsynse.org.uk
- Epilepsy Action LD booklet: ⌂ www.epilepsy.org.uk
- The Shaw Trust: ⌂ www.shaw-trust.org.uk

References

1. ⌂ www.jec.com—website of the Joint Epilepsy Council

2. ⌂ www.epilepsynse.com—website of the National Society for *Epilepsy*

3. ⌂ www.epilepsy.org.uk—website of Epilepsy Action

Neurocutaneous syndromes

- Skin and nervous system have a common embryological origin, and consequently there are a family of developmental conditions that preferentially affect both tissues—the so called *neurocutaneous syndromes*.
- The most common neurocutaneous syndromes associated with epilepsy are *tuberous sclerosis* and *Sturge–Weber syndrome*.
- Neurofibromatosis and epidermal nervus syndrome are less commonly associated with epilepsy.

Tuberous sclerosis—Bourneville disease, epiloia

Genetics

- Two genetic loci, on tumour suppression genes, *TSC1* and *TSC2* code for the proteins hamartin and tuberin respectively. In about one-fifth of those affected, the locus has not been found.
- *Prevalence:* 1 in 9700 individuals.
- *Inheritance:* sporadic mutation or autosomal dominant with 100% penetrance but wide range of expressivity.
- Normal parents of affected individuals should be tested for the disease with:
  - Physical examination, including skin examination with Wood's lamp and fundoscopy after pupil dilation.
  - MRI of head.
  - Renal ultrasound.
- If neither parent is affected, the risk of tuberous sclerosis in the next child is the same as in the general population.
- If either parent has the disease, the risk is 50%.

Clinical manifestations

- The classic Vogt triad (seizures, LDs, and facial angiofibroma) is seen in 29% of patients.
- Facial angiofibroma (adenoma sebaceum) is a nodular brown rash over the face—nasolabial folds, nose, cheeks and infraorbital regions (Fig. 5.1).
- Other associated abnormalities (which are *major diagnostic criteria*) include:
  - Facial angiofibroma.
  - Periungual fibroma.
  - Hypomelanotic macules—'ash leaf' spots.
  - Cortical tubers.
  - Shagreen patches.
  - Subependymal nodules.
  - Subependymal giant cell astrocytoma.
  - Multiple retinal hamartomas.
  - Multiple renal angiomyolipomas.
  - Lymphangiomyomatosis.
  - Cardiac rhabdomyoma.

Other less common findings (*minor diagnostic criteria*) are:
- Multiple randomly distributed pits in dental enamel.
- Hamartomatous rectal polyps.
- Bone cysts.
- Cerebral white-matter 'migration tracts'.

- Gingival fibromas.
- Nonrenal hamartoma.
- Retinal achromic patch.
- 'Confetti' skin lesions.
- Multiple renal cysts.

Other manifestations with diagnostic value include:
- Infantile spasms in 80%.
- Single retinal hamartoma.
- Subependymal or cortical calcifications.
- Bilateral renal angiomyolipomas or cysts.
- History of tuberous sclerosis in first-degree relative.

The following levels of *diagnostic certainty* have been described:
- *Definite:* either two major features or one major feature plus two minor features.
- *Probable:* one major plus one minor feature.
- *Suspect:* either one major feature or two or more minor features.

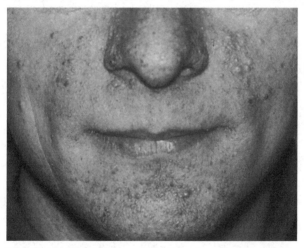

Fig. 5.1 Facial angiofibroma (adenoma sebaceum) in a patient with tuberous sclerosis and well-controlled complex partial seizures. (Reproduced with permission from Smith DF, Appleton RE, MacKenzie JM, *et al.* (eds.) (1998). *An Atlas of Epilepsy*. The Parthenon Publishing Group, New York and London.)

Neuroimaging (Fig. 5.2)

- Mainly cortical tubers and subependymal nodules. Histologically they are hamartomas
- Neuroimaging and neuropathological features of tubers are similar to those of focal cortical dysplasia, but are often multiple.
- Subependymal nodules are usually multiple, located along the ventrical surface of the caudate nucleus.
- Giant cell tumours can grow around foramen of Monroe—may induce hydrocephalus.
- 15% also have cerebellar tubers.
- Ventricular dilatation is common.
- Cortical heterotopia—islands of cortex within white matter—can also be seen, suggesting that tuberous sclerosis is a dysplastic process.
- Subependymal giant cell astrocytoma in up to 8%, perhaps arising from a subependymal nodule.
- Brain lesions progressively calcify causing nodular and curvilinear densities, particularly around the ventricular system and basal ganglia.

The term *forme fruste* of tuberous sclerosis refers to patients with single cortical tubers on neuroimaging and neither LDs nor other signs of the disease on brain or skin. On neuroimaging, lesions resemble focal cortical dysplasia. Apart from the presence of multiple lesions in tuberous sclerosis, it can be exceedingly difficult to distinguish focal cortical dysplasia and tuberous sclerosis on neuropathological or neuroimaging examination.

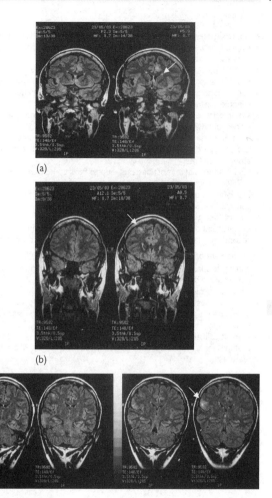

Fig. 5.2 Multiple cortical tubers (indicated by arrows) in a patient with tuberous sclerosis. (a) Left medial frontal tuber; (b) Right lateral frontal tuber; (c) Right suprasylvian and lateral temporal tubers.

Epilepsy, LDs, and EEG

- Approximately 80% of patients with tuberous sclerosis have epilepsy.
- Approximately 60% of patients with tuberous sclerosis have LDs, often associated with autistic features.
- LDs are particularly common if seizures start before the age of 2 years.
- Infantile spasms is the most common presenting seizure type (36–69%).
- Tuberous sclerosis is the cause of epilepsy in 25% of patients with infantile spasms.
- When seizures start after the age of 2, they are usually complex partial or secondarily generalized.
- Infantile spasms may evolve into Lennox–Gastaut syndrome.
- Other seizure types include focal motor, myoclonic, and atypical absence seizures.
- EEG is abnormal in most patients—up to 88%: epileptiform discharges in 75% and slowing in 13%.
- Epileptiform discharges can be focal (23%), multifocal (25%) or generalized (8%) and hypsarrhythmia is seen in 19%.
- 70% of focal discharges are temporal.
- Generalized discharges are probably secondarily generalized— secondary bilateral synchrony—which is often related to frontal tubers.

Management of epilepsy

- If infantile spasms present, as West syndrome—vigabatrin, corticosteroids, ACTH.
- AEDs according to seizure type.
- Surgical resection of tubers if seizures arise from a single focus. Sometimes a single tuber, among multiple existing tubers, is the source of seizures.
- Corpus callosotomy if drop attacks in Lennox–Gastaut syndrome.
- Multidisciplinary management is usually required in view of associated features.

Sturge–Weber syndrome (Sturge–Weber–Dimitri syndrome)

Clinical and neuroimaging manifestations

- *Cutaneous hemangioma* (port-wine stain or naevus flammeus): affecting the upper face, usually (72%) restricted to one side.
- *Naevi in extremities and trunk:* in 45%.
- No facial naevi: in 5%.
- *Facial naevi:* following the distribution of one of the trigeminal nerve divisions.
- *Supraorbital involvement:* is invariably associated with meningeal involvement.
- *Glaucoma:* is present in 47%, either congenital (buphthalmos) or developing before the age of 2 years.
- *Leptomeningeal venous angioma:* usually unilateral and ipsilateral to the facial naevus, with posterior predominance. Bilateral involvement in 15%.
- *Gyriform intracranial calcifications* ('tram-track appearance'): usually unilateral and posterior, appearing between age 2–7, best seen on CT or skull X-rays.
- *Epilepsy.*
- *Learning difficulties:* in 50–60%, particularly if epilepsy present.
- *Hemiparesis:* in 30% and hemianopia, due to progressive damage of the affected hemisphere.
- *Usually sporadic:* although inheritance has been reported.
- *Neurological manifestations:* are thought to result from chronic cortical ischaemia due to 'vascular steal' by leptomeningeal venous angioma. Contralateral hemiparesis may occur.
- *Leptomeningeal angioma:* best seen on after contrast injection on CT or MRI.
- *Forme fruste:* cerebral angioma with no skin lesions may occur.
- *Headache:* may occur.

Epilepsy and EEG

- After facial neavus, epilepsy is the most common presenting symptom.
- Epilepsy occurs in 71–89% of subjects.
- Seizures usually begin in the first year of life.
- Seizures are more likely if there are bilateral leptomeningeal angiomas.
- Seizures are usually focal motor or secondarily generalized.
- Visual auras are surprisingly uncommon.
- Abnormal EEG in 96%: unilateral attenuation of background activity (74%), epileptiform discharges without background abnormalities in 4%, epileptiform discharges in addition to background abnormalities in 22%.
- Bilateral or generalized epileptiform discharges have been reported but are rare.

Management

- AEDs.
- Chronic administration of low doses of aspirin has been suggested to prevent stroke-like episodes, but its use is controversial.
- Monitor vision to prevent complications from glaucoma.
- Cortical resection (if angioma limited) or hemispherectomy if frequent seizures in the context of hemiparesis. Seizure onset in first 5 years of life warrant early referral for surgical consideration.

Epidermal naevus syndrome

Epidermal naevi are congenital slightly raised, ovoid or linear, skin lesions, often located over the midline of the face. In children they are usually skin coloured and they become verrucous, orange, or brown with age. They affect the epidermis and not the dermis and include linear sebaceous naevus of Jadassohn, naevus verrucous, ichthyosis hystrix, and others. After puberty, they have a potential for malignant transformation.

Epidermal naevi can be associated with:
• Abnormalities of neuronal cortical migration.
• LDs.
• Seizures: often starting in the first year of life. They can be myoclonic, complex partial, partial motor, secondarily generalized seizures.
• Cortical atrophy.
• Hydrocephalus.
• Hyperkinesis.
• Porencephaly.
• Hemimegalencephaly.
• Hemimacroencephaly.
• Non-functioning cerebral venous sinuses.
• Infantile spasms.
• Hypsarrhythmia.
• Hemihysparhythmia.
• Hemiparesis.
• Ocular and skeletal abnormalities.
• Visceral malignancy.

Type I neurofibromatosis

Seizures occur in 3–5% of patients, about double the risk of the general population. Seizures can be complex partial seizures (the most common), infantile spasms, tonic–clonic convulsions, and absence seizures.

Other neurocutaneous syndromes

Incontinentia pigmenti (Bloch–Sulzberger syndrome)

In most cases, it is caused by mutations in a gene called *NEMO* (NF-kappaB essential modulator). Discoloured skin lesions are caused by excessive deposits of melanin. Most newborns with incontinentia pigmenti will develop discoloured skin within the first 2 weeks, involving trunk and extremities consisting of slate-grey, blue, or brown lesions, distributed in irregular marbled or wavy lines. Discolouration fades with age. Neurological problems include cerebral atrophy, small cavities in the white matter, and the loss of neurons in the cerebellar cortex. It is associated with:
• LDs—12%.
• Spasticity—11%.
• Seizures—13%.

Neurocutaneous melanosis

Hairy pigmented nevus (swimming-trunk naevus) is associated with seizures.

Hypomelanosis of Ito

Hypopigmented lesions with white or grey hair. Seizures and LDS are present in 66%. Other features include: corneal opacities, deafness, choroidal atrophy, hypotonia, hemihypertrophy, macrocephaly, cerebral atrophy, porencephaly, white matter heterotopias, abnormal cortical lamination. The last two features suggest a migration disorder. 📖 See Fig 5.3.

Urbach–Wiethe disease

Autosomal recessive transmission. Polymorphic papules, macular exudates, retinal pigmentation, malformations of the optic nerve head and tortuous renal vessels, calcification of hippocampus—associated with epilepsy in 15–40% of patients.

Multiple inherited cavernomas (cerebral cavernomatosis)

The condition is usually (80%) hereditary (autosomal dominant, with incomplete clinical penetrance). The genes have been identified (KRIT1, CCM2, CDCD10). There may be additional cavernomas outside the nervous system, e.g. skin, liver.

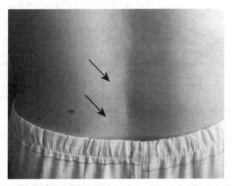

Fig. 5.3 Hypomelanotic lesions on the back of a patient with hypomelanosis of Ito.

Key reading

Kotagal P (1996). Epilepsy in the setting of neurocutaneous syndromes. In *The Treatment of Epilepsy: Principles and Practice*, 2nd edn, pp.646–53, Willie E (ed.). Williams and Wilkins, Baltimore.

Abnormalities of cortical development

Embryology
- The cortex originates from neurons that initially proliferate around the ventricular zone.
- Around the 6th postconceptual week, neurons start migrating towards more peripheral areas of the primitive nervous system, where they later organize, mature, and differentiate into the various neuronal types.
- Consequently, malformations of cortical development have been classified into malformations of *neuronal proliferation*, of *neuronal migration*, and of *cortical organization*.

Prevalence
- Severe malformations of cortical development are rare, having a prevalence of between 4–12 per million.
- Less severe malformations such as focal cortical dysplasia are relatively common, found in around 15–25% of patients assessed for epilepsy surgery.

Aetiology
Malformations of cortical development are developmental abnormalities *originating during intrauterine life*, of diverse aetiologies—acquired or genetic—but generally of unknown cause.

Many neuronal migration disorders have a genetic basis, and many genes have been discovered. Genotypes and phenotypes overlap. The same gene mutation can cause different phenotypes and mutations of different genes cause similar phenotypes. Genotypes are increasingly being considered as a criterion for classification.

Classification
- Malformations due to abnormal neuronal proliferation:
  - Microlissencephaly.
  - Megalencephaly.
  - Hemimegalencephaly.
  - Cortical dysplasia—with and without neoplastic changes.
- Malformations due to abnormal neuronal migration:
  - Classical lissencephaly and subcortical band heterotopia—agyria-pachygyria-band spectrum.
  - Partial lissencephaly—focal or multifocal agyria-pachygyria.
  - Cobblestone lissencephaly.
  - Other rare lissencephaly syndromes.
  - Diffuse heterotopia with normal cortex.
  - Focal heterotopia with normal cortex.
  - Focal or multifocal heterotopia with cortical dysplasia.
  - Excessive, single, ectopic white matter neurons.
- Malformations due to abnormal cortical organization:
  - Generalized polymicrogyria.
  - Bilateral and symmetrical focal polymicrogyria.
  - Asymmetrical polymicrogyria and schizencephaly.
  - Focal or multifocal cortical dysplasias.

The term **cortical dysplasia** has been applied as a general term to describe all developmental abnormalities described in this section. It is also used more specifically to refer to more specific abnormalities described as cortical dysplasia or focal cortical dysplasia. Throughout the text we will use the term 'cortical dysplasia' with the latter meaning.

Lissencephaly

- Lissencephaly means 'smooth brain' and is used to describe a marked reduction in number, magnitude, and complexity of the gyral and sulcal patterns existing on the surface of the hemispheres.
- The most extreme form of lissencephaly—where gyri and sulci are absent—is called agyria. It is equivalent to 'complete lissencephaly'.
- Pachygyria is the term to describe the presence of few, broadened, and flattened gyri. It is equivalent to 'incomplete lissencephaly'.

Lissencephalies have been classified into five types:
- Type I or classical lissencephaly.
- Type II or cobblestone lissencephaly.
- Type III or microlissencephaly or microcephalia vera.
- Type IV or radial microbrain.
- Type V or diffuse polymicrogyria.

Lissencephaly type I—classical lissencephaly

Classical lissencephaly and subcortical band heterotopia—agyria-pachygyria-band spectrum

Classical lissencephaly (generalized agyria-pachygyria) consists of a smooth cerebral surface, thickened cortex with only four layers, diffuse neuronal heterotopia, enlarged ventricles, and hypoplasia of corpus callosum.

Classical lissencephaly and subcortical band heterotopia (📖 see p.484) have been found in different individuals from the same families, and sometimes within the same patient, suggesting that they are different manifestations from the same condition (agyria-pachygyria-band spectrum).

Classical lissencephaly can occur in isolation (autosomal dominant or recessive, sometimes linked to chromosome 17) or in association with other syndromes: Miller–Dieker syndrome (prominent forehead, bitemporal hollowing, short nose, protuberant upper lip, and small jaw), Norman–Roberts syndrome, or X-linked (classical lissencephaly in hemizygous males and subcortical band heterotopia in heterozygous females).

Patients with classical lissencephaly can show apnoea, poor feeding, or hypotonia as newborns. Seventy five percent have seizures within the first 6 months. 80% present with infantile spasms and West syndrome within the first year. Seizure response to medical treatment is poor.

Neuroimaging shows the structural abnormalities already described. The EEG shows generalized spike-and-wave and/or multifocal EEG abnormalities.

Classical lissencephaly can also occur in association with cerebellar hypoplasia, neonatal death, T-cell deficiency, and other rare syndromes (Ramer syndrome, Winter–Tsukuhara syndrome).

Lissencephaly type II—Cobblestone lissencephaly

Cobblestone lissencephaly consists of cobblestone cortex, agyria, pachygyria, polymicrogyria, enlarged ventricles, small brainstem, small cerebellum, and cerebellar polymicrogyria. It is often associated with ocular malformations (unilateral or bilateral microphthalmia) and congenital muscular dystrophy. Extreme cases may show progressive hydrocephalus, Dandy–Walker malformation or occipital cephaloceles. It is usually inherited as an autosomal recessive trait.

It can occur in isolation or in association with various rare syndromes:

- Walker–Warburg syndrome: severe ocular malformations, posterior cephaloceles, congenital hypotonia.
- Fukuyama congenital muscular dystrophy: similar to Walker–Warburg syndrome, seen in patients of Japanese origin.
- Muscle–eye–brain disease.

Most patients have severe LDs and hypotonia, distal spasticity, and poor vision, and die within the first year of life from aspiration.

Lissencephaly type III—microlissencephaly, microcephalia vera

Rare malformation consisting of simplified gyral pattern and profound microcephaly. It is considered a disorder of neuronal proliferation in the germinal zone.

It can occur in isolation or associated with various syndromes:

- *Barth microlissencephaly syndrome:* lissencephaly, extreme microcephaly, cerebellar hypoplasia and neonatal death.
- *McCabe microlissencephaly syndrome:* lissencephaly, extreme microcephaly, cerebellar hypoplasia, cleft palate, congenital heart disease, hemivertebrae, genital malformations.
- *Neu-Laxova syndrome.*
- Microcephalic osteodysplastic primordial dwarfisms.

Most syndromes are autonomal recessive.

Lissencephaly type IV—radial microbrain

The brain is small and the cortex has normal thickness with an immature gyral pattern, despite patients being born at term and absence of brain destruction or gliosis. The number of cortical neurons are reduced by 30%.

Lissencephaly type V—generalized or diffuse plymicrogyria

Polymicrogyria is characterized by multiple small gyri separate by shallow sulci, slightly thickened cortex, heterotopia, and dilated ventricles. Several gyri may be fused and may appear as pachygyria. The most common cause is intrauterine cytomegalovirus infection, which is also associated with multiple calcifications. There is a familial form which is autosomal recessive.

Partial lissencephaly—focal or mutifocal agyria-paqyigyria

Partial lissencephaly tends to manifest as bilateral lissencephaly restricted to posterior regions (bilateral posterior pachygyria). Focal seizures start in infancy or early childhood and are associated with developmental delay.

Bilateral symmetrical polymicrogyria

This may be frontal, perisylvian, parietal, or occipital. The best characterized form is the congenital *bilateral perisylvian syndrome* which consists of bilateral polymicrogyria of the anterior Sylvian regions, prominent pseudobulbar paresis, dysarthria, and mild-to-severe developmental delay. Seizures (complex partial, atypical absence, atonic, tonic–clonic) occur in 85% of patients. The EEG shows generalized spike-and-wave activity and multifocal abnormalities.

Bilateral asymmetrical polymicrogyria

Asymmetrical polymicrogyria might be isolated or might be associated with white matter calcifications, particularly after intrauterine cytomegalovirus infection.

Schizencephaly and asymmetrical polymicrogyria

Schizencephaly (agenetic porencephaly) consists of grey matter-lined clefts that connect ependymal lining of the lateral ventricles with pial lining over the cortex. The cortex around the lips of the cleft might show dysplasia or polymicrogyria. The clefts might be unilateral or bilateral and tend to be located pericentrally (like cortical dysplasia). Schizencephaly can be further subclassified into schizencephaly with fused lips or with separated lips, depending on whether the walls opposing one another obliterate the CSF space.

Patients present with seizures, hemiparesis, and LDs if clefts are large or bilateral. In patients with bilateral clefts, blindness can result from optic nerve hypoplasia. On neuroimaging, the cleft is lined with abnormal, dysplastic grey matter or polymicrogyria, and may extend into the ventricle as subependymal heterotopia.

Schizencephaly might occur with asymmetrical polymicrogyria or with septo-optic dysplasia.

Heterotopia—singular: heterotopion

Regions of grey matter present in the white matter. Heterotopia can be *laminar* or *nodular*, depending on whether the ectopic grey matter forms lamina (layers) or nodules (round-shaped masses). Laminar heterotopia tends to occur within the centrum ovale. Nodular heterotopia tends to occur around the angles of the lateral ventricles. Heterotopia are often bilateral and may or may not be associated with LDs. Most patients present initially with seizures. In contrast to tumours, heterotopic nodules lack the surrounding oedema and do not take up contrast.

Subependymal (periventricular) nodular heterotopia

In periventricular nodules heterotopia, there are nodules of grey matter in the walls of the lateral ventricles. It can be unilateral or bilateral. It can occur in association with hypoplasia of the corpus callosum. Bilateral periventricular heterotopia can resemble the subependymal nodules seen in tuberous sclerosis but the latter are less extensive, often calcified, and show MRI features of white matter. Periventricular heterotopia with normal cortex occur in several syndromes: bilateral periventricular nodular heterotopia (X-linked), marginal glioneuronal heterotopia, leptomeningeal heterotopia, and bilateral cortical infolding.

Patients often present with normal development and seizures in the second decade that may be difficult to control, but in many patients epilepsy is not a prominent feature. The EEG often shows non-specific abnormalities or generalized epileptiform discharges.

Focal heterotopia

In this condition, there are subependymal or subcortical heterotopic nodules. Subcortical nodules sometimes appear to contain vessels which turn out to be CSF within infoldings form adjacent cerebral cortex.

Focal heterotopia with normal cortex can be seen in subependymal nodular heterotopia, subcortical nodular heterotopia, subependymal and subcortical nodular heterotopia, fetal alcohol syndrome, marginal glioneuronal heterotopia, cortical infoldings, and leptomeningeal heterotopia.

Focal or multifocal heterotopia in association with cortical dysplasia take the form of subependymal nodular heterotopia, subcortical nodular heterotopia, subependymal and subcortical nodular heterotopia, and can be seen in Aicardi syndrome (X-linked, agenesis of corpus callosum, pachygyria, polymicrogyria, mainly perisylvian, LD, epilepsy particularly with infantile spasms, retinal abnormalities and hemivertebrae, 📖 see Aicardi syndrome, p.464), Galloway–Mowat syndrome, metabolic disorders, cortical infoldings, marginal glioneuronal heterotopia, and leptomeningeal heterotopia.

Subcortical band heterotopia—double cortex syndrome

Subcortical band heterotopia (double cortex syndrome) consists of symmetrical circular bands of grey matter located under the cortex and separated from the cortex by a thin layer of white matter. The cortex overlying the band heterotopia may show various abnormalities.

As already mentioned, classical lissencephaly and subcortical band heterotopia have been found in different individuals from the same families, and sometimes within the same patient, suggesting that they are different manifestations from the same condition (agyria-pachygyria-band spectrum).

In contrast to patients with classical lissencephaly, patients with subcortical band heterotopia tend to show only mild-to-moderate developmental delay, mild pyramidal signs, and dysarthria. Seizures begin in childhood and are often of multiple types. The EEG shows generalized spike-and-wave and/or multifocal EEG abnormalities.

Cortical dysplasia (focal cortical dysplasia)

(☐ See Fig. 3c.7.) In this condition, lamination of the cortex is lost, there is a reduction in the number of normal neurons, and abnormally large neurons and 'balloon cells' are scattered throughout the cortex and may extend in small clusters into the subadjacent white matter. Aytrocytes with abundant cytoplasm, and lobulated, or multiple nuclei are frequent. Cortical dysplasia tends to occur around the Sylvian fissure. Cortical dysplasia may coexist with polymicrogyria, particularly after intrauterine cytomegalovirus infection. It can be associated with Aicardi syndrome. The findings resemble those seen in tuberous sclerosis but there is no cortical nodularity, calcification, subependimal lesions, or cutaneous or visceral manifestations.

The presence of balloon cells distinguishes cortical dysplasia type I (without balloon cells) from focal cortical displasia type II (with balloon cells, also called Taylor's type). Cortical dysplasia type I (without balloon cells) is thought to be an abnormality of cortical organization rather than migration. Cortical dysplasia type II (with balloon cells) is thought to be an abnormality of cortical migration (balloon cells deriving from migrated primitive neurons). On neuroimaging, the cortex appears thickened, with blurred limits between cortex and underlying white matter, and sometimes with thin radial tracks of grey matter extending into the white matter. Calcification is uncommon (<5%).

Focal cortical dysplasia is the most common cause of intractable epilepsy in children and is a frequent cause of epilepsy with onset in adulthood. Interesting, the first seizure in focal cortical dysplasia can occur with a long delay after birth, between 2 and 31 years of age.

Cortical dysplasia with abnormal non-neoplastic cells

It can present in isolation (usually focal, i.e. focal cortical displasia type II) or as part of tuberous sclerosis (usually multifocal).

Seizures usually start 2 or 3 years after birth, but sometimes in the second decade or shortly after birth. Seizures are focal and semiology depends on the location of abnormalities, which are often extratemporal, particularly frontal and peri-central. Neuroimaging shows thickened cortex with blurred distinction between affected cortex and underlying white matter. The EEG shows frequent epileptiform discharges, often in bursts or continuous.

Cortical dysplasia with neoplastic changes.

Several types of low-grade tumours (dysembrioplastic neuroepithelial tumour, ganglioglioma, gangliocytoma, hamartomas; ☐ see Epilepsy after cerebral tumours hamartomas, and neurosurgery, pp.486–488) occur in association with cortical dysplasia. They occur most frequently in the temporal lobes, usually in children and young adults.

Excess in single ectopic white matter neurons

Reported in post mortem specimens and in brain from resections after epilepsy surgery. They are more often in the temporal lobe.

Focal or multifocal cortical dysplasia

This includes cortical dysplasias without 'balloon cells' (Type I). The clinical manifestations of seizures depend on the location of the abnormalities. Clinical and neuroimaging features are similar to those of cortical dysplasias with 'balloon cells'. They require histological examination to confirm the diagnosis, and consequently they are usually only diagnosed in postsurgical specimens.

Hemimegalencephaly

(📖 see Fig. 3c.12, p.189.) One hemisphere is enlarged due to unduly thickening and disorganization of the cerebral cortex and is associated with cortical dysplasia. Heterotopias, enlarged ventricles, LDs, and epilepsy are often present. They present with seizures, often starting within the first 6 months of life, usually arising from the megalencephalic hemisphere. Infantile spasms and drop attacks may present in early childhood. Unilateral neurological signs such as hemiparesis and hemianopia are common. Neuroimaging shows enlargement of at least one lobe, but commonly all lobes are enlarged unilaterally. Affected cortex appears dysplastic, thickened, with flat gyri and shallow sulci (pachygyria), often with diminished underlying white matter. Polymicrogyria may be present. It should be distinguished from contralateral hemiatrophy by the finding that the hemimegalencephalic hemisphere shows abnormal cortex. Heterotopias and enlarged ventricles are often present, with straightening of the frontal horn which points superiorly and anteriorly. It can be part of neurocutaneous syndromes (📖 see Neurocutaneous syndromes, pp.470–477), in particular hypomelanosis of Ito and epidermal naevus syndrome. Seizure response to medical treatment is usually poor and hemispherectomy has been used to treat seizures if there is significant hemiparesis.

Microdysgenesis

Microdysgenesis is a microscopic malformation initially described in postmortem tissue from patients with generalized epilepsy. This constellation of subtle cyto-architectural abnormalities includes heterotopic neurons in the molecular layer, an excess of neurons in the white matter, and alterations in the cortical laminar architecture. Similar abnormalities have been described in temporal lobe surgical resections, suggesting that microdysgenesis also plays a role in temporal lobe epilepsy. Its role in epileptogenesis is debated, as mycrodysgenesis can be found in normal brains and in patients without epilepsy.

Key reading

1. Dobyns WB and Kuzniecky RI (1996). Normal development and malformations of the cortex. In *The Treatment of Epilepsy: Principles and Practice*, 2nd edn, Willie E (ed.), Williams and Wilkins, Baltimore. pp.93–105

Epilepsy after cerebral tumours, hamartomas, and neurosurgery

Cerebral tumours and epilepsy

Epidemiology

- Any brain tumour, primary or metastatic, can be a cause of seizures or epilepsy. Approximately 35% of patients with brain tumours have seizures (not necessarily chronic epilepsy).
- Certain tumour types (particularly low-grade benign tumours) are more likely to induce seizures: 92% of oligodendrogliomas, 70% of astrocytomas and meningiomas, 35% of glioblastomas.
- Nevertheless, the incidence of brain tumours in patients with chronic epilepsy is relatively low (3.5-4%), increasing to around 15–16% among those patients who develop epilepsy after the age of 25. The incidence is higher among patients undergoing surgery for epilepsy (10–17%), and even higher among children undergoing surgery (25–46%).
- The most common tumour types found in patients with chronic epilepsy are: low-grade astrocytoma, ganglioglioma, oligodendrogioma, mixed glioma, and dysembryoplastic neuroepithelial tumour.
- Although gangliogliomas and dysembryoplastic neuroepithelial tumours are relatively rare brain tumours, most patients with these tumour types suffer from epilepsy.
- Coexistence of brain tumours and cortical dysplasia occurs infrequently.

Clinical features

- The typical history of epilepsy in patients with brain tumours is that of gradually worsening focal epilepsy. However, many patients suffer stable seizure frequency with indolent or stable lesions.
- Around 40% of patients with seizures due to tumours have seizures as the first symptom.
- Seizure manifestations depend on tumour location.
- Physical examination is usually normal in benign tumours. Focal signs and papilloedema are rare unless there are mass effects.
- Headaches—other than postictal—are rare.
- EEG might be normal or show focal slowing of background activity related to tumour location. Sharp waves and epileptiform discharges are sometimes present, usually around the location of the tumour. Occasionally, temporal tumours can show bilateral independent sharp waves or epileptiform discharges, and mid frontal tumours may show (secondarily) generalized discharges.
- Neuroimaging may show tumour or may be normal if tumour is small, depending on the quality of the imaging
- A useful study of 300 new presentations showed, as expected, more epileptogenic lesions, including tumours, on MRI compared to CT, with 53% missed on CT alone.[1]

Treatment

- *Drugs appropriate for focal epilepsy:* anecdotal evidence seems to suggest that epilepsy due to tumours, especially if progressive, may be

poorly controlled by drugs but there is limited data to support this. While full seizure control is the goal, sometimes it is more realistic to aim for controlling more severe seizures, rather than, for example, auras.
- *Advice* on the use of rescue medication should be provided.
- *Surgery:* a few tips:
  - Seizures arise from area around tumour unless otherwise demonstrated.
  - It is unclear how much normal tissue around a tumour should be resected. Intraoperative electrocorticography may help to decide.
  - Functional mapping might be necessary for tumours close to speech, primary motor and somatosensory areas. It might be easier to carry out resection under local anaesthesia to allow for intraoperative functional mapping.
  - Approximately 41% of patients who undergo resections for the treatment of their epilepsy, with usually indolent tumours, become seizure free, and 29% enjoy a marked reduction in seizure frequency.
- *Consult* not only epilepsy driving regulations, also those related to brain tumours.

Hamartoma

A hamartoma is an area of normal cells in their normal site, arranged in a disorganized architecture. Hypothalamic hamartomas may present with gelastic seizures (seizures showing laughter), precocious puberty, and learning difficulties, or a combination of the three. On MRI, they usually appear as a mass in the interpeduncular fossa and may be associated with displacement of the surrounding tissue and of the third ventricle. T2-weighted images show an increased signal in the hypothalamus. In contrast to craniopharyngiomas and astrocytomas, the lesion appears homogeneous and confined to the hypothalamus. In addition to AED treatment, a number of interventions have been used for hypothalamic hamartomas, including resection, disconnection, radiosurgery, and thermocoagulation.

Neurosurgery and epilepsy

The average incidence of seizures occurring for the first time after supratentorial neurosurgery for reasons other than epilepsy is 17% after a 5-year follow-up.

The risk depends on the condition for which surgery was undertaken (the following figures are largely based on older series):
- 20% for aneurysm surgery.
- 50% for surgery for arteriovenous malformation.
- 20% for spontaneous intracerebral haematoma.
- 20% for surgery for meningioma without previous seizures.
- 15% for frontal surgery for pituitary adenomas or craniopharyngiomas.
- Nearly 100% for supratentorial abscess.
- 24% for ventricular shunts.

Of all patients who experience postoperative seizures, 37% do so within the first week, of whom 40% continue to have seizures beyond 1 week.

There is no evidence that prophylactic administration of AEDs will decrease the risk of chronic epilepsy.

References

1. King MA, Newton MR, Jackson GD, *et al.* (1998). Epileptology of the first-seizure presentation: a clinical, electroencephalographic, and magnetic resonance imaging study of 300 consecutive patients. *Lancet*, **352**, 1007–11.

Cerebrovascular disease

- Cerebrovascular disease (stroke, cerebral infarct or haemorrhage, subarachnoid haemorrhage) is becoming an increasingly common cause of epilepsy due to population aging.
- The incidence of epilepsy within one year after a cerebrovascular accident is 4% in patients suffering infarct, 18% after intracerebral haemorrhage, and 28% after subarachnoid haemorrhage.
- Cerebrovascular disease is associated with epilepsy in 15% of all newly diagnosed patients, and in >50% in the elderly.
- Seizures might be the first symptom of cerebrovascular disease or carotid occlusion, particularly in older patients.
- Occurrence of seizures within a week of stroke (acute symptomatic seizures) is not highly predictive of epilepsy.
- Epilepsy due to stroke is not restricted to the elderly or to those with primary cerebrovascular disease, for example:
  - In the syndrome of MELAS, patients tend to suffer occipital strokes and occipital epilepsy.
  - Intrauterine infarcts of the mid cerebral artery tend to cause massive necrosis in the territory supplied by this artery (porencephaly) which can be associated with epilepsy later in life. In around 80% of patients epilepsy starts before the age of 5 years.
  - CADASIL (**C**erebral **A**utosomal **D**ominant **A**rteriopathy with **S**ubcortical **I**nfarcts and **L**eukoencephalopathy) is associated with migraine headaches, transient ischemic attacks or stroke, usually occurring between 40–50 years of age. It is the most common form of hereditary stroke disorder and is thought to be due mutations on chromosome 19 (*Notch3* gene).
- Epilepsy occurs in 40–50% of patients with arteriovenous malformations and most commonly occurs in those with haemorrhage or who have undergone surgical treatment. Epilepsy is also associated with cavernomas (📖 see Neurocutaneous syndromes, p.477).
- Arteritic disorders can cause epilepsy: 17% of patients with systemic lupus erythematosis have seizures and 50% of patients with cerebral involvement in the context of systemic lupus erythematosis have seizures. There is an association between seizures and antiphospholipid syndrome (a disorder of coagulation due to the autoimmune production of antibodies against phospholipids, which causes blood clots in arteries and veins, in addition to pregnancy-related complications). More rarely, seizures can be a complication of systemic necrotizing vasculitis (polyarteritis nodosa), Behçet's disease and mixed connective tissue disease.
- Hypertensive encephalopathy and subacute bacterial endocarditis can also cause seizures.
- Posterior reversible encephalopathy syndrome was first described in 1996 and is characterized by headache, confusion, seizures, visual loss associated with bilateral cortical, and subcortical occipital oedema. It can be induced by abrupt elevation of blood pressure, fluid retention, renal failure, and immunosuppressive therapy.

Epilepsia partialis continua and Rasmussen's syndrome

Epilepsia partialis continua (Kojewnikow's syndrome) consists of very prolonged episodes of focal motor seizures, usually focal clonic or myoclonic convulsions involving unilaterally facial or hand muscle groups, sometimes associated with jacksonian march. The episodes can last for long periods (days, weeks, or even years) and often remain surprisingly focal for very long periods. In effect this is a type of focal motor (simple partial) status epilepcus. Overall it is a rare condition.

Two types of epilepsia partialis continua are distinguished:

Type I: often secondary to *Rasmussen's syndrome* which includes:

- Progressive unilateral chronic encephalitis (📖 see Fig. 5.4) of unknown cause (viral, autoimmune?).
- Age of onset between 2–10 years (peak at 6), although adult cases have been described.
- Focal motor seizures in addition to other seizure types.
- Progressive unilateral motor deficit.
- Mental deterioration.
- Asymmetrical slowing of EEG background activity.
- Numerous ictal and inter-ictal multifocal epileptiform discharges not restricted to the Rolandic area.
- Neuroimaging is normal at onset, but later shows progressive atrophy of only one hemisphere—cortical atrophy, enlargement of temporal horn, later massive ventricual enlargement and cortical destruction.
- Epilepsia partialis continua is present in only 56% of Rasmussen's syndrome.
- Histopathological examination shows chronic encephalitis

Other causes

Viral, renal, hepatic or paraneoplastic encephalitis, mitochondrial disorders.

Type II: secondary to a focal lesion of the motor cortex (vascular, tumour), often with the following features:

- Occurring at any age.
- Additional late focal myoclonic jerks of similar distribution to the focal clonic movements.
- Focal epileptiform discharges over motor-Rolandic area.
- No diffuse abnormalities of EEG background activity.
- No progressive evolution apart from that of the underlying focal lesion.
- Course and prognosis depending on aetiology.

Treatment

Management of type II depends on the underlying condition and follows the usual principles for the treatment of epilepsy.

Treatment of Rasmussen's syndrome is difficult and often unrewarding. AEDs can be used to treat seizures but do not affect the evolution of the disease. Corticosteroids, immunoglobulins, and more recently immunosuppressants, have variable results. Hemispherectomy has a high chance of seizure control but with inevitable functional consequences. The decision on when hemispherectomy may be appropriate in management will require careful evaluation considering progression of disease, possible cognitive consequences, and hemispheric dominance with the likelihood of relocalization of language.

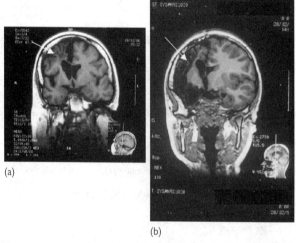

(a)

(b)

Fig. 5.4 Two patients with unilateral chronic encephalitis in Rasmussen's syndrome. Note: unilateral widespread atrophy (arrows).

Syndrome of hemiconvulsions–hemiplegia–epilepsy (HHE)

- Onset in infants between 6 months and 2 years.
- Hemiconvulsions initially develop during a febrile illness followed by hemiparesis.
- Chronic epilepsy develops 6 months to 6 years after the febrile illness.
- Jacksonian motor convulsions or temporal lobe seizures from the affected hemisphere.
- Secondarily generalized tonic–clonic seizures.
- *Causes*: meningitis, subdural effusions, trauma, often unknown.
- *Incidence* has been declining over the years, possibly the result of more prompt treatment of prolonged seizures.
- It has been suggested that this syndrome represent an extreme form of the syndrome of mesial temporal sclerosis.

Epilepsy and cerebral trauma

Cerebral trauma or traumatic brain injury is very common with an overall incidence in developed countries of 200 per 100,000, with a peak in the 15–24 year old age group. Men are affected 3–4 times more than women.

- Traumatic brain injury is often associated with the development of seizures.
- The greater the severity of the injury, the greater the risk of developing seizures.
- Most civilian injuries are as a result of road traffic accidents, falls or recreational injuries.
- The highest incidence occurs following a penetrating injury.
- Approximately 2–12% of all cases of epilepsy result from civilian head injuries
- Post traumatic seizures can be broadly categorized into
  - Immediate seizures.
  - Early seizures.
  - Late seizures.

Immediate—'concussive convulsion'

If this occurs at the time of impact, there is no increased risk of developing epilepsy. These do not require treatment.

Early seizures—acute symptomatic

- Occur within the first 7 days of the injury.
- They are most common in children, with an incidence of 2–6%.
- There is an overall risk of developing late onset epilepsy in 25% of persons experiencing early seizures.
- Early seizures usually require treatment in their own right.

Treatment

If the child or adult has only experienced one early seizure there is no indication for long-term AED therapy.

Late seizures/epilepsy

- >50% of those who develop late seizures have their first within 12 months of the injury.
- Seizures can, however, develop even 10–15 years after the injury.
- The greater the severity of the injury, the greater the risk of epilepsy.
- There is usually a latency period between injury and onset of epilepsy.

Risk of developing epilepsy

The following factors increase the risk of developing epilepsy:

- Depressed skull fracture.
- Intracranial haematoma.
- >30min of post-traumatic amnesia.
- Penetrating injury.
- Cerebral contusion.
- Family history of epilepsy.
- Focal neurological signs.
- Early seizures.

Treatment

- In the majority, treat, as per guidelines for new onset epilepsy with focal seizures (🕮 see Choosing an AED in partial epilepsy, p.270).
- *There is no evidence for use of prophylactic AED use following a traumatic brain injury.*

Further information

Prophylaxis guidelines for head injury: ⊕ www.ann.com

NICE guidelines for head injury: ⊕ www.nice.org

Key reading

1. Temkin N (2003). Risk factors for post-traumatic seizures in adults. *Epilepsia*, 44 (Suppl.10), 18–20.

2. Hauser WH and Anngers FJ (1997). Epidemiology of acute symptomatic seizures. In *Epilepsy: A Comprehensive Textbook*, Engel Jr J and Pedley.T (eds.), pp.87–91. Lippincott-Raven, Philadelphia.

Epilepsy and dementia

- Seizures occur in association with dementia from a variety of causes
- Those with a neurodegenerative disorder associated with cognitive impairment are at increased risk of epilepsy.
- Epilepsy in dementia can have prognostic implications, including in relation to independence, greater risk of injury and higher mortality.
- The presence of pre-existing dementia should not preclude investigating for other symptomatic causes of seizures.
- In a study from the Mayo clinic, 3.6 % of patients with Alzheimer's had epilepsy, often complex partial seizures. A proportion had imaging evidence of epileptogenic lesions. The response to AED therapy was excellent in 79%, but about one third had dose-related side-effects.[1]
- Myoclonic jerks may occur in Alzheimer's, usually late in its course, as in the phase of cognitive decline and dementia associated with Down's syndrome. In this situation broad spectrum AEDs are preferred.
- As those with dementia are often elderly, this has implications to the choice of AEDs and doses used (□ see 3b, Seizures in the elderly pp.152 –154)
- Cognitive impairment, particularly memory deficits, occur in chronic epilepsy

Aetiology

The underlying aetiology of dementia and epilepsy—not infrequently associated with other features—can represent a diagnostic challenge. An accurate diagnosis is important particularly with younger onset presentations, where the differential diagnosis is large. Some conditions are reversible and others may have implications to family members. The term dementia is not commonly applied to early childhood disorders associated with developmental regression. Dementia is commonly defined as a decline in intellectual functioning, often with personality change, severe enough to interfere with the ability to perform routine activities. A detailed discussion is beyond the scope of this handbook, but some categories are listed below:

- Neurodegenerative, such as Alzheimer's Disease. This is common and likely to become more so with changing demographics.
- Infective, such as HIV or neurosyphilis.
- Autoimmune: Examples include limbic encephalitis, Hashimoto's encephalopathy, and anti-NMDA receptor associated encephalitis. Limbic encephalitis (LE) classically presents with a rapidly progressive dementia and seizures. The syndrome may be paraneoplastic or primary autoimmune. Paraneoplastic cases are often associated with circulating anti-neuronal antibodies (particularly anti-Hu) whereas primary autoimmune cases are often associated with circulating anti-voltage gated K channel antibodies (AVGKCA). A minority of paraneoplastic cases are also associated with AVGKCA. Non-paraneoplastic AVGKCA-associated LE oftens responds to immunomodulatory therapy. Paraneoplastic LE may respond to removal of the tumour. Cognitive decline and seizures may also be associated with connective tissue disorders, such as Systemic Lupus Erythematosis.

- Inflammatory/ demyelinative: The incidence of seizures is reportedly increased in demyelination; the latter can be associated with cognitive decline. Seizures and cognitive deficit may also occur in neurosarcoidosis
- Prion Disease: Dementia is a cardinal feature of Creutzfeldt-Jakob disease (CJD) (sporadic, familial or new variant). Startle myoclonus occurs commonly particularly as the disease progresses. Partial seizures and status epilepticus have also been reported. Epilepsy has been reported as a feature of some forms of Gerstmann-Sträussler-Scheinker disease, an inherited prion disese.
- Inherited/genetic conditions: These are many. Examples include some progressive myoclonic epilepsies (📖 see p.99) which are usually but not always associated with dementia (e.g. in Unvericht Lundborg disease there is relative sparing of cognition). Kuf's disease (adult-onset neuronal ceroid lipofuscinosis) presents with progressive myoclonus epilepsy, dementia, pyramidal and extrapyramidal signs. Occipital seizures may also occur. Epilepsy is a prominent feature of many mitochondrial disorders.
- Toxicity from exogenous agents, e.g. alcohol, aluminium salts, immunosuppressive therapy.

References

1. Rao SC, Dove G, Cascino GD, Petersen RC (2008). Recurrent seizures in patients with dementia: Frequency, seizure types, and treatment outcome. *Epilepsy Behav.* [Epub ahead of print]

Epilepsy, alcohol, and drug abuse

Alcohol and seizures
There is a strong relationship between alcohol and seizures. Two categories exist:
- Alcohol abuse, including alcohol withdrawal seizures.
- Those with a diagnosis of epilepsy who drink alcohol.

Alcohol abuse
- The number of persons drinking above the recommended weekly amount is rising in the UK, and increasing numbers of the population are becoming alcohol dependant.
- The prevalence of alcohol dependence in the UK overall is 3.6% (6% of men and 2 % of women).
- 1.1 million people nationally have alcohol dependency in the UK.

Alcohol withdrawal seizures
Seizures are a frequent complication of alcohol withdrawal and a common symptom of delirium tremens (DTs):
- Seizures are associated with acute drop of ethanol levels in chronic alcoholics.
- Seizures usually occur between 6–72 hours after cessation of alcohol.
- Tonic–clonic seizures are typical.
- Seizures usually occur in the early phases of DTs after tremulousness and transient hallucinations, and are followed by motor and autonomic hyperactivity
- Seizures singular event or clusters of seizures, lasting no >12 hours.
- 3% are present with status epilepticus.
- Withdrawal seizures most commonly occur in middle aged men.
- The greater the alcohol intake the greater likelihood of seizures.
- Episodes of detoxification and hospitalization are associated with increased seizure risk.
- Family history of epilepsy increases risk of withdrawal seizures (lowers seizure threshold).
- *15–20% of patients presenting with withdrawal seizures have a non-alcohol, non-trauma related cause for their seizures.*
- Given that patients who experience alcohol withdrawal seizures are at greater risk of head trauma, they can go on to develop focal epilepsy as result of traumatic brain injury.

DTs—other symptoms:
- Fever.
- Tachycardia.
- Raised blood pressure.
- Increased respiratory rate.
- Vivid visual and tactile hallucinations, acute confusional state, anxiety.
- Fluctuating level of consciousness.
- Tremor.

Treatment

- *DT has a 15% mortality rate and always warrants admission.*
- Benzodiazepines are the safest and most effective and safest drugs for withdrawal seizures.
- If a convulsive seizure lasts >5min, follow the protocol for the management of status epilepticus (📖 see Management of convulsive seizures status epilepticus in adults, pp.297–401).
- CT/MRI scan should be considered if a focal lesion is suspected or if this is a first seizure.
- Treat as per local DTs protocol.

If chronic seizures persist, some neurologists advocate long-term therapy but practice varies. This patient group does not often adhere to treatment, thus increasing the risk of seizures if treatment is discontinued abruptly by the patient. This group is often very difficult to manage.

Ultimately, these patients are likely to continue to experience withdrawal seizures unless they choose to pursue long-term alcohol abstinence.

People with epilepsy who drink alcohol (Box 5.3)

- Certain patients can be very sensitive to alcohol consumption, resulting in seizures, particularly those with an idiopathic generalized epilepsy syndromes such as juvenile myoclonic epilepsy.
- Often alcohol in the young can be associated with staying out late— both alcohol and sleep deprivation are significant seizure precipitants.
- Seizures tend to occur the morning or day after alcohol consumption.

Box 5.3 Practical advice for patients

- Patients with a diagnosis of epilepsy should be advised about the relationship between alcohol and seizures.
- A maximum of 1–2 units of alcohol are recommended per sitting if patients with epilepsy choose to drink alcohol, but individual tolerance varies.
- Patients should be advised that although there is an interaction with their AED they must take their medication—some patients are anxious about taking medication after drinking alcohol and will often do not take their medication on days that they have taken alcohol. This increases the risk of seizures.
- Binge drinking must be avoided.
- If possible, alcohol is best avoided.
- In those on polytherapy and high doses of AEDs, tolerance to alcohol may be reduced.

Recreational drug use

Seizures are commonly associated with recreational drug use. There are two significant categories:

- Drug dependence.
- Social/recreational drug users.

The mechanisms behind seizures are the same in both categories although management may differ. In order to manage those with drug dependence, a detoxification programme should be pursued. Acute recreational drug adverse reactions will place a person at risk of an acute symptomatic seizure. Drugs associated with seizures include:

Cocaine

This drug is the recreational drug most commonly associated with seizures. An adverse reaction to cocaine can cause tremors and generalized seizures. Seizures can occur immediately after drug administration. In some cases seizures and death occur shortly after overdose. A higher incidence of seizures is thought to occur after 'crack cocaine' use.

Amphetamines

This can cause seizures, usually tonic–clonic seizures occur following IV administration of large doses. Acute overdose of amphetamines causes:

- Excitement.
- Chest pain.
- Hypertension.
- Tachycardia.
- Delirium.
- Hallucinations.
- Hyperpyrexia.
- Seizures.
- Coma.

Methamphetamine

This is associated with seizures. There is limited experience in the UK although the drug is increasing in popularity. Toxic effects are similar to amphetamines.

Ecstasy MDMA (methylenedioxymethamphetamine)

This can cause seizures in association with rhabdomyolisis and hepatic dysfunction.

Heroin

Generalized tonic–clonic seizures can occur as an adverse reaction to heroin, but heroin use is often associated with concurrent administration of alcohol and other recreational drugs which can also cause acute seizures.

Barbiturate and benzodiazepines

These drugs are occasionally used for recreational purposes often in conjunction with other drugs and alcohol. Abrupt withdrawal can induce tonic–clonic seizures. Barbituates can aggravate delirium.

Marihuana

This is not known to be associated with an increased risk of seizures. It should be avoided due to increased risk of psychiatric morbidity.

General observations

- Usual seizure type—generalized tonic–clonic seizure/serial tonic–clonic seizures and rare cases of status epilepticus.
- Seizures seem to be independent of route—i.e. oral or intravenous.
- Seizures tend to occur shortly after administration of recreational drug.
- Seizures affect chronic and occasional users equally.
- Long-term AED treatment is *not* indicated.
- Drug counselling should be offered to patients.

Support organizations for alcohol addiction in UK

- Addaction: Tel: 020 7251 5860. ⌁ www.addaction.org.uk Email: info@ addaction.org.uk
- Al-Anon & Alateen: Tel: 020 7403 0888. ⌁ www.alanonuk.org.uk
- Alcohol Advisory Service: Tel: 020 7530590.
- Alcohol Concern: 020 79287377. ⌁ www.alcoholconcern.org.uk Email: contact@alcoholconcern.org.uk

Support organizations for drug addiction in UK

- Addaction: Tel: 020 7251 5860. ⌁ www.addaction.org.uk Email: info@ addaction.org.uk
- FRANK: Tel: 0800 776600 ⌁ www.talktofrank.com Email: frank@ talktofrank.com
- Narcotics Anonymous: Tel: 0207 730 0009 ⌁ www.helpline@ukna.org Email: helpline@ukna.org

Epilepsy and the developing world

Incidence and prevalence

- Epilepsy affects >50 million people worldwide.
- 80% of people with epilepsy live in developing countries.
- Epilepsy is more prevalent in developing countries, where incidence ranges from 49–190 per 100,000 population.
- Higher incidence rates are thought to be as a result of parasitosis, HIV, trauma, perinatal morbidity, and consanguinity.
- Prevalence is higher in rural areas.
- Epilepsy accounts for 1% of the global burden of disease.

Common causes in the developing world

- Trauma—most common aetiology in developing countries.
- Parasitosis—neurocysticercosis.
- Cerebral tuberculosis.
- Cerebral malaria.
- HIV.
- Antenatal and perinatal risk factors.
- Cerebral vascular disorders.
- Idiopathic aetiology.

Investigations and treatment

- Diagnostic facilities may be limited, e.g. in Africa. MRI access is limited although EEG is available in >80%.
- 90% of people with epilepsy in developing countries are not receiving treatment, although most cases could be easily and cheaply treated.
- Phenobarbital is the drug of choice to treat those in the developing world—where cost of other medication is prohibitive—because it is a cheap, broad spectrum drug which is easily available.
- Phenytoin, carbamazepine, and valproic acid are also available in most developing countries although usually at a far greater cost than phenobarbital
- There is wide disparity in the availability of drug treatment.
- It has been estimated that the direct cost of treating a patient with phenobarbital for a year could be as low as ~\$2.60 (~£1.40).

Social care

- People with epilepsy in developing countries are often unable to maintain employment.
- Disability benefits are available in only ~15% of low income/ developing countries compared with 82% of developed/high income countries.

Prevention

- The most common causes of epilepsy in the developing world are preventable, for example by:
  - Reduction of trauma—e.g. through enforcement of traffic regulations.
  - Improvement of perinatal care.
  - Improved medical services—vaccination/immunization against communicable diseases.

Cultural beliefs and stigma

- Stigma remains a significant problem in the developing world with damaging belief systems held about epilepsy often causing social isolation and community exclusion (see Stigma, social prejudice and self image, pp.538–539).
- Traditional medicine is often used instead of conventional treatment such as AEDs.

International organizations and programmes

- World Health Organization (WHO).
- International League Against Epilepsy (ILAE).[1]
- International Bureau for Epilepsy (IBE).[2]
- *The Global Campaign Against Epilepsy: 'Out of the Shadows'*[3] was established in 1997 by WHO, ILAE, and IBE with the following objectives:
  - Increase public and professional awareness of epilepsy as a universal, treatable brain disorder.
  - Raise epilepsy to a new plane of acceptability in the public domain.
  - Promote public and professional education about epilepsy.
  - Identify the needs of people with epilepsy on a national and regional basis.
  - Encourage governments and departments of health to address the needs of people with epilepsy including: awareness, education, diagnosis, treatment, care services, and prevention.

Project Atlas[4]

Ongoing since 2000, this was established by WHO, and involves, data from 160 countries for 97.5% of the world's population. This study collects and disseminates crucial data about worldwide epilepsy care and management. The core objectives are to obtain information about:

- Aetiology of epilepsy.
- Budget and financing.
- Epidemiology.
- Lay associations.
- Availability of treatment—e.g. AED use.
- Number of health professionals delivering care.
- Training of epileptology.

Bridging the treatment gap in developing countries

The WHO, IBE, and ILAE recommend the following actions to bridge the epilepsy treatment gap:

- Fostering public commitment.
- Improving access to care for those with epilepsy.
- Arranging educational and training programmes.
- Developing adapted guidelines for those with epilepsy management.
- Considering the cultural environment in any epilepsy health plan.
- Facilitating collaboration with traditional healers and community leaders.
- Ensuring integration of epilepsy prevention in public health interventions.
- Providing appropriate support and care.

References

1. ILAE: ☝ www.ilae.org;

2. IBE: ☝ www.ibeltd.com

3. WHO—The Global Campaign Against Epilepsy: 'Out Of The Shadows'. ☝ www.who.int

4. Project Atlas:—epilepsy care in the world: ☝ www.who.int

Consequences of having epilepsy

Consequences of epilepsy in childhood

The aim of management is for epilepsy to have as little consequence on everyday life as possible. However, inevitably such a diagnosis does have an impact, if only in psychological adjustment for the individual and family to come to terms with such consequences. The impact of course, will also vary according to the age of the child, severity of the epilepsy, and prognosis for seizure control, both with regard to consequences on day-to-day living as well as with regard to co-morbidity.

At diagnosis, advice needs to be given with regard to safety; it is advised that children do not partake in an activity if it could be of danger should they have a seizure. In many circumstances this does not involve prohibition from undertaking the activity altogether which could be carried out with supervision and care. For example, independent climbing should be prohibited but the situation would be different in a controlled-roped environment. Riding a bicycle is possible if not in traffic, as is swimming with one-to-one supervision. Older children, particularly teenagers, may find it difficult to adapt to such advice, and experience a loss of independence particularly through the teenage years. However, it is important that the development of independence is not inhibited. Some parents tend to become excessively involved and this can inhibit independence. In this situation, it may be preferable to engage the child's peers, e.g. a buddy system for swimming or showering. The use of SOS bracelets to be retained on the person may also be advisable.

Cognition

Often of great concern to families is the impact the condition or treatment may have on learning and behaviour. However, the majority of children who develop epilepsy—particularly in mid to late childhood—will become seizure free, and their epilepsy will have little impact on cognition. However, some parents tend to believe that antiepileptic medication is the only factor of importance. This may be reinforced by under informed medical professionals and teachers. Any impact that epilepsy has on learning in an individual case will be multi-factorial; there may be an influence from the underlying aetiology, ongoing seizures, and ultimately medication in a proportion. The difficulty will be the perceived idea that medication will inevitably have an impact, often reinforced by teachers and medical professionals who do not know about the disorder. It is important to assess all possible factors, and consider the possibility that specific learning difficulties may have antedated the presentation with epilepsy but not have been manifest. Unrecognized problems with learning where a child is struggling at school may have an impact on behaviour in and out of school.

Idiopathic epilepsy by definition does not have associated brain lesion. There are some studies to suggest that subtle cognitive problems may exist in certain individuals with idiopathic epilepsy, perhaps with frequent seizures or frequent discharges on EEG, but in general the majority do not have overt problems.

Early onset epilepsy carries a poorer prognosis in terms of developmental and behaviour difficulties. The majority of epilepsies presenting in the first 2 years of life have a high rate of long-term cognitive and behaviour problems. In particular, the epileptic encephalopathies present as a group where a deterioration or plateau in cognition is seen at presentation—by definition it is presumed that this is related in some way to ongoing seizures and epileptiform activity, although this may not be the whole cause. This aside, the goal must be to carefully assess the likely contribution from the epilepsy, and try and achieve optimal control of seizures. In the majority, overt seizure control is the target; in some (e.g. Epilepsy with continuous spike-and-wave during sleep, p.120) to improve the EEG may be desirable, with specific targets with regard to improvement in cognition and development.

Depending on the degree of difficulty, a Statement of Special Educational Needs may be warranted;[1] a document is produced with contribution from parents and all professionals involved, stating the needs of a child in school with agreement of funding required. All children with difficulties are entitled to this from the age of 2 years, although in many cases it is not suggested until school age unless profound difficulties are manifest. Once agreed the statement is reviewed annually. The majority are drawn up in view of learning difficulty and the need for teaching support for an individual, but, physical and behavioural difficulties may also warrant a statement in view of the need for support. If seizures are frequent enough to be a safety issue in school this may also need to be considered.

It may often be advisable to involve the child's school and education authorities. In the UK, a Statement of Special Educational Needs may be warranted.

Behaviour

The issue of associated behaviour problems is a little more complex. Most young people with epilepsy lead apparently normal lives, and the average child with epilepsy will not have behavioural problems. However, there is a significant minority of children with epilepsy, usually those who have continuing seizures despite treatment, or who have an underlying brain disorder or syndrome of which epilepsy is a part, who may run into serious difficulties with emotions and behaviour with a resultant impact on daily functioning.

Although the prevalence of behaviour problems is greatest amongst those with more severe epilepsy, it is still of higher prevalence amongst those with idiopathic epilepsies compared to other ongoing chronic diseases unaccompanied by seizures. The Isle of Wight, an epidemiological study[2] of psychiatric disease reported in 1970 showed a prevalence of behavioural problems in 7% in the general population, 12% in disorders not involving the CNS, 29% in those with idiopathic seizures, 38% in those with structural brain abnormalities, and 58% in those with epilepsy and structural brain abnormalities. More recently, a study—almost 30 years later—reported similar rates of psychiatric disorder despite a greater range of treatments for epilepsy over this time. Data from the British and Adolescent Mental Health Survey[3]—a study of 10438 British children aged 5–15 years—compared 67 children with epilepsy with 47 with diabetes, and showed DSM IV disorder in 37% children with epilepsy (56% with 'complicated' epilepsy versus 26% 'uncomplicated' epilepsy), 11% with diabetes, and 9% control children. In addition, behaviour problems not seem limited to children with ongoing active epilepsy; other studies have shown that behaviour difficulties appear in children early following diagnosis if not before the emergence of seizures.

The likelihood is that the cause of any ongoing behaviour difficulty will be multi-factorial (📖 see Fig. 6.1). Of course medical factors will have an impact, such as ongoing seizures, underlying pathology and medication, but other factors will also play a role—including learning ability, developmental stage of life, as well as family and peer relationships. Whenever a child with epilepsy is reported as having behaviour difficulty, a full history and assessment as to the nature, circumstances, and timing of the behaviour must be sought, as well as control of epilepsy, medication, educational progress, and family relationships (Box 6.1). Often acknowledgement of the problem is the first step toward management. There is no reason why many of the behaviours seen in epilepsy should not be treated in the same evidence-based way as similar difficulties seen in other children without epilepsy; this includes behaviour modification packages as well as medication. Involvement of specialist child and adolescent health services may need to be sought.

> **Box 6.1 Assessment of behaviour**
>
> - Epilepsy review.
> - Psychiatric review.
> - Behavioural analysis.
> - Family review.
> - Educational review.

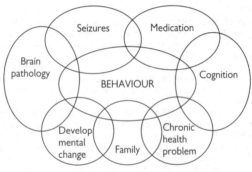

Fig. 6.1 Inter-relationships at play influencing behaviour in a child with epilepsy.

Involvement of family and school

Communication is key to those involved in the day-to-day life of an individual to enable as much understanding and to minimize consequences of seizures for the individual. There may be a reluctance to inform those around a child about the diagnosis, but a greater knowledge leads to greater understanding and will dispel myths. The family should be advised to fully inform a school or preschool; a clear plan may be useful with regard to what to do should the child have a seizure and expectations with regard to learning should be discussed—many presumptions are made about medication and expectations of a child may be inadvertently lowered.

There should be no reason why, with the correct support and advice, a child should not participate fully in school activities. In September 2000 the Disability Discrimination Act was extended to make it unlawful to discriminate against disabled pupils in all aspects of school life (without justification). The principle behind the legislation is that wherever possible disabled children should have the same opportunities as those without disabilities in their access to education.

Impact of epilepsy in the family

The impact a diagnosis of epilepsy has on the family differs according to the age of the child, severity of the epilepsy, and the stage at which the child is at in the natural history of the disorder. At presentation, however benign and whatever the prognosis, the family, especially parents, may find it difficult to come to terms with the diagnosis. Adjustment will need to be made in the acceptance of not only the diagnosis but also the need to take medication, and any restriction that may need to be considered on activity. The exact impact will vary between individual families and discussion adjusted accordingly.

The impact on day-to-day family life may of course depend on the degree of control of the seizures. A child who has had a catastrophic onset with frequent seizures that are poorly controlled may limit the ability of the family to participate in activities as a whole, and strain relationships previously considered to be strong. One parent may find the situation 'easier' than another, particularly if taking the major caring role, or may feel isolated and unsupported putting strains on relationships. Financial strain may be aggravated by periods of time off work, or the need to remain at home by one parent. Siblings may feel that more care is required of the individual, and/or feel 'left out' of the family situation as a whole. Any adverse behaviour manifest by a child with epilepsy may be directed toward siblings or parents and add to further discord. All this may also have an impact on the child with epilepsy who may feel responsibility or blame for the family's strife; alternatively they may have no insight into the situation as a whole.

References

1. ⬧ http://www.direct.gov.uk/en/EducationAndLearning/Schools/SpecialEducationalNeeds)

2. Rutter M, Graham P, and Yule W (1970). A neuropsychiatric study in childhood. *Clinics in Developmental Medicine, 35/36.* Heinemann Medical, London.

3. Davies S, Heyman I, and Goodman R (2003). A population survey of mental health problems in children with epilepsy. *Dev Med Child Neurol,* **45**, 292–5.

Depression and epilepsy

Depression is probably the most common psychiatric morbidity experienced by those with a diagnosis of epilepsy. Between 8–48% of those with a diagnosis of epilepsy will experience an episode of depression[1] (📖 see also Epilepsy and mental health-prescribing AEDs in psychiatric conditions, pp.359–363).

General Practice studies have shown that depression is under-diagnosed in the epilepsy population

The cause of depression in this group of patients is usually complex but the following are thought to play a role:

• Genetic vulnerability.
• Psychological impact of chronic condition.
• Effect of AED.
• Underlying aetiology of epilepsy/complex epilepsy e.g. temporal lobe seizure disorders.

Depression must be considered in the context of proximity to seizures:

• Pre-ictal—prior to the seizure.
• Ictal—during seizure.
• Post-ictal—immediately following the seizure.
• Inter-ictal—between seizures.

Pre-ictal depression

• Symptoms can occur hours or even days before a seizure—irritability, poor concentration or feelings of hopelessness.
• Symptoms usually resolve after the seizure.

Ictal depression

The person's mood may suddenly change. He/she may experience:

• Sadness.
• Fear.
• Anxiety.
• Suicidal ideation.
• Helplessness/hopelessness.

These symptoms are usually brief, representing a simple partial seizure, often followed by impairment of consciousness leading to a complex partial or secondarily generalized tonic–clonic seizure.

Post-ictal depression

Low mood/depressive symptoms are very common post seizure. In some patients these symptoms are present after every seizure. Post-ictal depressive symptoms most commonly occur in those who have drug resistant focal epilepsy syndromes. Symptoms commonly last 12–24 hours. Symptoms include:

• Tearfulness.
• Hopelessness.
• Irritability.
• Suicidal ideation.
• Sleep disturbances.

- Anxiety.
- Appetite disturbance.

Treatment of pre-ictal, ictal, and post-ictal depression are aimed at gaining better seizure control with AED therapy, although individuals may also require supervision and support during the period of depression.

Occasionally people with recurrent and debilitating pre and post ictal depression could benefit from an anti-depressant.

Inter-ictal depression

Although the symptoms of depression are similar to those found in the general population, such as inability to find pleasure in activities or problems with sleep, some characteristics are found in to approximately 50% of epilepsy patients diagnosed with depression:

- Symptoms of irritability.
- Frustration/poor tolerance
- Labile mood.

Risk factors

- Temporal lobe partial seizures—seizures arising from the left temporal lobe possibly more at risk.
- Family history of psychiatric disorder.
- Past history or depression/psychiatric morbidity.

Treatment

Inter-ictal depression will require assessment by a psychiatrist and use of an antidepressant should be considered.

Box 6.2 Treatment summary

- Although the literature suggests antidepressants can lower one's seizure threshold, we do not see this frequently in clinical practice with currently used antidepressants.
- Depression is a significant clinical problem that should be treated.
- Risk of seizures is related to high doses of tricylic antidepressants (📖 see Epilepsy and mental health-prescribing AEDs in psychiatric conditions, pp.359–363).
- People with epilepsy are 5 times more at risk of suicide than the normal population. Most common form of suicide attempts involve overdose of antiepileptic drugs.
- Some antiepileptic drugs may affect mood; care with use is required, with adjustments made to medication should this occur.

References

1. Hermann BP, Seidenberg M, and Bell B (2000). Psychiatric co-morbidity in chronic epilepsy: identification, consequences and treatment of major depression. *Epilepsia*, **41**(Suppl2), S31–41.

Further information

🔗 www.nice.org.uk—website of The National Institute for Health and Clinical Excellence:

—Depression: management of depression in primary and secondary care (Dec 2004)

—Depression in children and young people (Dec 2004)

🔗 www.depressionalliance.org.uk—website of Depression Alliance UK

🔗 www.samaritans.org—Samaritans' website

🔗 www.rcpsych.ac.uk—website of The Royal College of Psychiatrists

Anxiety and epilepsy

Anxiety is frequently reported by patients who experience seizures and occurs most commonly as an inter-ictal phenomenon, but is also a feature of ictal and post ictal phases.

Inter-ictal anxiety/primary anxiety

Primary anxiety includes:
- Panic disorder.
- Agoraphobia.
- Social phobia.
- Specific phobia.
- Generalized anxiety disorder.

The lifetime prevalence of anxiety in the normal population is approximately 10–20%.

Over 30% of people with epilepsy experience anxiety. Some believe that the figure is probably nearer to 50% in those with drug resistant epilepsy.

Similar to depression, anxiety is probably under-diagnosed in the epilepsy population.

Inter-ictal anxiety disorders have varying underlying causes including:
- Adjustment to diagnosis.
- Side effects of drugs.
- Fear of seizures/'loss of control'.
- Underlying depression.
- Social isolation.

Panic disorder and anxiety/panic attacks

Panic disorder involves frequent, usually brief, discrete anxiety attacks. Anxiety or panic attacks include a combination of the following symptoms:
- Sudden onset.
- Palpitations.
- Sweating.
- Trembling and shaking.
- Sensations of shortness of breath/hyperventilation.
- Feeling of choking.
- Chest pain or discomfort.
- Nausea.
- Abdominal discomfort.
- Dizziness/feeling faint.
- Derealization or depersonalization.
- Fear of losing control.
- Fear of dying.
- Numbness/tingling.
- Chill or hot flush.

Panic attacks can co-exist with epilepsy!

Agoraphobia and social phobia

- Patients experience a morbid dread of open spaces or dread of social contact.
- Often agoraphobia and social phobia co-exist.
- Usually more prevalent in those with drug-resistant epilepsy.
- Thought to be associated with the patient's fear of further seizures, particularly in public.

Specific phobia

- A specific phobia is an overwhelming, irrational fear of a specific situation or object that poses no real danger.
- Diagnosis can be made when the dread and fear interfere with a person's daily life or activities.
- When the patient is exposed to the feared item they experience severe anxiety which can lead to a panic attack.

Generalized anxiety disorder

- Excessive worry.
- Feelings of often constant anxiety.
- Restlessness.
- Sleep disturbance.
- Concentration difficulties.
- Fatigue.
- Irritability.

Diagnosis

- Diagnosis is dependent on the type of anxiety disorder.
- Ask patients open-ended questions about their general well being.
- Use of screening questions can be helpful, e.g. 'Are you a particularly nervous or anxious person?' 'Do you or people who know you well think of you as a "worrier"?'
- The Hospital Anxiety and Depression (HAD) scale[1] can be a very useful diagnostic tool. It is quick and easy for patients to use. It can be obtained from: ⌒ http://www.depression-primarycare.co.uk/ (go into 'useful links' and then click 'depression protocol').

Treatment

Psychology review for cognitive behavioural therapy (CBT) or cognitive group behavioural therapy (CGBT).

Medication

- *First line* (if associated with depression): SSRI, e.g. citalopram.
- *Second line*: Benzodiazepines—usually short term, maximum 4 weeks' use. Caution in view of habituation.
- Some AEDs may have beneficial effects. Pregabalin is licensed for use in generalized anxiety disorder and can be used as a first-line treatment if there is no associated depression and psychological intervention is not suitable.

Ictal anxiety, panic attack, or seizure?

Simple partial seizures arising from the temporal lobe can be similar to panic attacks and may be misdiagnosed.

Table 6.1 Differential diagnosis between panic attacks and seizures[*]

Panic attack	Seizure
Can range from 30 seconds to 10 minutes or more.	Usually very brief lasting up to 60 seconds.
Feeling of severe anxiety/fear can feel sudden fear of dying.	Fear and anxiety. Rare to have feelings of dying.
Usually aware of surroundings and is responsive.	Fear may be followed by loss of awareness, may experience automatisms and will be amnesic of event if it develops into complex partial seizure.

[*]Adapted from Holzer JC and Bear DM(1997). Psychiatric considerations in patients with epilepsy. In: The comprehensive evalution and treatment of epilepsy, Schacter SC and Schorner DL (ed.) pp.131–48. Academic Press, SanDiego, California, copyright 1997, with permission from Elsevier.

Post-ictal anxiety

Feelings of anxiety are common after a seizure—these can last minutes or even up to 24 hours, rarely for days. The anxiety is often associated with the fear of a further seizure. Often these post-ictal symptoms of anxiety are associated with a degree of post-ictal depression.

References

1. Zigmond AS and Snaith RP (1983). The Hospital Anxiety and Depression Scale. *Acta Psychiatr Scand,* **67,** 361–70.

2. Holzer JC and Bear DM (1997). Psychiatric considerations in patients with epilepsy. In *The comprehensive evaluation and treatment of epilepsy,* Schacter SC and Schomer DL (eds.), pp.131–48. Academic Press, San Diego, California.

Further information

⌁ www.nice.org.uk—website of The National Institute for Health and Clinical Excellence:

— Anxiety-management of anxiety (panic disorder, with or without agora-phobia, and generalized anxiety disorder) in adults in primary, secondary and community care. (2004)

— Management of panic disorder and generalized anxiety disorder in adults-Information for people with panic disorder, their families and careers and the public (Dec 2004)

Support and advice for patients

National Phobics Society: 339 Stretford Road, Hulme, Manchester M15 4ZY. Tel: 0870 7700456. Stress Management:'Fox hills', 30 Victoria Avenue, Shanklin, Isle of Wight PO376LS.
  The Thanet Phobic Group: 47 Orchard Road, Westbrook, Margate, Kent CT9 5JS. Tel: 01843 833720.
⌁ www.rcpsych.ac.uk/info/help/anxiety—website of The Royal College of Psychiatry.

Personality and epilepsy

Historically, neurologists and psychiatrists alike have felt that there was an 'epileptic personality'. In modern medicine this is actively denied. The origin of this concept may relate to the huge stigma attached to epilepsy in decades and centuries past. It should be noted that bromides and barbiturates first used in the treatment of epilepsy produced varying degrees of cognitive and behavioural side effects, which may have also accounted for altered personality.

Research by Geshwind in the 1940s suggested certain personality traits for those with temporal lobe seizures. Later in the 1950s, Janz described a group of personality traits seen in those with JME. One of the most detailed reviews of personality and epilepsy was published by Bear in the 1970s, identifying 18 personality traits thought to be over represented in those with temporal lobe epilepsy. These traits included emotionality, manic tendencies, altered sexuality, and aggression. Since this study, other authors have failed to support these findings—which remain controversial—with a suggestion that some patients, particularly those with severe drug resistant temporal lobe epilepsy, may have a higher degree of personality disorders.

While not subscribing to the theory of an epileptic personality, we recognize the complexities of neuropsychopathology associated with the epilepsies.

If a patient with epilepsy exhibits traits suggesting a personality disorder review by a psychiatrist is recommended.

References

1. Waxmon SG, Geshwind N(1975). The interictal behaviour syndrome of temperal lobe epilepsy. *Arch Gen Psychiatry* **30**, 1580–1586.

2. Janz D, Christian W. Impulsive Petit Mal In: Malatosso A, Genton P, Hirsch E, Maroscaux C, Broglin D, Bernasconi R (eds) Idiopathic generalized epilepsies: *clinical experimental and genetic aspects* (1994) 229–251.

3. Bear D, Fedio P (1977), Quantitative analysis of interictal behaviour in temporal lobe epilepsy. *Arch Neurol* **34**, pp.454–467.

Psychoses in epilepsy

Post-ictal and inter-ictal psychoses are the most common forms of psychotic episodes seen in patients with epilepsy. Pre-ictal and ictal psychoses are rare. Prevalence of psychoses in epilepsy ranges from 2–9%. There is no internationally recognized classification for psychoses in epilepsy.

Ictal psychotic symptoms may mimic simple partial or complex partial status epilepticus (📖 see Diagnosis of status epilepticus, pp.198–205).

Psychosis can occur following withdrawal of any AED which has mood stabilizing properties.

Post-ictal psychosis

- Most common in people with recurrent partial and generalized seizures/status.
- More common in patients who have had seizures for 10–15 years.
- Often follows clusters of tonic–clonic seizures/complex partial seizures.
- Usually there is a period of lucid/normal behaviour for 1–6 days after a cluster of seizures, before symptom onset.
- Accounts for 25% of psychoses in epilepsy.

Symptoms

- Insomnia.
- Thought blocking/sudden interruption in thought.
- Intrusive thoughts.
- Formed and unformed hallucinations.
- Paranoid, grandiose and religious delusions.
- Confusion—can fluctuate.

Investigations

EEG often shows deterioration with increased epileptiform activity, as well as slow wave activity.

Treatment

- Psychiatric review.
- Symptoms often spontaneously remit within days or weeks.
- In many cases no treatment is required other than observation to ensure safety.
- Use of antipsychotic treatment for the short period of psychosis may be warranted, depending on severity.
- Admission to a psychiatric unit is often necessary.

Inter-ictal psychosis

- Occurs between seizures, without a clear association with seizures/ clusters of seizures and their onset/offset.
- Can be associated with an affective disorder.
- Strongly associated with temporal lobe onset seizures—left sided seizure onset thought to increase risk.
- Thought to be more prevalent in females.
- Mean onset usually 11–15 years after the diagnosis of epilepsy.
- More prevalent in those with severe drug resistant epilepsy.

Symptoms

Similar to idiopathic schizophrenia although the following differences can be identified:

- Intact affect.
- Unimpaired ability to relate to others.
- Lack of chronic deterioration.
- Relative absence of negative symptoms, therefore do not display a lack of initiative.
- No family history.
- No pre-morbid traits.
- Paranoid delusions and hallucinations are prominent.

Investigations and assessment

- Psychiatric review.
- EEG: there are no EEG changes beyond the patient's baseline interictal EEG findings.

Treatment

- Psychiatric review and management.
- Anti-psychotic drug therapy—those taking enzyme-inducing AEDs show lower serum levels of anti-psychotic drugs, therefore may require higher doses. Caution: anti-psychiatric drugs can reduce seizure threshold (📖 see Epilepsy and mental health—prescribing AEDs in psychiatric conditions, pp.359–363).
- AEDs with neuropsychiatric side effects should be avoided where possible.
- Regular review and management by a community mental health team may be required.

Key reading

1. Trimble MR and Schmitz B (1997). The Psychoses of epilepsy/schizophrenia. In *Epilepsy: a Comprehensive Textbook*, Engel Jr J and Pedley TA (eds.) Lippincott-Raven, Philadelphia.

Further information

🖱 www.rcpsych.ac.uk/info/help/anxiety—website of The Royal College of Psychiatry.

Aggression and epilepsy

Aggressive behaviour has for centuries somewhat inappropriately been associated with people who have a diagnosis of epilepsy. Only a small number of those who suffer from epilepsy exhibit aggressive behaviour, and these incidences can be spilt into the ictal, post-ictal, and inter ictal states.

Ictal aggressive behaviour

It has been suggested that ictal aggression is more prevalent in those with temporal lobe epilepsy, although frontal lobe seizures can involve dramatic motor activity which inadvertently appear to be aggressive in nature total aggression.

- Usually occurs in complex partial seizures.
- Is brief in duration.
- Is unintentional.
- Involves no evidence of directed violence.
- Is associated with an abnormal EEG.

Management

- Stay calm.
- Talk gently to the person.
- *Do not restrain.*
- Remove dangerous objects from person/area.

Post-ictal aggressive behaviour

- Post-ictal aggression is more common than ictal aggression. The management of a person after their seizure plays a significant role in their responses and potential for aggressive behaviour.
- Most patients are very confused after a seizure. They may be disorientated, and will often not recognize familiar faces e.g. family members. This acute post-seizure confusion can be very alarming for patients.
- Post-ictal aggression can occur if the person is restrained, although some patients will exhibit aggressive behaviours without being restrained.
- The person may appear confused, irritable, depressed, or in pain.
- An episode of aggressive behaviour is usually very brief.
- Usually the person will have no or limited memory of the aggressive behaviour.

Management

- Avoid restraint or loud commands e.g. 'stop that'.
- Try and contain the person but avoid approaching him or her if possible e.g. ensure he or she does not walk out of the house/room.
- Talk calmly and stay with the person.
- Partners/families should avoid issues of guilt. Patients after an event may feel very embarrassed and remorseful.
- This aggression or violence is not intentional.

Inter-ictal aggressive behaviour

It is important to distinguish between irritability which is often described as aggression, and true aggressive outbursts, which are rare in those with epilepsy.

Often the psychiatric definition of irritability and the term aggression are used interchangeably. Irritability in this context refers to easily angered and short tempered, sometimes with aggressive verbal outbursts, rather than directed physical violence.

Irritability can be an adverse side effect of AEDs and is a common complaint of those with seizures.

Causes

The underlying aetiology in the small group of patients who exhibit aggressive inter-ictal behaviours is complex.

Often aggressive behaviour is not associated with the epilepsy but related to a person's social history. Patients who are at greater risk of developing aggressive behaviour include those with:

- History of physical abuse in childhood.
- History of sexual abuse.
- History of conduct disorder.
- Drug or alcohol abuse problems.

Treatment

In those patients who show evidence of aggressive inter-ictal behaviour a review/referral to a psychologist or psychiatrist is advised. These patients must also be assessed for anxiety and depression.

Key reading

1. Blumer D and Altshuler (1997). Affective disorders. In *Epilepsy: a Comprehensive Textbook*, Engel Jr J and Pedley TA (eds.). Lippincott-Raven, Philadelphia.

2. Holzer JC and Bear DM (1997). Psychiatric considerations in patients with epilepsy. In *The comprehensive evaluation and treatment of epilepsy*, Schacter SC and Schomer DL (eds.), pp.131–48. Academic Press, San Diego, California.

Further information

⌂ www.rcpsych.ac.uk/info/help/anxiety—website of The Royal College of Psychiatry.

⌂ www.angermanage.co.uk —website of the British Association of Anger Management.

Epilepsy and sexual dysfunction

Sexuality and epilepsy have been linked for centuries—Hippocrates wrote that 'complete abstinence from, and excessive indulgence of intercourse could cause epilepsy'. In fact this assumption was the rationale behind the use of bromides in the 1900s to treat 'hypersexuality'. It was thus by chance, that this compound which was known to cause impotence also aborted seizures. The age of AED treatment was born.

Later in the 1950s Gastaut reported the opposite, namely hypo-sexuality in those with a diagnosis of seizures. Controversy remains, but there is evidence to suggest a degree of sexual dysfunction in a minority of persons who develop epilepsy. It is generally considered that those with epilepsy are more likely to experience global hyposexuality.

The three most commonly accepted mechanisms for reduced sexual interest or sexual dysfunction in those with epilepsy are:

- Psychosocial impact of epilepsy.
- Impact of brain dysfunction caused by epilepsy, which may interrupt the mechanisms for sexual interest.
- Effects of AEDs.

Psycho-social impact of epilepsy (Box 6.3)

- It is thought that those who develop epilepsy from childhood may be at greater risk of sexual dysfunction as a result of the psychosocial impact of the diagnosis.
- Experiencing stigma associated with seizures from a young age may go on to interfere with developing and maintaining relationships.
- Marriage rates are lower in those with a diagnosis of epilepsy.

Box 6.3 The psycho-social impact of epilepsy

- Potential for social embarrassment.
- Difficulties developing and maintaining relationships.
- Lowered social status—e.g. employment/education.
- Impact on self worth.
- Helplessness.
- Potential for dependent relationships.
- Fear of experiencing a seizure during sexual intercourse.

Impact of epilepsy-originated brain dysfunction on sexual function

- Sexual dysfunction is more common in those who experience complex partial seizures, particularly those arising from the temporal lobe.
- Side effect of neurotransmitters, e.g. GABA (inhibitory neurotransmitter), may inhibit sexual behaviour.
- 1/3 of men complain of lack of spontaneous morning penile tumescence, anorgasmia and erectile difficulties.
- 1/3 of women report dyspareunia, vaginismus, and lack of vaginal lubrication.

Effect of AEDs
- Free testosterone is reduced by AEDs, and therefore may contribute to sexual dysfunction in men.
- Many AED have been associated with impotence.

There remains controversy in this field
- A number of patients experience difficulties, but the underlying cause for sexual dysfunction is related to multiple factors, probably both physiological and psychological.
- More recent studies, performed using sexological methods, have neither shown hyposexuality, nor in general, significant sexual dysfunction in either men or women with a diagnosis of epilepsy.[1,2]

Investigation and treatment
Explore all possible psychological causes for sexual dysfunction—e.g. marital problems, stress etc.

Sexual dysfunction can be a signal that a person may be developing depression!

Psychological causes of sexual dysfunction can be addressed therapeutically by appropriate referral to:
- Marriage guidance.
- Local counselling..
- Psychology review—e.g. CBT or psychotherapy.

Thorough physical and neurological examination is required. Check as appropriate:
- Medication.
- Thyroid function.
- Testosterone.
- Oestrogen,LH,FSH.
- Prolactin.
- FBC.
- Fasting glucose.

Consider referral to urologist or gynaecologist!

References

1. Jensen P Jensen, SB, Sorensen, PS et al. (1990). Sexual dysfunction in male and female patients with epilepsy. A study of 86 outpatients. *Archives of Sexual Behaviour* **19**, 1–14.

2. Kuba R, Pohanka M, Zakopcan J, et al. (2006). Sexual dysfunctions and blood hormone profile in men with focal epilepsy. *Epilepsia* **47**, 2135–40.

Further information
⁂ www.sda.uk.net—Sexual Dysfunction Association. Tel: 0870 7743571.

Counselling in people with epilepsy

A new diagnosis can instil feelings of fear, anxiety, frustration and even anger. It is common for people to experience a feeling of loss or bereavement when the diagnosis of a chronic condition is made. Fortunately the majority of people diagnosed with epilepsy will respond well to treatment, and thus are rendered seizure free. Despite a good prognosis in most people, a person's fear of experiencing a seizure in the future can be debilitating. Patients are usually worried about their family's and friends' reactions to the diagnosis as well as public witnessing of seizures. Early intervention can limit a person's fears and anxieties.

NICE, UK, recommends that adults and children as well as their carers/parents should receive appropriate information and education about all aspects of epilepsy, listing the following topics:

- Epilepsy in general.
- Diagnosis and treatment options.
- Medication and side effects.
- Seizure type(s), triggers, and seizure control.
- Management and self-care.
- Risk management.
- First aid, safety and injury prevention at home, school, or work.
- Psychological issues.
- Social security benefits and social services.
- Insurance issues.
- Education and healthcare at school.
- Employment and independent living for adults.
- Importance of disclosing epilepsy at work, if relevant—if further information or clarification is needed, voluntary organizations should be contacted.
- Road safety and driving regulations.
- Public transport concessions for those who do not satisfy driving regulations.
- Prognosis.
- SUDEP.
- Status epilepticus.
- Lifestyle, leisure, and social issues—including recreational drugs, alcohol, sexual activity and sleep deprivation.
- Family planning and pregnancy.
- Voluntary organizations, such as support groups and charitable organizations, and how to contact them.

There is some controversy about how appropriate it is to discus SUDEP after an initial diagnosis. Some neurologists feel this is better explored in subsequent consultations (📖 *see p.528). It is important, however, even at the first consultation to emphasize the importance of avoiding and preventing seizures because of the risks associated.*

Counselling can be provided by a:
- Consultant neurologist.
- Epilepsy specialist nurse.
- Trained epilepsy counsellor.
- General practitioner.
- General practice nurse.

Specialist counselling is an essential aspect of the patient's management. The following should be considered:
- Specialist counselling should where possible be provided by the neurologist or epilepsy specialist nurse.
- People must be given adequate time and support to cope with the new diagnosis.
- Several sessions may be required to go through all of this information in detail, particularly complex issues such as preconception counselling.
- A checklist can be a useful way to ensure all information has been provided and documented.
- Information should be provided in a timely fashion, dependent on the security of the diagnosis.
- Information provision should be in an appropriate format taking into consideration age, gender, language, and cultural differences.
- Where possible, all verbal information should be followed by some written literature or details of local and national support organizations.
- It is advisable to involve family members, e.g. parents/partners during these sessions, while keeping the individual the main focus. The families' reactions play a significant role in adjustment to the diagnosis.

Support and counselling for the drug-resistant patient

On-going seizures that are resistant to drug treatment have major psychological and social ramifications.

Patients can experience the following:
- Perceived and real stigma.
- Social isolation.
- Low self-esteem.
- Loss of control.
- Anxiety disorders.
- Depression.

The psychosocial impact of a poor prognosis has far reaching consequences for:
- Relationships—social integration, dependency issues in partnerships.
- Schooling/education—low expectations of patient and family.
- Employment—difficulties in maintaining or obtaining employment due to seizures. Low employment expectations/under-employment.

If a person is identified to have adjustment difficulties and requires counselling, consider referral to the following:
- Epilepsy specialist nurse.
- Trained epilepsy counsellor—in the UK, these are often only available in specialist epilepsy centers.
- Local psychology services for initial assessment, who may then refer to local counselling services attached to general practice.

If depression or anxiety disorders are suspected, refer to a psychiatrist for assessment—remember that those with drug resistant epilepsy are at a far greater risk of developing anxiety disorders or depression.

Genetic counselling—risk to offspring

Prospective parents with epilepsy will want to know how likely they are to pass the epilepsy on.
- *Where there is a known inherited condition:* such as some of the syndromes outlined in Chapter 3b, specific estimates can be given based on the condition and pedigree. Prenatal diagnosis may be possible and referral to a genetic clinic is advised.
- *If there is no clear family history in someone with remote symptomatic epilepsy:* for example epilepsy secondary to a severe head injury or stroke, the chance of passing the epilepsy is unlikely to be significantly increased over the general population risk.
- *If the epilepsy is idiopathic and there are many affected family members:* Mendelian inheritance should be considered and, where appropriate, advice from a genetic clinic sought. In autosomal dominant or recessive pedigrees, the risks of passing the epilepsy on are 50%, and 25% respectively. Penetrance may be reduced and phenotypes vary. It is not be possible to predict the severity of the epilepsy in the offspring based on that of the parent. In general, however, idiopathic epilepsies tend to be less severe than symptomatic epilepsies although this is by no means always the case.
- *If the epilepsy is idiopathic without a strong family history:* complex inheritance is assumed. Overall the risk is <10%. The risk if the parent has partial seizures is less than with generalized seizures. Older studies also suggest that the risk to offspring is greater if the mother is affected, although not all studies have shown this. Table 6.2 gives broad estimates of risk to offspring or siblings. If both parents have epilepsy the risk is likely to be significantly higher than the risks quoted below but are difficult to quantify.

General practical advice for patients
- Use of local and national support groups and organizations such as NSE[4] and Epilepsy Action[5] is encouraged.
- Self management plans can be provided and patients with poorly controlled seizures can be encouraged to complete an Expert Patient Programme.[6]

Table 6.2 Broad empiric risk to offsprings or siblings in epilepsy[1-3]

Individual affected	Risk
Primary generalized epilepsies*	4–10% offspring risk (similar risk in siblings)
Partial and secondary generalized epilepsies†	2–4% offspring risk (similar risk in siblings)
Febrile seizures (FS)	10% of offspring in whom 2/3 have only FS

Notes:

* Risk towards upper half of quoted range in some syndromes e.g. CAE, where there is also a clearly elevated risk of febrile seizures.

† Risk likely to greater in those with idiopathic partial epilepsies.

These estimates are guidance for use only in the case of likely complex (presumed polygenic/multifactorial) inheritance, and is not applicable if there is a clear Mendelian history or syndrome with known genetic defect, where individual genetic assessment is indicated.

Approximate background population risk by age 20 years of 1%.

Overall risk in first degree relative 2.6%.

Overall, family risk is highest in idiopathic generalized epilepsies. It is also higher in idiopathic epilepsies in general compared to symptomatic. Generally, there is some concordance for the broad epilepsy syndrome rather than the specific subtype.

Some but not all studies quote a higher inherited risk of seizures from the mother compared to the father.

If both parents are affected, the risk is considered to be significantly higher but it is difficult to give an accurate estimate.

In those with febrile seizures, there is an increased risk in relatives not only of febrile seizures but also of epilepsy.

References

1. Blandfort M, Tsuboi T, and Vogel F (1987). Genetic counseling in the epilepsies. *Hum Gen*, **76**, 303–31.

2. Bianchi A, Viaggi S, Chiossi E; LICE Episcreen Group (2003). Family study of epilepsy in first degree relatives: data from the Italian Episcreen Study. *Seizure*, **12(4)**, 203–10.

3. Doose H and Maurer A (1997). Seizure risk in offspring of individuals with a history of febrile convulsions. *Neuropediatrics*, **156** (6), 476–81.

4. The National Society for Epilepsy: ⓦ www.epilepsynse.org.uk

5. Epilepsy Action: ⓦ www.epilepsy.org.uk Email: www.epilepsy@epilepsy.org.uk

6. NHS Expert Patient Programme: ⓦ www.expertpatient.nhs.uk

Further information

The National Institute for Health and Clinical Excellence: ⓦ www.nice.org.uk

—The epilepsies: the diagnosis and management of the epilepsies in adults and children in primary and secondary care (2004).

— Epilepsy: the diagnosis and management of epilepsy in children and adults (2004).

Mortality in epilepsy

The epidemiology of excess mortality in epilepsy has been discussed in Chapter 1 (☐ see Mortality, pp.8–11). In this section, we briefly discuss patient information about mortality risk.

There has been debate on the advisability or otherwise of discussing risk of death routinely with patients with epilepsy and, indeed, a questionnaire survey of UK neurologists showed only 31% discussed SUDEP with all or most patients.[1] More research is needed, and individual risk is difficult to estimate.

Those against such discussions argue that:
- This may harm the patient for no benefit.
- The patient has a right not to know.
- Patients with 'mild' epilepsy are at very low risk.
- This should be addressed only with those with severe epilepsy.

Those for informing patients, including the self-help group Epilepsy Bereaved (⊕www.sudep.org), argue that:
- Those with epilepsy, as with other conditions, have the right to know risks associated with their diagnosis.
- Such information provision is within NICE guidelines.
- While risk is lower with less severe epilepsy, SUDEP can occur in patients with a history of generalized tonic–clonic seizures.
- It is likely that SUDEP is largely related to generalized tonic–clonic seizures and that some epilepsy related deaths including SUDEP are preventable, by seizure prevention and response to seizures.

Balanced information provision of risks associated with epilepsy helps keep them in perspective, and aids both the patient and clinician in making decisions about treatment and lifestyle. Risks associated with epilepsy can be addressed at any stage of diagnosis in patients with mild or severe epilepsy and tailored to individual need. For example, in discussing advantages and disadvantages of long-term treatment in new onset epilepsy, one can include in the discussion that such treatment, where successful, prevents seizures—this being an advantage, as severe epileptic seizures carry a small risk not only of serious accident or injury but also to life if severe.

References

1. Morton B, Richardson A, Ducan S. (2006) Sudden unexpected death in epilepsy (SUDEP): don't ask, don't tell? *J Neurol Neurosurg Psychiatry* **77(2)**: 199–200.

Lifestyle

Epilepsy can have potentially far-reaching effects on a person's psycho-social functioning. In the past, healthcare professionals have over-emphasized what a person can't do, rather than the current view of ensuring that a person's life, within reasonable safety margins and while avoiding seizure triggers, is not restricted by their seizures. The appropriate lifestyle advice can be provided, but ultimately it is the person's choice to lead his or her life in a way that they desire. Lifestyle choices will be influenced by the following:

- Seizure type.
- Seizure frequency.
- Seizure pattern.
- Severity of the epilepsy.

For the majority of patients who are well controlled, awareness of potential risks is essential but usually the diagnosis should not have a major impact on their day-to-day life. All patients should receive basic information and literature about safety issues after a first seizure or new diagnosis ([book icon] see Counselling in people with epilepsy, pp.524–527). Some patients will require more in-depth counselling and risk assessment.

Home safety

Can I take a bath?

- A shower is recommended rather than taking a bath if the person experiences seizures associated with functional deficit or loss of awareness, due to the risk of drowning whilst bathing.
- If a person has only ever experienced brief simple partial seizures the risk is minimal (patients should be aware that any person who experiences brief partial seizures may be at risk of a more severe seizure in the future).
- If patients choose to bathe we would recommend a shallow bath.
- Where possible, the patient is advised to take a bath when someone else is in close proximity.
- Remember it does not take long to drown!

Toilet and bathroom doors should not be locked and ideally doors should be fitted to open outwards.

Can I cook?

The simple answer is yes. The risk from seizures when cooking usually involves minor injuries such as burns. To avoid injury we recommend:

- Cook using the back hobs.
- Do not have long flexes in the kitchen i.e. kettle flex.
- Carry food on a tray.
- If at high risk of seizures, carry food in sealed containers.
- Use of a microwave is probably the safest way to prepare food for those with frequent seizures.
- Cook when someone else is in the house if possible.
- Electric hobs are felt to be safer than gas.

Do I need to change anything in my house?

As a general rule, few adaptations are required. Severity and frequency of seizures will affect this, but the majority need not make any changes to their home.

Living room
- Open fires/gas fires should have a protective shield/fire guard.
- Radiator guards can be installed.
- Avoid sharp edged furniture or glass furniture e.g. glass coffee tables.
- For high-risk patients, unbreakable glass should be installed into windows and doors.

Kitchen
- Gas or electric stoves can be protected by a low shield top.
- Hot taps can be fixed with a temperature control device.

Bathroom
- Door made to open from the outside, and where possible made to open outwards.
- Install shower facilities.
- Shower screens made with unbreakable glass.
- Hot taps can be fixed with a temperature control device.

Bedroom
- Avoid sharp edges e.g. sharp corners on bedside tables.
- If seizures involve falls out of bed, consider low bed/futon.
- Padded sides are rarely used/required but can be fitted for those with severe frequent nocturnal seizures.

Are there any foods that I should avoid?

- Generally, people with epilepsy do not require any specific dietary change.
- A healthy balanced diet is recommended.
- Dehydration and a poor diet should be avoided.
- There are no specific foods that can trigger seizures.
- Alcohol should be taken in moderation. In some syndromes, alcohol is a seizure trigger even in moderation, especially if coupled with sleep deprivation.
- Avoid excess caffeine/stimulants which may alter sleep patterns and may possibly trigger seizures in those susceptible.
- Avoid excess diet drinks as aspartate has been reported to precipitate seizures.
- It has been suggested that the association between seizures and evening primrose oil in older reports is spurious.
- St Johns Wort is thought to induce cytochrome P450s and drug transporter P-glycoprotein and thus may interact with some AEDs.

In children, a high fat diet (the 'ketogenic diet') may be used in certain cases (💻 *see The ketogenic diet, p.249). Some have tried modified ketogenic or Atkin's diets in adults. However, the role of such diets is still to be established.*

Can I work?

The majority of employment options are open to people with epilepsy. It is essential to consider the seizure type and frequency when discussing employment. In the UK, legislation prevents people with epilepsy from pursuing the following professions:

- Aircraft pilot.
- Ambulance driver.
- Merchant seaman.
- Large goods vehicle (LGV), passenger carrying vehicle (PCV), or taxi driver.
- Train driver.
- Armed service.
- Fire brigade.
- Police.

Some jobs may involve a degree of risk and require assessment. Examples include:

- Working at heights—e.g. scaffolder, window cleaner.
- Working with dangerous machinery—e.g. factory work, carpentry.
- Catering.

Often people are anxious that they will lose their employment following a seizure or the diagnosis of epilepsy. It is generally recommended that employers are informed of the epilepsy in order to allow them to fulfil their obligations under the Health and Safety at Work Act. Reassurance should be given that it is unlawful to terminate employment due to disability (Disability Discrimination Act).

Employment should be encouraged and can have a profound and positive impact on a patient's general well-being and self worth. Many agencies are available to assist patients gain appropriate employment, training and advice. For example:

Contacts

- Disability Employment Officer: ✆ www.jobcentreplus.gov
- Learn Direct: ✆ www.learndirect.co.uk
- The National Federation of ACCESS Centers: ✆ www.nfac.org.uk
- Disability Rights Commission (DRC): ✆ www.drc-gb.org
  Tel: 0845 7622 633
- Health and Safety Executive (HSE): Tel: 0845 300 3142

Driving

The information in this section applies to the UK. It is correct at the time of writing but driving regulations are regularly updated (consult ✋ www. dvla.gov.uk regularly):

- Blackouts require the person to inform the Driver and Vehicle Licensing Agency (DVLA).
- Seizures are the most common cause of blackout at the wheel of a car.
- It is the patient's legal responsibility to inform the DVLA.
- Ensure advice is documented in medical notes.
- Consider that associated diagnosis may also have bearing on driving restrictions (e.g. arteriovenous malformation or brain tumour).

Any seizure will revoke a person's licence in the UK—even small brief attacks such as a brief simple partial seizures or myoclonic jerks.

Patients who do not fulfil the regulation in Box 6.4 must surrender their driving licence and are at risk of prosecution if they drive. Their insurance will be invalid and they may be criminally liable in the case of an accident.

Box 6.4 Driving regulations and epilepsy, UK

First epileptic seizure

- Group 1 licence: 1 year banned from driving with medical review before restarting driving.
- Group 2 licence: demonstrate 10 years' seizure freedom without AED medication.

Withdrawal of anti-epileptic medication

- A 6-month period of abstinence is recommended after withdrawal, and during the period of withdrawal.
- Patients should be advised of the degree of risk of re-emergence of seizures within the first year.
- MRC study shows 41% rate of seizure recurrence by year 2 after withdrawal, compared to 22% in those randomized to continue treatment. [2] 📖 See also How to withdraw an AED, pp.281–282.

Nocturnal seizures

Group 1: a person who has suffered an attack whilst asleep must also refrain from driving for 1 year from the date of that attack, unless they have only had attacks whilst asleep for >3 years, and have not had any attacks whilst awake during this period.

Learning to drive

The regulations in Box 6.4 apply also to provisional driving licences. Even if the person's epilepsy is well controlled, it is important that they declare this on the provisional licence application form.

Loss of freedom

- The loss of a driving licence can be very upsetting for patients, particularly for those in rural areas, those with children, or those who need to drive as part of their employment.
- These patients can apply for free travel passes as available from their local authority.
- The Disabled Persons Railcard provides a third off all rail travel for the person and a companion.

Reapplying for a licence

- Usually the DVLA will provide a 3-year licence upon reinstatement.
- If a person is seizure free for 7 years a full licence may be issued and will be valid until the age of 70 years.
- A history of seizures/epilepsy must be declared.

Contacts

- ◌ www.disabledpersons-railcard.co.uk Tel: 0191 218 8103.
- DVAL: ◌ www.dvla.gov.uk Tel: 08702 400 009.
- Association of British Insurers: ◌ www.abi.org.uk Tel: 0207 600 3333.

Leisure

Generally leisure activities are perfectly acceptable for those with a diagnosis of epilepsy, and a fit and healthy lifestyle is recommended.

There are no major contraindications to sport and leisure activity except for dangerous sports such as:

- *Scuba diving:* the British Sub-Aqua Club recommends that people should be seizure free and off antiepileptic medication for 5 years.
- *Rock climbing:* suitability will depend on type and severity of epilepsy.
- *Bungee jumping.*
- *Sky diving.*
- *Boxing.*
- *Swimming:* people with epilepsy should be advised to swim in company or let the swimming pool lifeguard know about their risk of seizures.
- *Sailing and other water sports:* waterskiing, sailing, and windsurfing should be assessed depending on seizure control/type. Buoyancy aids are recommended with the reservations mentioned for canoeing and kayaking).
- *Canoeing and kayaking may pose a risk:* buoyancy aids may keep the person pressed under the kayak if it capsizes.
- *Cycling:* a helmet is recommended. If a person has poorly controlled seizures, cycling with a friend is ideal while avoiding busy roads.
- *Horse riding:* an approved riding helmet should be worn. If a person has poorly controlled seizures then we would advise riding with a person who can manage their seizures. For those with severe epilepsy and learning disability some riding schools provide special sessions with harnesses. Contact Riding for the Disabled.[2]
- *Alcohol and drugs:* minimal alcohol intake is recommended as is avoidance of recreational drugs (◻ see Epilepsy, alcohol and drug abuse, pp.498–501).
- *Night clubs:* going to night clubs should not be a problem. Some people are worried about photosensitive epilepsy. Only a small number of people are photosensitive. An EEG can easily identify this. Covering one eye can reduce the effect. Avoid significant sleep deprivation.

- **TV and video games:** most TV programmes/films do not cause a flash rate that would induce a seizure in someone who is photosensitive. Computer games are generally safe. There have been reports of seizures in those with diagnosed photosensitive epilepsy. The general advice is to watch TV or play video games in a well-lit room and take regular breaks.
- **Medical tags:** some people, especially those with poorly controlled seizures wear a medical tag. There are two main companies in the UK (Medic Alert® and Medi-Tag®)[3,4] that produce a selection of wearable items such as pendants, bracelets, and watches. They provide medical data about the person's condition, medication, and a next-of-kin contact number.

Can I fly?

- There are usually no difficulties in flying as a passenger.
- Some airlines may request a letter from the patient's GP confirming that he/she is safe to fly.

What to remember when going on holiday

- Obtaining adequate travel insurance is essential. Some companies (although this should not occur) may penalize people with disabilities such as epilepsy. Shop around, or contact NSE[5] or Epilepsy Action[6] who are often able to advise.
- Medical costs abroad can be very expensive, so it is important to ensure medical cover is fully comprehensive.
- Ensure you take your medication in your hand luggage where possible—unfortunately bags can be lost sometimes and may take several days to retrieve.
- Minor adjustments may be required to accommodate changes in time zones for long-haul travel.
- A letter stating the type of epilepsy and list of medications is often useful.
- Make sure you have booked the appropriate accommodation—i.e. ground floor if you have severe, frequent seizures.
- Make sure you have a full supply of your medication in their boxes—it is always useful to bring a few days' extra supply in case your flight is delayed.
- Do you take any special tablets to abort clusters of seizures (e.g. clobazam)? If so, ensure you have a small supply of this.
- Do you require rectal diazepam or buccal midazolam? If so, ensure you have brought a supply with a doctor's letter confirming this.
- Seek advice about antimalarial prophylaxis. Some antimalarial are contraindicated in epilepsy.
- Avoid stress and sleep deprivation before or after travel.
- As far as possible, sleep deprivation and excess alcohol should be avoided. Patients may need advice about how to adjust timing of drug doses in relation to time zone shifts.

References

1. (1991). Antiepileptic drug withdrawal—hawks or doves? *Lancet*, **337**, 1193–4.
2. ⊖ www.riding-for-disabled.org.uk—Riding for the Disabled Association.
3. Medic-alert Foundation. Tel: 0207 8333034. Email: info@medicalert.co.uk
4. Medi-Tag. Tel: 0121 200 1616. Email: info@medi-tag.co.uk
5. The National Society for Epilepsy: ⊖ www.epilepsynse.org.uk
6. Epilepsy Action: ⊖ www.epilepsy.org.uk Email: www.epilepsy@epilepsy.org.uk

Epilepsy and the law

Are patients legally responsible for their actions during a seizure?

- It is extremely rare for a person to commit a directed act of violence during or after a seizure unless provoked (e.g. if restrained).
- An act of physical violence is defensible if the person can reasonably prove that the violent act occurred during a seizure, and that they were not aware of their actions.
- It is usually at the discretion of the judge whether the defendant goes free or is under the care of a mental health/hospital facility.
- In the UK, one can use the defence of automatism but this categorizes the defendant as insane. This is stigmatizing but remains the practice in current law.
- A violent act occurring in the post-ictal phase can be more difficult to defend. If the person has experienced post-ictal psychosis this will be defined as mental illness.
- As a general rule the majority of incidences when a crime is committed as a consequence of the seizure, a good defence can be secured.

Unfortunately, there are some individuals who may claim to have epilepsy/seizures in order to avoid conviction. Based on consultant psychiatrist Peter Fenwick's work, the following questions should be considered:[1,2]

- Did the defendant have a secure diagnosis of epilepsy before the offence was committed?
- Was the offence premeditated in any way?
- Was the defendant confused after the episode?
- Did the defendant seek help after the episode?
- Did the defendant conceal evidence after the episode?
- Does the defendant have any memory of the event? (They should be amnesic for the duration of the event.)
- Can witnesses confirm the defendant was in a state of confusion during or after the event?

Inappropriate arrest of patients

A far more common problem for those with a diagnosis of epilepsy, particularly males, is inappropriate arrest by police (Box 6.5). People who experience complex partial seizures and post-ictal confusion can be mistaken as:

- Being under the influence of alcohol.
- Being under the influence of recreational drugs.
- Having a psychiatric illness.
- Displaying inappropriate behaviour.

In many countries special training packages have been developed to assist police to identify those experiencing seizures (Australia and USA).

In cases where patients experience frequent seizures we would advise that they carry a card stating they have epilepsy, wear an SOS talisman, medic alert pendant, or bracelet.

Box 6.5 Case example

Mr B was on a London underground tube on his way to work. He had a diagnosis of temporal lobe epilepsy. His habitual complex partial seizures involved automatisms including disrobing. Mr B has post-ictal confusion including amnesia for at least 20min after the majority of his seizures.

A member of the public was concerned about his behaviour after witnessing a seizure (but did not recognize it as a seizure) and called the police. The British Transport Police attempted to arrest and restrain him. Because he was confused post-ictally he tried to get away from the police resulting in an injury to a police officer.

Mr B was subsequently arrested and charged with assaulting a police officer (three officers tried to restrain him). The charge was dropped by the police after his consultant provided confirmation of the diagnosis, and his video telemetry report clearly showed a seizure followed by prolonged post-ictal confusion.

References

1. Fenwick P and Fenwick E (1985). *Epilepsy and the Law*. Royal Society of Medicine International Congress and Symposium Series, No. 81. Royal Society of Medicine, London.

2. Fenwick P (1990). Automatism, medicine and the law. *Psychol Med*, **20**(17), 1–27.

Stigma, social prejudice, and self image

Historical context

Stigmata were the symbols used by the Greeks to mark slaves and other people considered less desirable. In modern language, 'stigma' designates an attribute associated with social disgrace. Stigma can lead to social disqualification for those with attributes that are viewed as undesirable.

Hippocrates, as well as biblical texts, make references to seizures. Texts right up to the last century usually associate epilepsy with negative attributes or behaviours. Some of the common themes wrongly associated with seizures and epilepsy are:

- Demonic possession.
- Criminal behaviour.
- Insanity.
- Immoral behaviour.

Fortunately the majority of modern society does not hold these beliefs, but people with epilepsy continue to feel stigmatized and discriminated against. Listed here are some of the probable causes for social stigma:

- Impact of previous perceptions—e.g. parental beliefs/religious beliefs.
- Public fear of seizures—educating the public, e.g. talks at schools, employers etc. can go some way to address this.
- Social exclusion/isolation—this can potentially occur from a young age at school. Educating staff and pupils will help minimize this.
- Fear of developing and maintaining relationships—marriage rates are lower, especially in men, with a diagnosis of epilepsy. Disclosure of the diagnosis is often described as a difficult issue for patients.

Examples of cultural impact on stigma

Consider a person's cultural beliefs and place of origin. Many cultures still hold strong and often damaging views about seizures and epilepsy.

- *Europe:* historically associated with witchcraft and insanity.
- *Africa:* attributes are country dependant but particularly in east and north Africa, epilepsy is thought to be contagious, resulting in drastic social consequences e.g. social isolation, difficulty in marrying.
- *Asia:* in India epilepsy is regarded as 'insanity' in legal terms.
- *China:* negative attitudes cause social stigma that affects the entire family.

Real and perceived stigma

There is little doubt that there has been significant discrimination and stigma against those with epilepsy. Modern studies however, highlight the importance of the person's perception of stigma, identifying that some people with epilepsy experience 'perceived stigma' or 'felt stigma'. Perceived/felt stigma is the feeling that a person is being stigmatized without a definite example of true discrimination/stigma.

Both real and perceived stigma exist to a greater or lesser extent. The health professional may identify and reduce the impact of either real or felt stigma.

Real stigma

- Consider the cause of stigma.
- Educate family, friends, and colleagues.
- Provide written information.
- Provide supportive letters for employment, schooling, etc.
- Consider the social ramifications of investigations or treatment—e.g. cognitive effects of AEDs or time off work.
- Ensure the patient and family are aware of support groups and voluntary organizations related to epilepsy.
- Ensure the patient and family are aware of legal aspects e.g. Disability Discrimination Act.

Perceived stigma

- Listen to and validate the person's concerns.
- Explore their beliefs and feelings about the diagnosis.
- Ensure the patient is well informed about epilepsy/seizures.
- Encourage independence.
- Encourage social activities.
- Consider local counseling or referral to a psychologist.

Self image

- Perceived/felt stigma is thought to be strongly associated with the individual's own perception of epilepsy.
- Many people report feelings of embarrassment, shame, and fear when diagnosed with epilepsy.
- A diagnosis instils feelings of helplessness, loss of control, and anxiety. It is very upsetting and embarrassing for patients to experience seizures in public.
- A small number of people can go on to develop agoraphobia or social phobia so it is essential the psychological impact of the diagnosis is always addressed.
- It is normal that a short period of adjustment to the diagnosis is required, and patients may experience feelings similar to bereavement such as shock, anger etc.

Healthcare and economics

Guidelines and implications for practice: NICE and SIGN, UK

NICE, the National Institute for Clinical Excellence, was set up in 1999, and replaced by the National Institute for Health and Clinical Excellence (also called NICE) in 2004. Its role is to provide guidance in three areas of health: public health, health technologies, and clinical practice. Guidance applies to England and Wales; the Scottish Intercollegiate Guidelines Network (SIGN) sets out guidelines for practice in Scotland. Topics for guidance for public health and technology appraisals are commissioned by the Department of Public Health. Topics for NICE guidance however, are suggested by various bodies including health professionals, parents, carers, and the general public. Once published, NICE states that health professionals and organizations that employ them are expected to take its guidelines fully into account.

There are several excellent NICE documents that relate to epilepsy; Guidance for the Diagnosis and Management of the Epilepsies in Adults and Children in Primary and Secondary care (2004); Health Technology Appraisals on the Newer Anticonvulsant drugs (2005); and Vagal Nerve Stimulation (2004). SIGN developed guidelines initially for management of adults (first published in 2003, revised 2005) and subsequently in parallel with NICE for epilepsy in children, published in 2005. The methodology for the development of the SIGN and NICE guidelines remain different but are complementary in format.

The guidelines provide a framework with which we can attempt to standardize care. They provide information on which care pathways for individuals can be based, from first seizure to presentation to tertiary care. Guidance is provided on who should look after the individuals, when and what should be investigated, when to consider treatment as well as advice as to information that should be provided for individuals and carers. Within the guidance are tables about medication, with cross reference to the Health Technology Appraisal for newer AEDs. They should not be seen as a set of rules, but a basis on which to structure services and audit practice. However what they also illustrated was the need for further study and evidence base not presently in existence in support of many of the recommendations made.

Key reading

1. NICE (2004). Guidelines for the management of epilepsy in adults and children in primary and secondary care. Available at: ⬚ www.NICE.org.uk/CG20

2. Epilepsy Action (2004). The epilepsies: you, epilepsy and the NICE guideline. Available at: ⬚ www.epilepsy.org.uk/news/niceguideline.html

3. NICE (2004). Vagus nerve stimulation for refractory epilepsy in children. Available at: ⬚ www. NICE.org.uk/IPG050

4. NICE (2004). The clinical effectiveness and cost effectiveness of newer drugs for epilepsy in adults. Available at: ⬚ www.NICE.org.uk/TA76

5. NICE (2004). The clinical effectiveness and cost effectiveness of newer drugs for epilepsy in children. Available at: www.NICE.org.uk/TA79

6. SIGN (2003). Diagnosis and Management of Epilepsy in adults. Available at: ⬚ http://www.sign. ac.uk/guidelines/fulltext/70/index.html

7. SIGN (2005). Diagnosis and management of epilepsies in children and young people. Available at: ⬚ http://www.sign.ac.uk/pdf/sign81.pdf

8. Dunkley C and Cross JH (2006). NICE guidelines and the epilepsies – how should practice change? *Archives of Disease in Childhood*, **91**, 525–8

General practice and epilepsy—the UK experience

The government's health strategy is currently focused on the primary care setting, with GPs playing a pivotal role in commissioning of health and social services. This includes an emphasis on management of chronic conditions, such as epilepsy within the primary care setting.

- Management of chronic conditions is a significant part of the GP's role
- Epilepsy is the most common chronic disabling condition of the nervous system, affecting about 456,000 people in the UK.
- The average GP has a patient list ranging from 1500–2000 patients.
- The expected caseload of patients with epilepsy may vary, but is thought to be between 8–12 people with a known diagnosis of epilepsy, of whose 2 or 3 will be attending a paediatric clinic. The majority are likely to be well controlled on one AED, but there may be one or more complex cases.
- A GP will often see only one or two new diagnoses of epilepsy each year.
- For those with drug-resistant epilepsy, GP support enables families to adjust and adapt to the condition. These patients are expected to generate a greater number of consultations and telephone contacts. Ongoing monitoring is essential, in conjunction with a treatment plan from secondary care.

Within a shared care approach the GP would:

- Monitor all patients with a diagnosis of epilepsy. This includes a register/record of seizure type, frequency, and medication.
- Make a provisional diagnosis in new patients; provide appropriate information, such as safety and driving regulations, and refer to a specialist centre.
- Monitor seizures, aiming to improve control by adjusting medication—usually with specialist guidance—refer to hospital services.
- Minimize side effects of medications and effects of their interactions.
- Facilitate structured withdrawal from medication where appropriate and if agreed by patient, who must be well-informed regarding risks of withdrawal.
- Introduce non-clinical interventions and disseminate.
- Address specific women's issues and needs of patients with learning disabilities.
- Ensure patients are aware of voluntary support organizations and local groups.

The GP contract (Table 7.1) recognizes the importance of monitoring epilepsy and encourages a joint management plan for patients with close liaisons between secondary and primary care. The development of specialist GPs is allowing the development of community-based epilepsy services. The vast majority of services for epilepsy remain in secondary and tertiary care.

Table 7.1 General Medical Services (GMS) contract

	Indicator	Points	Payment stages
Epilepsy 1	The practice can produce a register of patients receiving drug treatment for epilepsy	2 points	
Epilepsy 2	The percentage of patients aged ≥ 16 years, on drug treatment for epilepsy who have a rewcord of seizure frequency in the previous 15 months.	up to 4 points	25–90%
Epilepsy 3	The percentage of patients aged ≥ 16 years, on drug treatment for epilepsy who have a record of medication review in the previous 15 months.	up to 4 points	25–90%
Epilepsy 4	The percentage of patients aged ≥ 16 years, on drug treatment for epilepsy, seizure free for the last 12 months recorded in the previous 15 months.	up to 6 points	25–70%
Records 7	The medicines that a patient is receiving are clearly listed in his or her record	1 point	
Records 8	There is a designated place for the recording of drug allergies and adverse reactions in the notes and these are clearly recorded	1 point	
Records 9	For repeat medicines, an indication for the drug can be identified in the records (for drugs added to the repeat prescription with effect from 1 April 2004)	4 points	Minimum standard 80%
Medicines 9	A medication review is recorded in the notes in the preceding 15 months for all patients being prescribed repeat medicines	8 points	Minimum standard 80%

The GMS contract points allocated for epilepsy are relatively small in comparison with other chronic conditions such as asthma but the targets are easily achievable. We hope in the future additions can be made. If a practice wants to develop epilepsy services, the following could be considered:

- GP with a Special Interest in Epilepsy.
- Joint outreach GP/consultant clinic.
- Joint outreach/epilepsy clinical nurse specialist clinic.
- Practice nurse-led epilepsy clinic for monitoring of seizure frequency.
- Display patient leaflets: ⏚ www.epilepsynse.org; ⏚ www.epilepsy.org.
- Advertise local epilepsy support groups.
- Agree individualized general or shared care protocols with specialist services.

General Practitioner with a Special Interest (GPwSI)

A GP with a Special Interest has been defined by the Department of Health and Royal College of General Practitioners as follows: 'General Practitioners with special interests supplement their important generalist role by delivering a high quality, improved access service to meet the needs of a single primary care trust (PCT) or group of PCTs. They may deliver a clinical service beyond the scope of normal general practice, undertake advanced procedures, or develop services. They will work as partners in a managed service not under direct supervision, keeping within their competencies. They do not offer a full consultant service and will not replace consultants or interfere with access to consultants by local general practitioners'.

Key attributes of GPwSI
- Work in general practice.
- Usually employed/commissioned by PCT.
- Receive referrals direct from GPs.
- Usually, but not exclusively community based.
- Needs-based appointment.
- Defined role.
- Accreditation:
  - Knowledge and skills framework.
  - Educational contract.
  - Appraisal.
- Local flexibilities within a National Framework.
- Evaluation of practitioner and service.

GPwSI in epilepsy
The DOH has produced 'Guidelines for the appointment of General Practioners with Special Interests in the Delivery of Clinical Services-Epilepsy' (April 2003).[1]

Activities will include:
- Provision of clinical services including care to special groups i.e. learning disabilities and women.
- Education and liaison.
- Service development/leadership.

Competencies:
- Has the ability to take a full medical and neurological history.
- Understands the psychosocial aspects of epilepsy.

- Understands the natural history of epilepsy.
- Has a sound knowledge of the pharmacological treatments of epilepsy e.g. side effects, interactions, terotegenic effect, etc.
- Understand co-morbid factors influencing seizure control.
- Understand use of and make appropriate referral to, appropriate specialist investigations.
- Able to establish epilepsy register and use it for call, recall, audit, and outcome.
- Understands the role of the voluntary sector and other support organizations.
- Able to provide information about support organizations and legal aspects, e.g driving.
- Able to understand the networks of carers and services involved in the provision of care to patients with seizures

Evidence of training:
- Royal College of General Practitioners.
- Supervision by specialist clinician i.e. epileptologist.
- Recommended number of sessions with the specialist: 40–50.
- Personal development portfolio.
- Attendance of relevant courses.
- An annual appraisal.

Accreditation:
- At present this is agreed locally by the primary care organization.
- In the future the Joint Neurosciences Council in conjunction with the Association of British Neurologists plan to develop appropriate neurosciences training for GPwSI in neurosciences.
- Currently there is no formal list of GPwSI in epilepsy in the UK.

References

1. Department of Health/Royal College of General Practitioners (2002). Implementing a scheme for general practitioners with special interests. DH/RCGP, London. Available from: ⌨ www.dh.gov. uk/en/Publicationsandstatistics/index.htm

Key reading

1. SIGN (2003). Diagnosis and Management of Epilepsy in adults. Available at: ⌨ http://www.sign. ac.uk/guidelines/fulltext/70/index.html

Further information

⁀ www.nice.org.uk—website of NICE

—The epilepsies: the diagnosis and management of the epilepsies in adults and children in primary and secondary care (2004)

—Newer drugs for epilepsy in adults (2004)

⁀ www.sign.ac.uk—website of the Scottish Intercollegiate Guidelines

⁀ www.abn.org.uk—Association of British Neurologists (ABN)

⁀ www.gpwsi.org.uk— General Practitioners with a Special Interest

Residential care and special centres for epilepsy

Although the vast majority of persons with epilepsy are able to maintain an independent lifestyle despite their diagnosis, one in five has learning or intellectual disabilities. Many also suffer varying degrees of physical disability. Most people in these circumstances will have their specific needs met within local communities, some in well supported frames with supervision from trained resident carers, with an emphasis on independence where appropriate.

All patients, depending on needs, should have access to:
- Social work services.
- Learning disability services, including community psychiatrist and community learning disability nurse.
- Occupational health.
- Physiotherapy.
- Practical social care—shopping and house work.
- Physical social care—washing and dressing.

For a small minority of people with poorly controlled epilepsy, usually in conjunction with severe physical and intellectual disabilities, residential care is required.

The JEC published a document entitled 'UK providers of residential services for children and adults affected by epilepsy'.[1] This document summarizes the work and services available at six specialist residential centres across the UK (Table 7.2). All of these services are hoping to expand and diversify their activities to include smaller more community based centres.

Is a residential centre the right choice?

The possibility of a residential centre should be discussed at length with the person with epilepsy and their family/carers. The majority of day services for people with learning disabilities have experience and training in the case of people who experience seizures. Integration with the wider community is the ideal and residential care should only be considered when no other options are suitable. In a minority of cases, however, a patient's quality of life can be significantly improved as a result of the care options available at a specialist residential centre (Table 7.2), e.g.
- Supported Living Projects (NSE).
- Residential Schooling (DLC, NCYPE, SEC).
- High Dependency units (DLC, NSE).
- Social and Working Enterprises (NSE, SEC).

Table 7.2 UK providers of residential services for children and adults affected by epilepsy.

Organization	Location	Age range	Residential places
David Lewis Centre (DLC)	Cheshire	7 upwards	296
The Meath Epilepsy Trust	Surrey	18 upwards	64
NCYPE	Surrey	3–25	200
NSE	Buckinghamshire	18 upwards	230
Quarriers	Renfrewshire	All	500
St Elizabeth Centre (SEC)	Hertfordshire	5 upwards	172

Referral

- Usually referrals are made by health professionals, e.g. a GP, consultant neurologist, or specialist nurse, but some centres will accept self referrals.
- Written referrals are generally preferred.
- If the child or adult with epilepsy meets the specific centre's criteria, usually an application form is sent to the person/carers.
- After the application has been processed, assessments, which may be carried out at the person's home or within the residential centre, will be performed. Each centre will have their own policy and protocol for referrals.
- There may be a waiting time for the assessment and a potentially long waiting list for these centres due to the small number of places available.

Cost

- Residential centres can be expensive due to the specialist nature of the services provided.
- Costs of residential care will vary from centre to centre, but local authorities will usually only consider funding these specialist services if no local alternative can be found.
- Funding must be agreed with the local health authority.

Respite care

Respite care is often essential for families and carers of those with severe epilepsy, particularly if they have severe physical or intellectual disabilities. Most local authorities can provide some respite services. Specialist respite can be provided at a residential epilepsy centre. All potential candidates will require assessment and need to secure funding from their local authority.

Contacts

- David Lewis Centre: email: moira@davidlewis.org.uk Tel: 01565 640176
- The Meath Epilepsy Trust: email: gordan@meath.org.uk Tel: 01483 415095
- NCYPE: email: ngee@ncype.org.uk Tel: 01342 831 273
- NSE: email: Karen.lane@epilepsynse.org.uk Tel: 01494 601300
- Quarriers: email: enquiries@quarriers.org.uk Tel: 01505 612224
- St Elizabeth's Centre: email: clemencea@stelizabeths.org.uk Tel: 01279 844230

References

1. JEC (2005). UK providers of residential services for children and adults affected by epilepsy. Available from: ⌁ www.jointepilepsycouncil.org.uk (brochure)

Organizations and support services for people with epilepsy

- There are many national and local support services for those with a diagnosis of epilepsy.
- Ensure those with a diagnosis of epilepsy—including partners, family, and carers—are made aware of local and national services available.
- These organizations provide essential support, advice, and information.

The following services are available:
- Information leaflets.
- Specialist packs—e.g. on learning disability.
- Helpline.
- Educational tools—e.g. videos.
- Online support—e.g. chat rooms.
- Online information leaflets to download.
- Training for employers/health professionals.
- Local support group meetings.

Epilepsy Bereaved provide support and guidance through bereavement related to epilepsy and campaign to raise awareness of excess mortality related to epilepsy, particularly SUDEP.

UK and Ireland services

- Epilepsy Action Helpline: Tel: 0808 800 5050 International +(44) 113 210 8850. www.epilepsy.org.uk
- National Society for Epilepsy 01494 601 400. www.epilepsynse.org.uk
- Epilepsy Scotland: Tel: 0808 800 2200 ww.epilepsyscotland.org.uk
- Brainwave—The Irish Epilepsy Association: +(353) 1455 7500. Email: info@epilepsy.ie
- Epilepsy Wales: Tel: 0845 741 3774. www.epilepsy-wales.co.uk
- Epilepsy Bereaved: 01235772850; www.sudep.org
- ILAE—UK Branch contact: Membership secretary 0207 8373611. www.ilae.org/visitor/chapter/uk/index.cfm

Local support groups

The majority of national organizations will have a list of local support groups. Many local support groups meet monthly.

Professional bodies and charities associated with epilepsy

- Epilepsy Research UK: Tel: 02089954781. www.epilepsyresearch.org.uk
- Joint Epilepsy Council: Tel: 01943 871. www.jointepilepsycouncil.org.uk/
- Neuroeducation: www.neuroeducation.org.uk

International organizations

- ILAE-International League Against Epilepsy: www.ilae.org
- IBE-International Bureau for Epilepsy: www.ibe-epilepsy.org
- International Epilepsy Resource Centre: www.ierc.ch
- Epilepsy Foundation of America: www.epilepsyfoundation.org

Please note there are many epilepsy support organizations that are not listed here. The authors do not have preference regarding local, national, or international support organizations.

'Epilepsy week' is usually the second week of May in the UK.

Specialist nurse programmes and epilepsy in UK

The role of the Epilepsy Specialist Nurse (ESN) has developed and flourished since the late 1980s. There are now over 150 ESNs across the UK. An ESN can act as the cornerstone of care, liaising with all professionals involved in patients' management to ensure a seamless care pathway. The ESN can improve quality of care and efficiency. The role of the ESN may vary depending on local needs. ESNs can work in primary, secondary or tertiary care, or occupy a joint post between organizations e.g. primary and secondary care. Roles and responsibilities may include the following:

- Provision of information and advice to patients and carers covering all aspects of epilepsy care and psychosocial issues.
- Provide advice and act as a resource to GPs and other members of the multidisciplinary team.
- Educational support to schools and employers.
- Liaise with other members of the multidisciplinary team to provide a smooth care pathway.
- Develop and provide local epilepsy training.
- Establishment of nurse-led clinics including specialist clinics e.g. LD, VNS, and women's.
- Manage a case load-review of patients within their own home or hospital environment, taking direct referrals from GPs and other health care professionals.
- Monitoring: medication and seizure management via face-to-face and telephone consultations (Helpline service).
- Appropriate arrangement of tests e.g. EEG blood serum monitoring
- Accident and emergency service for review and smooth transition to first seizure services.
- Epilepsy surgery/VNS counselling.
- Play a strategic role in health planning and commissioning for epilepsy in local, and in some cases national, service development.
- Prepare general and individualized protocols for rescue medication and shared care pathways.
- Audit aspects of epilepsy care.
- Research.
- ESNs may also have nurse prescribed role within national guidelines.

The RCN has recently published a competency framework and guidance for practice for developing paediatric epilepsy specialist nurse services (2005). A similar document for adult services is currently being developed (🖰 www.rcn.org.uk).

Funding for ESN

Many areas do not have epilepsy nursing services. One of the main constraints to setting up a service is usually financial. A proposal/business plan is submitted to the employing organization(s). This is usually led by a key professional such as a consultant neurologist. In order to compile a proposal, the benefits for the patient, primary and secondary care must be highlighted, particularly quality of care and efficiency/cost effectiveness. For example:

- Reduction of general neurology waiting times—ESNs can provide ongoing review, allowing consultant neurologists more time to see new patients.
- Prevention of admission to A&E and unnecessary use of ambulance services by empowering patients to manage seizures in the community.
- Reduction of patients' hospital stays by prompt assessment, advice and information to medical teams.
- Provision of education and advice to primary care, reducing unnecessary referrals to secondary care.
- Providing telephone advice where appropriate, thus reducing clinic attendance.

Epilepsy Action has provided support and funding for many ESNs with the 'sapphire nurse scheme'. It is important to bear in mind that funding is usually only provided for 1 year by the charity, while the employer must honour ongoing payment of salaries. This must be agreed in writing before establishment of the post.

Epilepsy Action provides a helpful pack to assist campaigning for a sapphire nurse. Available at: www.epilepsy.org.uk

ESN Training and Educational Programmes

- For training requirements in paediatrics, refer to 'A competency framework and guidance for practice for developing paediatric epilepsy nurse specialist services' Royal College Nurses (RCN), UK, 2005.
- Currently there are no formal guidelines for minimum training requirements in adults, but the forthcoming competency framework for adults is expected to rectify this.
- All ESNs should have specialist training and experience in the field of epilepsy.

Professional bodies

Epilepsy Specialist Nurses Association—ENSA.

ESNA is a professional organization whose membership consists of nurses and other health professionals working to support people with epilepsy. ESNA acts as a resource and networking opportunity for all ESNs. It organizes annual conferences and runs a network of local groups who meet regularly, whilst also providing up-to-date professional advice to ESNs and raising the profile of epilepsy in the public and political arena (www.esna-online.org.uk).

Contacts

- British Association of Neuroscience Nurses BANN. www.bann.org
- World Federation of Neuroscience Nurses—WFNN. www.wfnn.nu

Links between hospital and GP services in epilepsy

Specialist Centres, Tertiary Referral Centres, and Epilepsy Clinics

- Usually patients can be well managed by local neurologists and primary care services.
- Cases involving those with ongoing seizures, potential need for epilepsy surgery and issues surrounding diagnosis and classification may require referral to a specialist centre (📖 for referral criteria, see When to refer patients to secondary or tertiary centres, pp.238–241).

📖 Tables 7.3 and 7.4 list national epilepsy clinics and specialist centres. These lists have been obtained with the permission of the NSE and is not exhaustive. There may be other epilepsy clinics in your area.

Table 7.3 Some UK epilepsy clinics and specialist centres for children

Royal Preston Hospital Sharoe Green Lane Fulwood Preston PR2 9HT Tel: 01772 716565	Great Ormond Street Hospital for Children Great Ormond Street London WC1N 3JH Tel: 020 74059200
Royal Manchester Children's Hospital Hospital Road Pendlebury Manchester M27 4HA Tel: 0161 7944696	Royal Liverpool Childrens Hospital (Alder Hey) Eaton Road West Derby Liverpool L12 2AP Tel: 0151 2284811
Park Hospital for Children Old Road Headington Oxford OX3 7LQ Tel: 01865 226213	The John Radcliffe Hospital Headley Way Headington Oxford OX3 9DU Tel: 01865 741166
King's College Hospital Denmark Hill London SE5 9RS Tel: 020 77374000	Addenbrookes Hospital Hills Road Cambridge CB2 2QQ Tel: 01223 245151
Guys Hospital 8 St Thomas Street London SE1 9RT Tel: 020 79555000	Leeds General Hospital Great George Street Leeds LS1 3EX Tel: 0113 2432799
Southern General Hospital 1345 Govan Road Glasgow G51 4TF Tel: 0141 2011100	University Hospital of Wales Heath Park Cardiff CF14 4XW Tel: 01222 747747
Ryegate Children's Centre Sheffield Children's Hospital Tapton Crescent Road Sheffield S10 5DD Tel: 0114 267 0237	Queens Medical Centre Derby Road Nottingham NG7 2UH Tel: 0115 9249924
The National Centre for Young People with Epilepsy St Piers Lane Lingfield Surrey RH7 6PW Tel: 01342 832243	David Lewis Centre for Epilepsy Mill Lane Alderley Edge Cheshire SK9 7UD Tel: 01565 640000
St Elizabeth's School South End Much Hadham Herts SG10 6EW Tel: 01279 843451	

Table 7.4 Some UK epilepsy clinics and specialist centres for adults

The National Hospital for Neurology and Neurosurgery (affiliated to NSE) Queens Square London WC1N 3BG Tel: 020 7837 3611	University of Birmingham Seizure Clinic Queen Elizabeth Psychiatric Hospital Mindelson Way Edgebaston Birmingham B15 2QZ Tel: 0121 678 2000
Special Centre for Epilepsy York District Hospital Wigginton Road York YO3 7HE Tel: 01904 631 313	University Hospital of Wales Heath Park Cardiff CF4 4XW Tel: 01222 747 747
David Lewis Centre Mill Lane Alderley Edge Cheshire SK9 7UD Tel: 01565 640 000	Addenbrookes Hospital Hills Road Cambridge CB2 2QQ Tel: 01223 245 151
Burden Neurological Hospital Burden Centre Frenchay Hospital Frenchay Park Road Bristol BS16 1JB Tel: 0117 918 6710	Doncaster Epilepsy Services Doncaster Hospital Tickhill Road Balby Doncaster DN4 8QL Tel: 01302 796 217
Centre for Epilepsy Kings College Hospital Denmark Hill London SE5 9RS Tel: 020 7346 8331	Walton Centre Lower Lane Liverpool L9 7LJ Tel: 0151 525 3611
Maudsley Hospital Neuro-psychiatry department Denmark Hill London SE5 8AZ Tel: 020 7703 6333	Radcliffe Infirmary Neurology Department Woodstock Road Oxford OX2 6HE Tel: 01865 311 188
Royal Hallamshire Hospital Glossop Road Sheffield S10 2JF Tel: 0114 271 1900	Kent and Canterbury Hospital Ethelbert Road Canterbury CT1 3NG Tel: 01227 766 877
Derriford Hospital Derriford Road Crownhill Plymouth PL6 8DH Tel: 01752 777 111	Hope Hospital Stott Lane Salford M6 8HD Tel: 0161 789 7373
Southampton General Hospital Tremona Road Southampton SO16 6YD Tel: 02380 777 222	The Royal London Hospital PO Box 59 Whitechapel London E1 1BB Tel: 020 7377 7381

Table 7.4 Some UK epilepsy clinics and specialist centres for adults
(*continued*)

Leicester General Hospital Gwendolen Road Leicester LE5 4PW Tel: 0116 249 4040	Queens Medical Centre Derby Road Nottingham NG7 2UH Tel: 0115 924 9924
Newcastle General Hospital Westgate Road Newcastle Upon Tyne NE4 6BE Tel: 0191 233 6161	Quarriers Quarriers Village Bridge of Weir Renfrewshire PA11 3SD Tel: 01505 616 006
Ninewells Hospital PO Box 120 Dundee DD1 9SY Tel: 01382 660 111	Southern General Hospital 1345 Govan Road Glasgow G51 4TF Tel: 0141 201 1100
Western Infirmary Dumbarton Road Glasgow G11 6NT Tel: 0141 211 2534	Atkinson Morley Regional Neurocience Centre Atkinson Morley Wing St Georges Hospital Blackshaw Road Tooting London SW17 0QT Tel: 020 8672 1255

Health economics and epilepsy—the UK experience

In today's political climate, health professionals cannot disregard the financial aspect of patient management. Our healthcare service provision continues to change rapidly with the advent of GP commissioning and tight financial constraints on both acute and primary care trusts. Although the UK government continues to report increasing expenditure on healthcare, the reality is that accessing funds is difficult and often we are competing against other specialties. The effect of the 'credit crunch' is yet to unfold.

- The UK government spent £80.6 billion on healthcare in 2005, 7.7% of gross domestic product.
- The annual cost of established epilepsy in the UK has been estimated at approximately £4500, although other studies suggest a lower cost of about $3000 (£1604) per person in Europe and the USA.
- The economic burden of epilepsy is complex, ranging from cost of care and treatment to social care (direct costs), mortality, and impact on employment (indirect costs).
- 58,900 people with epilepsy in the UK are claiming disability living allowance (DLA) costing £184 million per year.
- The greatest economic burden is from those with active epilepsy, accounting for more than half the total cost, although this group represents less than a quarter of the total number of those with epilepsy.
- Only 1% of grants from the UK government's Medical Research Council funded epilepsy research in 2002/2003.

The following play a role in the overall cost of those with epilepsy:
- Financial impact on the national economy—primarily through unemployment, resulting in loss of manpower hours of both skilled and unskilled workers.
- Financial impact on the individual and family—e.g. main wage earner is unable to work due to seizures, or family members may need to give up work to care for those suffering from epilepsy.
- Cost of treatment—this includes assessment/diagnosis, investigations.
- Drug treatment—the cost of AED treatment, particularly the newer generation drugs.
- Cost of misdiagnosis.
- Cost of impact of the diagnosis—depression, anxiety disorders.
- Cost of admission to hospital—following seizure and seizure induced injuries.
- Social care where there is associated illness or deficit—support for activities of daily living.

Reducing costs

Education

Providing appropriate education to patients and carers can have a dramatic impact on general health costs nationally. For example, the call-out cost for an ambulance is approximately £500. Ensuring parents, carers, day centres, schools and employers are able to manage seizures appropriately can have a major impact on the overall cost. This would impact on unnecessary A&E admissions and reduced GP emergency calls.

AEDs

Newer AEDs are more expensive. There is no good evidence to advocate their routine use as first-line treatment in newly diagnosed epilepsy, although they may be used in individual cases. Cheaper first-line AEDs such as carbamazepine and valproate have proven to be as efficient with minimal difference in tolerability. It has been estimated that if all newly diagnosed patients were treated with one of the newer drugs the extra annual cost would exceed £15 million. In intractable cases or in those with medication related side effects, new AEDs are useful. Valproate should be avoided as first line in women of reproductive age.

Misdiagnosis

If a misdiagnosis of epilepsy is incorrectly made in between 20–31% of all cases, as has been reported, this equates to up to 105,000 people receiving AEDs who do not have the condition.

Comparative burden

A study performed in 1992/93[1] showed that epilepsy is a significant financial burden in comparison to other conditions (Table 7.5).

Table 7.5 Comparative cost of epilepsy versus other conditions

Condition	Total expenditure
Asthma + COPD	£347.1 m
GI ulcers	£264.2m
Diabetes	£216.9m
Epilepsy	£193.6m
Hypertension	£163.2m
Parkinson's disease	£160.2m

References

1. NHS Executive (1996). Burden of disease: a discussion document. Department of Health.

Key reading

1. Cockerell OC, Hart YM, Sander JWAS, *et al.* (1994). The cost of epilepsy in the United Kingdom: An estimation based on the results of two population based studies. *Epilepsy Research*, **18**, 249–60.

2. Joint Epilepsy Council (1999). The Epilepsy Task Force, Burden of Epilepsy; a health economics perspective. Available at: www.jointepilepsycouncil.org.uk

Training courses

MSc/Diploma in Epilepsy (2-year part-time/1-year full-time course)

To obtain information about the course, contact:

Dr Gonzalo Alarcon

Senior Lecturer and Honorary Consultant in Clinical Neurophysiology

Department of Clinical Neuroscience

Institute of Psychiatry

PO 43

16 De Crespigny Park

London SE5 8AF

Email: gonzalas.alarcon@iop.kcl.ac.uk, MSc.epileptology@iop.kcl.ac.uk

⌐ http://www.iop.kcl.ac.uk/courses/?id=49

Professional Certificate/Diploma /MSc in Epilepsy Practice /(distance learning)

To obtain information about this course, contact:

Course Administrator

Centre for Community Neurological Studies

Leeds Metropolitan University

Leeds LS1 3HE

Tel: 0113 283 5198

Email: J.Buckingham@lmu.ac.uk

BA (Hons) Practice Development (Epilepsy) (part-time)

BSc Hons or Diploma in Epilepsy Care (2-year part-time course)

Course based at the National Society for Epilepsy (NSE). To obtain information about this course, contact:

Course Leader—Michael Farquharson (Lecturer)

Department of Health Studies

Bucks Chiltern University College, Chalfont Campus

Bucks, HP8 4AD

Email: m.farqu01@bcuc.ac.uk

Epilepsy and the arts

A museum in Germany dedicated to epilepsy was opened in 1998. That the first museum is located in Germany is perhaps no coincidence. Although discrimination against those with epilepsy was by no means unique to the Third Reich, epilepsy or 'hereditary falling sickness' was one of the conditions for which sterilization could be performed under the 'Law for the Prevention of Offspring with Hereditary Diseases'. Interested readers may wish to visit the museum's website (🖰 http://www.epilepsiemuseum.de)

The subject of art and epilepsy may be considered under the following headings:

Famous people with epilepsy

This is of interest for many reasons. For some, it demonstrates that people with epilepsy are capable of great achievements. There is also the consideration of how the life and artistic work of those affected may have been influenced by their condition. Many famous people are said to have had epilepsy with varying degrees of supportive evidence. These include Flaubert, Dostoyevsky, and van Gogh.

How epilepsy is represented in art, including visual arts, literature, drama, music and cinema

In the Middle Ages and Renaissance period, religious art represented as healers both Christ and Patron Saints of Epilepsy, of whom St Valentine is perhaps the best known.[1] The invocation of supernatural forces, in the treatment of epilepsy, still has an echo in exorcism.

Epilepsy is a common condition and it is thus not surprising that it is represented in literature and other forms of art, particularly given the loss of control and sometimes dramatic nature of epileptic fits. Demonic characterization in some works is balanced by the not infrequent portrayal of the person with epilepsy as good or as a victim. George Eliot's Silas Marner's life is forever shaped by being wrongly accused of theft, a crime committed by another, who took advantage of Silas's epilepsy. The epilepsy later resulted in him being known, following a witness' account, as a 'dead man come to life'. A minor character in Forester's Hornblower's book series, convulses during a covert mission, and is sacrificed, to avoid the mission failing should the noise alert the enemy. The media is said to portray epilepsy in an alarmist and inaccurate manner, as indeed does cinema. Social exclusion without treatment is the portrayed fate, albeit in affluence, of the son of Idi Amin's fourth wife in the acclaimed film *The Last King of Scotland*.

How people with epilepsy, both adults and children[2] may express themselves or their predicament using art

Dostoyevsky is perhaps one of the best known examples. He suffered from late onset epilepsy and reportedly felt enriched by the experience. In his writing, he created a number of characters, some considered autobiographical figures, with the condition. The following poem has been written by one of our patients who suffers from seizures (reproduced with permission from Justine Camille).

Suffering because of silence
by Justine Camille

Ancient yet unknown, there's plenty to uncover,
It is not my friend and surely not my lover.
It's an enemy still trying to wreck my life
Because old stories cause more struggles, stress and strife.
Roughly once a week this enemy appears;
Has my nerves in tremor, my tongue in great tears.
I get lost in a battle unknown to me,
People think I'm an addict with no will to be free.
And what makes it worse, they shrink back in tension
Afraid to approach once this enemy's mentioned.
It then leaves a world of loneliness and jumble
Where negative thoughts continue to rumble.
There's always some help but very little knowledge
Which will take little time, no need to go to college …
For thousands like me have shared these words I utter;
Yet sadly our pleas just melt like heat to butter!

References
1. www.desitin.no/index.php/article_html/detail/5
2. www.desitin.no/index.php/artgallery/detail/1326

Index